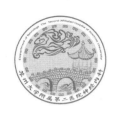

尿酸与帕金森病的
基础临床研究

主审　包仕尧

主编　罗蔚锋　胡丽芳　刘春风

U0395829

苏州大学出版社
Soochow University Press

图书在版编目（CIP）数据

尿酸与帕金森病的基础临床研究/罗蔚锋，胡丽芳，
刘春风主编. —苏州：苏州大学出版社，2023.12
ISBN 978-7-5672-3520-5

Ⅰ.①尿… Ⅱ.①罗… ②胡… ③刘… Ⅲ.①帕金森
综合征—诊疗—研究 Ⅳ.①R742.5

中国版本图书馆 CIP 数据核字（2022）第 035543 号

书　　名：尿酸与帕金森病的基础临床研究
NIAOSUAN YU PAJINSENBING DE JICHU LINCHUANG YANJIU

主　　编：罗蔚锋　胡丽芳　刘春风
策　　划：刘　海
责任编辑：刘　海
装帧设计：刘　俊

出版发行：苏州大学出版社（Soochow University Press）
出 版 人：盛惠良
社　　址：苏州市十梓街1号　邮编：215006
印　　刷：苏州工业园区美柯乐制版印务有限责任公司
网　　址：www.sudapress.com
E - mail：Liuwang@ suda.edu.cn　　QQ：64826224
邮　　箱：sdcbs@ suda.edu.cn
邮购热线：0512-67480030
销售热线：0512-67481020

开　　本：718 mm×1 000 mm　1/16　印张：16.25　字数：275 千
版　　次：2023 年 12 月第 1 版
印　　次：2023 年 12 月第 1 次印刷
书　　号：ISBN 978-7-5672-3520-5
定　　价：68.00 元

凡购本社图书发现印装错误，请与本社联系调换。服务热线：0512-67481020

目 录

概　述

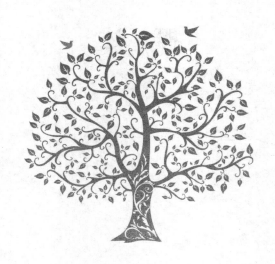

帕金森病

一、介绍

　　帕金森病（Parkinson's disease，PD）是一种渐进性的神经系统退行性病变，属于锥体外系疾病，60 岁以上的人群 PD 发病率为 1%～2%，是继阿尔兹海默病（Alzheimer's disease，AD）之后的又一大神经退行性疾病。病理特征是大脑黑质致密部（compact part of substantia nigra，SNpc）多巴胺能神经元的丢失和错误折叠 α-突触核蛋白（α-synclein，α-syn）的积累，这些蛋白存在于细胞质内的包涵体中，称为路易体（Lewy body，LBS）。其典型症状包括静止性震颤、肌肉僵直、运动迟缓，同时伴有智力减退、痴呆及记忆障碍。运动障碍协会于 2015 年对"Parkinsonism"重新进行定义，去除了四个典型特征中的姿势异常特征。目前，PD 起病隐匿、潜伏期长，且缺乏可靠的 PD 早期临床诊断指标，导致临床诊断延迟，发现 PD 时往往已经错过最佳治疗时机，严重影响患者生活质量，同时也增加了家庭和社会的负担。

　　2003 年，H. 布拉克（H. Braak）等提出 PD 的病理进程可依照路易体的出现时间分为 6 期：1 期主要为嗅球、嗅核前部和迷走神经背侧运动核受累，临床表现为嗅觉障碍、便秘；2 期以下位脑干的病理改变为主，影响脊核、蓝斑、脑桥其他核团，继而产生快速动眼睡眠行为障碍、抑郁、自主神经功能失调、疲惫等症状；3 期、4 期时患者向上发展影响中脑的黑质及其他深部核团和端脑，跨越了 PD 运动症状前期和运动症状期的界限，临床表现有运动症状并被确诊；5 期、6 期的病理改变与路易体累及边缘系统、新皮质有关，临床表现为精神症状（认知损害、视幻觉）。目前，PD 根据症状的严重程度可细分为 3 类人群：45～50 岁的年轻发病人群，表现为强烈的震颤，很少有非运动性运动障碍；50～70 岁的发病人群；≥70 岁的高龄发病人群，有严重的运动缺陷，快速进行性疾病。根据遗传分布可分为家族性 PD（familial Parkin，sons disease，fPD）和散发性 PD（sporadic Parkinson's disease，sPD），其中 sPD 占 90%左右。

二、PD 疾病的历史

　　1817 年，詹姆斯·帕金森（James Parkinson）通过观察 6 名患者的临床症状,首次在其论文 *An Essay on the Shaking Palsy* 中将 PD 描述为神经退行性疾病。由此,PD 正式进入大众视野。当时的 PD 还被称作"shaking palsy",直到 1872 年才被重新命名为"Parkinson's disease"。

我国的《黄帝内经·素问》也曾对 PD 症状及其治疗进行过详细描述和记载。

金·马丁·查科特(Jean Martin Charcot)在 Parkinson 的基础上独立列出 PD 的四项核心症状。随着研究的深入,学者们不断丰富着 PD 的概念,越来越多的人集中研究 PD 的发病机制。

1893 年,布洛克(Blocq)和马瑞内斯库(Marinescu)发现某病人表现出的症状与 PD 类似,经深入研究,发现他患有结核性肉芽肿,肉芽肿压迫到同侧的黑质。这一发现提示了布瑞索德(Brissaud),他认为黑质可能是 PD 的发病区域关键所在。康斯坦丁·特列季亚科夫(Konstantin Tretiakoff)观察到患者大脑黑质有明显褪色,因此支持布瑞索德的说法。随着技术的提升,研究者发现了该病病变的更多细节,比如黑质致密部的不均匀病变,年龄的增加让黑质部分的细胞缺失更加明显等,而且 PD 的病变并不仅仅如此,还涉及其他部位。

1912 年,弗雷德里克·亨利·路易(Frederic Henry Lewy)在 PD 患者神经元中检出一种特殊的异常嗜酸性蛋白小体。1919 年,特列季亚科夫在 PD 患者黑质中发现该物质并将其命名为"路易体"。但在路易体的首次报告中,它存在于迷走神经背核和无名质。正因为如此,有学者如塞季·普兹德波斯基(Serge Przedborski)表示,也许黑质不是 PD 的发病区域,纹状体才是。而罗夫·海斯勒(Rolf Hassler)于 1938 年证实了特列季亚科夫的猜想,即黑质退化是帕金森病的致病原因。

20 世纪中期,研究者们陆续发现 PD 患者黑质、蓝斑等神经核团存在路易体,逐渐确定了 PD 的病理学特征。卡尔森(Carlsson)发现多巴胺(dopamine,DA)与运动相关,即 DA 水平下降导致运动障碍,DA 与利血平对运动的作用相反。后续证据也表明,PD 患者的脑部黑质和纹状体内多巴胺减少。同时,有研究者发现左旋多巴可以减轻 PD 患者的部分症状,但随后长期服用左旋多巴的患者表现出各种副作用。虽然左旋多巴是治疗 PD 的金标准,但由于其副作用,研究者便通过临床试验开发新药物和新疗法,如左旋多巴的新形式,新的服用药物方式,利用病毒载体或细胞运送 DA,脑内注射或载体运送神经营养因子等。1995 年,有研究者发现深部脑刺激

（deep brain stimulation，DBS）可以治疗 PD 患者，随后有研究者提出通过源于多巴胺能神经元的多能干细胞移植来治疗 PD，但是其临床风险和技术上的障碍使 DBS 目前无法被取代。

近年来，PD 的发病机制涉及两大类：一是基因，PD 的遗传性；二是环境对 PD 的影响。大量的流行病学数据及全基因组性状分析证明了 PD 具有遗传性的可靠性。风险因子的发现也让 C.坦纳（C.Tanner）等研究者对 PD 有了更全面的认识。普兹德波斯基认为，PD 是慢性病，急性暴露在毒性因子下并不会立即发作，但它会造成基因突变，随着暴露时间的加长，突变基因累积，直至机体生命系统崩坏。

三、PD 的流行病学研究

1. 发病率

PD 主要发生在 60 岁以上中老年人群，50 岁之前的患者不常见，以 65 岁为节点，65 岁以上人群 PD 发病率显著增长，并且随年龄增长呈现逐年增高的趋势。PD 的发病率在 5/100 000～35/100 000。2005 年，张振馨等对北京、西安、上海的 79 个农村和 58 个城市社区的 29 454 例居民（>55 岁）进行评估，确诊 277 例 PD 患者，其中年龄>65 岁的老年人群 PD 的发生率为 1.7%。2007 年，仅全美 PD 患者人数就达 100 万人。2014 年，基于中国 1983—2009 年报道的 PD 流行病学调查结果的 Meta 分析显示，我国全人群 PD 患病率为 190/100 000。1990—2015 年的数据显示，全球的 PD 患者增加了 118%，直达 620 万人。随着时间的推移，数据不断变化，预计 2040 年 PD 患者数将增长到 1 200 万人。正因如此庞大的人口数据，以及其所产生的经济负担，部分研究者将 PD 称为"PD 大流行"。如果没有有效的临床治疗手段，PD 将成为全国乃至全球的社会、经济负担。

2. 性别差异

通常在 PD 的患病率中发现性别差异，以前的几项研究结果表明，男性更有可能发生 PD。从患病风险来看，男性患 PD 的风险是女性的 1.5 倍；从患病人数来看，男性患 PD 的人数是女性的 2 倍。这些性别差异与雌激素、大脑性别二态性、多态性、DNA 甲基化甚至 X 染色体失活是否有关仍不清楚。

3. 环境

在几十年来全世界人口的研究中，接触农药如灭草剂、灭虫剂、百草枯、鱼藤酮、二硫代氨基甲酸盐类、有机氯（三氯乙烯、四氯乙烯、四氯化碳）等有害化学物质,从事农业工作或在农村居住与 PD 风险增加有关。虽然以上农药中有一部分已经停止使用,但它们仍存在于土壤、空气和水流中。同样的,部分职业接触者或住宅靠近有害化学物质制造工厂的居民患 PD 的风险更大。而且长时间暴露在铁、锰等金属下也会增加患 PD 的风险。交通中的环境总悬浮粒子也与 PD 风险增加有关。

个人生活质量同样与患 PD 的风险有关。良好的卫生习惯、健康的饮食可防止部分有害物质对机体的侵蚀。多吃蔬菜水果和谷物也会降低患 PD 的风险。有学者表示,适当的体育锻炼也会降低患 PD 的风险。适当的饮食和运动在一定程度上是可能限制神经老化的进展的。

2015 年,F.斯凯普简(F.Scheperjans)等人比较风险因素后发现,吸烟人士患 PD 的风险较不吸烟人士降低了约 40%,结合 H.Chen 等人的研究结果——吸烟的持续时间是吸烟与 PD 相关的基础可以得出,较长时间持续抽烟的居民在一定程度上减少了 PD 风险,但二者是否有因果关系并不清楚。与此同时,被动吸烟与无烟烟草的使用同样与患 PD 的风险有关。

咖啡或咖啡因的摄入也会降低 PD 风险;部分研究报道,喝茶也有可能降低 PD 风险。

总胆固醇、LDL-C 和甘油三酯的高水平与 PD 低风险相关。GBA、SMPD1 或 SREBF1 突变导致脂质积累的上升,此现象与 PD 高风险有关。血脂代谢平衡障碍可能是 PD 的风险因素。甲状腺功能减退症患者患 PD 的风险增加。

4. PD 风险易感基因

目前,基于全基因组的关联分析已经发现了 80 多个 PD 易感位点,其中包括亚洲人群的 11 个 PD 风险基因位点:PARK16,ITPKB,MCCC1,SNCA,FAM47E-SCARB2,DLG2,LRRK2,RIT2,FYN,SV2C,WBSCR17;以及欧洲人群的 87 个 PD 风险基因位点:FCGR2A,VAMP4,KCNS3,KCNIP3,LINC00693,KPNA1,MED12L,SPTSSB,LCORL,CLCN3,PAM,C5orf24,TRIM40,RIMS1,FYN,RPS12,GS1-124K5.11,FAM49B,UBAP2,GBF1,RNF141,SCAF11,FBRSL1,CAB39L,MBNL2,MIPOL1,RPS6KL1,CD19,NOD2,CHRNB1,UBTF,FAM171A2,BRIP1,DNAH17,ASXL3,MEX3C,CRLS1,DYRK1A,GBA,NUCKS1/SLC41A1,SIPA1L2,TMEM163/CCNT2,STK39,CHMP2B,MCCC1,TMEM175/DGKQ/FAM200B/CD38,FAM47E,SNCA,HLA-DRB6/HLA-DQA1/KLHL7,NUPL2/GPNMB,MICU3,BAG3,

DLG2，MIR469，LRRK2，OGFOD2，GCH1，TMEM229B，VPS13C，ZNF646/
KAT8， ARHGAP27/CRHR1/SPPL2C/MAPT/STH/KANSL1， SYT4， LSM7，
DDRGK1，ITPKB，IL1R2，SCN3A，SATB1，NCKIPSD/CDC71，ALAS1/TLR9/
DNAH1/BAP1，PHF7，NISCH，STAB1，ITIH3，ITIH4，ANK2，CAMK2D，
ELOVL7， ZNF184， CTSB， SORBS3/PDLIM2/C8orf58/BIN3， SH3GL2，
FAM171A1，GALC，COQ7，TOX3，ATP6V0A1/PSMC3IP/TUBG2。其中最新
发现的亚洲 PD 风险基因中有 7 个与欧洲 PD 风险基因相同（GBA-SYT11，
BST1，TMEM175-GAK-DGKQ，ZNF184，FGF20，VPS13C 和 ASXL3）。虽然目
前并无证据证明 PD 在地域、人种方面的差别，但在 PD 风险基因方面欧洲
人群和亚洲人群是有共通之处的。

　　大规模的流行病学研究也揭示了一些支持遗传假设的证据，包括编码
τ 的 MAPT 中的单核苷酸多态性即与 PD 易感性有关。此外，一项全基因组
复杂性状分析显示，PD 的可遗传成分至少为 30%。

四、PD 病的病理生理机制

1. 病理特征

病理特征主要是基底神经节中脑黑质致密部多巴胺能神经元的大量退
化和进行性缺失，导致多巴胺能神经元大量减少，形成以 a-syn 为主要成分
的路易体，最终引起运动迟缓、肌肉僵直、静止性震颤等行为功能障碍。

传统上，PD 的概念定义是以黑质致密部多巴胺能神经元为中心，但在
系统对比大量死亡后 PD 患者脑部的表征后，研究者认为路易体是 PD 的典
型标志。

同时，PD 患者不仅仅表现出多巴胺能神经元的退化和缺失，5-HT 能神
经元也呈现出进展性、非线性损伤。

一些研究者发现，PD 患者的脑细胞表现出低血糖和低氧化代谢速率。

2. 发病机制研究

虽然有关 PD 的确切病因至今未完全阐明，但我们已知 PD 涉及多种途
径和机制，包括老化、α-syn 的失衡、氧化应激、线粒体功能障碍、钙稳态紊
乱、轴突转运和神经炎症、金属紊乱、溶酶体功能障碍等。

（1）老化

研究表明，年龄是神经退行性疾病（阿尔兹海默病、帕金森病等）的主
要风险因子。PD 是一种衰老依赖性神经退行性疾病，PD 的流行病学数据

表明,随着年龄的增长,PD 的患病率和发病率明显上升。全球预期寿命的延长是导致疾病发病率上升的主要原因,大部分患者一般在疾病晚期死亡,在疗养院或医院去世,这给患者、保健系统和社会造成了经济负担。

（2）炎症

研究表明,肥大细胞、小胶质细胞、T 细胞、少突胶质细胞与这些细胞的相互作用在免疫功能和预防神经退行性疾病上具有重要作用。早在 1988 年,麦克·吉尔(Mc Geer)等人就发现,神经发炎、小胶质细胞的激活和促炎介质的持续升高与 PD 有关。反应性胶质增生和神经炎症是 PD 的完整特征。炎症会随着年龄的增长而上调,而不受控制的、持续的炎症会导致阿尔兹海默病和 PD。PD 患者死后其大脑图像显示严重的神经发炎现象。基因表达结果表明了炎症在神经退行性疾病中的重要性。慢性炎症,小胶质细胞的持续激活,促炎介质的持续升高和氧化应激的增加与神经退行性疾病有关。而且肠道和嗅觉系统中的组织炎症可引发一定程度的 α-syn 错误折叠,α-syn 聚集可诱导固有和适应性免疫。目前的证据已经表明 α-syn 在激活免疫中的作用,并已证明激活的小胶质细胞直接吞噬 α-syn。越来越多的证据表明,炎症是 PD 的主要介质,炎性应答机制涉及小胶质细胞和白细胞的激活。

（3）线粒体功能障碍

研究者首次发现 PD 发病机制可能与线粒体相关始于几个年轻人自发注射 1-甲基-4-苯基-1,2,3,6-四氢吡啶 (1-methyl-4-phenyl-1,2,3,6-tetrahydropyridine,MPTP) 后引发的急性症状与 PD 类似,因此将研究方向转向 MPTP 的毒性作用。

众所周知,线粒体是体内能量加工厂,机体 80% 的能量来源于此,其中大脑神经元放电、记忆、情感和机制等需要大量能量。除此之外,线粒体还参与了脂质生物合成、钙信号、细胞凋亡等生命活动,这些都是神经退行性疾病发展的中心过程。因此一旦线粒体受到损伤,其所参与的生命活动都会受到冲击。众多研究结果表明,线粒体功能障碍是许多神经退行性疾病的发病机制。比如线粒体 DNA(mtDNA) 的突变、线粒体动力学(如形状、大小、分布、分裂融合、运动) 受损、电子传递链复合物(electron transfer complex,ETC) 异常、线粒体三磷酸腺苷(Adenosine triphosphate,ATP) 产生的部分抑制导致自由基的过量产生,这会导致脂质、蛋白质、DNA 等生物大分子损伤、神经发炎、组织受损和中枢神经系统中连续的细胞凋亡,以上是神经退行性疾病的标志物。研究者发现,PD 患者脑部黑质神经元中存在线粒体 DNA 缺失和骨骼肌中线粒体呼吸链异常。大量的流行病学、病理学和遗传学证据都指向线粒体功能障碍是 PD 发病机制中的核心驱动因素。阿米特·沙玛（Amit Sharma）等人对 PD 女性患者 mtDNA 血清浓度相关研究的结果进一步加强说明了线粒体功能障碍与氧化应激是 PD 的发病机制。线粒体功能障碍与突变在多种神经退行性疾病的发病机制和衰老中起重要作用。比如线粒体的分布与运动在脑源性神经营养因子（glial cell line-derived neurotrophic factor，BDNF）介导的突触传递和可塑性中至关重要，如果线粒体功能障碍，则会影响突触传递和可塑性。线粒体介导的内外凋亡途径出现障碍，如 Bcl-2 家族抗凋亡和促凋亡失衡也会影响神经细胞死亡和神经退行性疾病。线粒体自噬是选择性降解功能失调的线粒体调节线粒体功能的过程。目前在 PD 致病基因中，PINK1、PARKIN、DJ-1、LRRK2 都参与了线粒体自噬的调控过程。同时，研究还发现，PD 患者中黑质和杏仁核线粒体存在自噬功能缺陷。激活线粒体自噬功能可以减轻神经退行性疾病中的风险因子——炎症。同时费文森（Fivenson）发现，线粒体自噬功能不足会导致神经退行性疾病。

（4）α-syn

α-syn 是由 SNCA 基因编码的蛋白，主要有 α，β，γ 这三类蛋白。α-syn 是 $14×10^3$ 的小分子酸性可溶性蛋白，主要位于神经突触前末梢，在突触囊泡循环、递质储存和分类中具有重要作用，它与囊泡和膜结构有关。在正常生理状态下突触核蛋白与膜结合，一旦膜或蛋白受到损伤，两者不能结合，同时蛋白质控制质量系统功能受损，无法降解多余或损伤的蛋白，则蛋白聚集形成路易体。

α-syn 在生理条件下是非折叠水溶性蛋白，在病理条件下异常聚集形成沉淀。目前研究发现，α-syn 聚集和沉积的第一步是其氨基端结构域和细胞膜发生结合，形成 α 螺旋结构，在此基础上进一步发生错误折叠和聚集，形成 β-片层结构，成为寡聚体和不溶性的纤维。异常累积的 α-syn 会导致损害线粒体、溶酶体和蛋白酶体功能，损伤生物膜和细胞骨架，改变突触功能，引起神经元变性。

神经元可以释放 α-syn，与胶质细胞受体结合，触发促炎反应，并且它可以在星形胶质细胞中积累。研究表明，胶质细胞可能暴露于细胞外 α-syn，有机会减轻神经元释放 α-syn 的传递。有研究提出，病理性 α-syn 聚集体更倾向于以朊蛋白样方式进行传播，Rey 等观察到注射了 α-syn 的小鼠存在

α-syn 的跨神经元转运。α-syn 可能起源于胃肠道。

（5）基因：PD 相关遗传致病基因

1997 年，斯皮兰提尼（M. G. Spillantini）首先发现了 α-syn 基因点突变 A53T 与家族性常染色体显性遗传 PD 有关，SNCA 突变涉及 α-syn 的错误折叠，积累后产生毒性，导致神经元的死亡。PARKIN 基因产生的 PARKIN 蛋白属于 E3 泛素连接酶，发生突变后导致自噬障碍，引起氧化应激和神经元缺失。

UCH-L1 表达泛素 C 端水解酶 L1，在单体形式下具有生成和稳定自由泛素单体的作用，使泛素循环利用，当其发生突变时会影响泛素蛋白酶体途径。

PINK1 是遗传性 PD 中较为常见的突变基因，编码的蛋白位于线粒体外膜，具有 Ser/Thr 激酶活性，发生突变会导致线粒体自噬异常。

DJ-1 在调节线粒体钙通量（内流/释放）方面起着至关重要的作用，保护细胞免受多巴胺能神经元的 pace-making activity 和多巴胺毒性产生的氧化应激损伤。

LRRK2 突变干扰自噬，减缓 α-syn 的降解，是 α-syn 聚集和路易体产生的原因。

ATP132A 突变决定溶酶体功能障碍并引起年轻人的帕金森病（Kufor-Rakeb 综合征），而其在特发性 PD 存活的多巴胺能神经元中的表达上调，提示其神经保护作用。

GBA 是一种 β 葡萄糖脑苷脂酶，其缺陷导致戈谢病（Gaucher disease，GD），是目前已知的 PD 重要的遗传风险因素。在 PD 患者中，GBA 突变十分普遍。GBA 与 PD 发病机制有关：
α-syn 积累、内质网应激和线粒体功能障碍。

GIGYF2 在我国汉族迟发型散发性 PD 人群中的突变频率为 2.7%。

omi/HtrA2 编码的蛋白位于线粒体，具有促进凋亡的作用。

PLA2G6 突变与小儿营养不良、脑内铁沉积有关。

FBX07 遗传性 PARK15 型 PD 又称 PD-锥体束综合征。

GAK 编码的蛋白具有 Ser/Thr 激酶活性，通过修饰 α-syn 的表达和毒性水平影响 PD 的发病率。

HLA-DRA 患者中大部分为白种人。

VPS35 属于 PARK17，是重组人液泡分拣蛋白基因，目前有两个假设通路可能与 VPS35 诱发 PD 有关：（1）wnt信号传导通路；（2）二价铁转运体

（DWT1）调节铁离子跨膜转运途径。

NR4A2：编码核受体超家族成员的 NR4A2 对黑质多巴胺能神经元的分化至关重要。NR4A2 突变导致转染细胞系和受影响个体淋巴细胞 NR4A2 mRNA 水平显著降低。此外，NR4A2 的突变影响编码酪氨酸羟化酶的基因的转录。以上表明，NR4A2 的突变可能导致多巴胺能功能障碍，与 PD 有关。

CHCHD2 基因编码的 CHCHD2 蛋白是一种具有成对的半胱氨酸-x9-半胱氨酸结构的小分子蛋白，位于线粒体的内膜。具有半胱氨酸-x9-半胱氨酸结构的蛋白一般具有合成调节线粒体呼吸链相关的酶的功能，因此 CHCHD2 突变可能导致 CHCHD2 蛋白功能的异常，增加线粒体的氧化应激水平，从而导致多巴胺能神经元退变，促进 PD 的发生、发展。

到目前为止，已发现的与家族性 PD 明确有关的致病基因有 9 个，SNCA，LRRK2，VPS35，UCH-Ll 和 GIGYF2 为常染色体显性遗传，PARKIN，PINK1，DJ1 和 ATP13A2 为常染色体隐性遗传。散发性和家族性 PD 可能有着共同的潜在机制（免疫机制和相关基因）。

尽管某些特定基因的突变导致 PD 发生，但在 5%～10% 的例子中，大部分 PD 患者并无基因突变的发生。研究数据表明，10% 的患者携带导致 PD 的单基因突变，但 90% 以上的患者无家庭、遗传因素影响。虽然这些变异风险可能作用很小或者十分罕见，但是它们可以帮助我们进一步了解驱动 PD 的基因和途径。同时某些研究利用单卵子和合卵子双胞胎评估 PD 的遗传性，结果反映 PD 风险部分与环境和行为因素相关。因此我们可以理解虽然突变基因对 PD 有影响，但目前大部分的证据表明 PD 的发生发展更多与环境和行为相关。

（6）钙稳态

钙通道阻断剂可用来抵抗 PD。$Ca^{2+}/cAMP$ 参与控制神经递质的释放和神经元死亡。神经-遗传毒性效应可能是 cAMP 通路下调引起的，除了细胞内 Ca^{2+} 的上升外，主要是因为 $Ca^{2+}/cAMP$ 信号反应失衡。$Ca^{2+}/cAMP$ 调节障碍可能是由于以下原因：细胞内 Ca^{2+} 的升高；Ca^{2+} 通过 VACC 内流；通过线粒体上的理阿诺受体和 IP3-Ca^{2+} 储存的 Ca^{2+} 释放。这些失调可能导致 SNpc 中 DA 的退化和死亡。

（7）金属沉积

接触金属包括铅、锰、锌、铁和铜等，工业产品和污染物，杀虫剂与线粒体功能障碍、金属稳态改变和蛋白聚集有关。有学者表示，暴露在金属离子环境下与 PD 发生风险存在正相关关系。研究表明,过量金属会通过氧化应激损伤线粒体功能,导致细胞死亡,诱发神经退行性疾病。金属离子的神经毒性作用常与中枢神经系统的线粒体障碍、酶活性的下降、蛋白质的聚集和氧化应激有关,导致多巴胺能神经元变性和死亡。

① 铁

铁在机体血浆内以 Fe^{3+} 形式结合蛋白存在,在细胞里,游离铁以二价铁形式构成铁池,为胞浆、细胞核中的二价铁依赖酶提供铁离子作为辅助因子。在生理状态下,血脑屏障高度调节选择性运输系统限制铁离子,避免脑中铁过载。如果脑中铁过载,会造成氧化应激和细胞死亡。铁过载造成的氧化应激十分危险,因为它会促进机体内含铁蛋白进一步释放铁,形成破坏性的正反馈,加重铁危害。在 PD 患者黑质中观察到铁的局灶性沉积。随着老化,不同的铁复合物在特定脑区积累。在 PD 中,局部铁稳态的改变导致细胞内铁的累积和分布改变,最终导致神经毒性。在机体内,结合铁在一定程度上是安全的,但游离铁可能与周围的分子交换电子,产生自由基,然后自由基又与大脑中的氧分子及其他分子作用,形成更多的自由基。我们知道羟自由基可以攻击蛋白质、DNA 和脂质膜,这一过程可能破坏细胞的完整性和功能,最终导致氧化应激和细胞凋亡。

以上说明的是铁过载,如果铁不足,同样与 PD 有关。因为铁的转运载体 DMT-1 也可以吸收其他二价金属,当铁缺乏时会上调小肠中 DMT-1 的水平,增加对锰的吸收,从而产生神经毒性。因此,铁不足会导致脑内锰的积累增加。

外周铁代谢紊乱可能参与了 PD 非运动症状中快动眼睡眠行为障碍、淡漠及抑郁的发生、发展,铁蛋白、转铁蛋白可能是 PD 快动眼睡眠行为障碍、淡漠及抑郁发生的外周血指标。α-syn 可能参与铁代谢功能障碍,研究发现,α-syn 通过调节 DMT1 蛋白的稳定性,改变细胞的铁摄取来影响脑内铁稳态。

研究证明,大脑中的几种必需金属之间存在共同稳态关系,不仅仅是铁和锰。总之,由于铁离子的促氧化特性,研究者认为它在 PD 的发病机制中具有重要作用。

② 锰

锰是正常生长、发育和细胞内稳态所必需的微量元素。一般锰的接触途径包括饮食、皮肤接触和呼吸。过量接触锰会使锰在大脑中积累。虽然锰诱导的 PD 与典型 PD 在病理和临床上有所差异,但两者都具有广泛而相似的病理生理机制。在大脑星形胶质细胞中发现了更高水平的锰聚集,因此认为星形胶质细胞是锰运输到脑的重要靶细胞,以及在神经元应激和损伤期间启动炎症的信号。所以星形胶质细胞是锰在大脑中的主要稳态调节剂及储存场所。同时,小胶质细胞直接累积锰并通过释放 IL-6、TNF-α、CCL2 和 CCL-5 形成混合炎症表型。线粒体是细胞内锰的储存场所,锰的含量增加会干扰线粒体氧化磷酸化,导致线粒体功能障碍。锰与激活参与氧化应激的信号通路有关(AP-1 和 NF-kB),锰还可以通过激活蛋白酶 C(PKC-δ),以 caspase-3 依赖的方式触发多巴胺能神经元凋亡,并通过细胞色素 c 释放和 caspase 激活的线粒体途径导致星形胶质细胞凋亡或死亡。

③锌

锌主要分布在人体的睾丸、肌肉、肺和大脑中。锌稳态是大脑正常功能所需要的,锌对病原体或组织损伤做出反应,发挥抗炎、抗氧化作用。对比 PD 患者和对照组的锌水平,发现 PD 患者的锌水平明显下降。研究发现,它是发生发展神经退行性疾病的关键因素。过量的锌会抑制铜和铁的吸收,促进线粒体活性氧(reactive oxygen species,ROS)的产生,破坏代谢酶的活性,并激活凋亡。锌会影响多种细胞类型中多种炎症细胞因子的产生和信号传递。对 PD 患者补充锌可降低促炎细胞因子的表达、减少其产生。

④铜

在生理条件下,胞浆中过量的铜离子与金属硫蛋白结合从而减少游离的铜,避免游离铜引起毒性。而铜的神经毒性效应是二价铜离子固有的氧化还原特性导致中枢神经系统中 ROS 的产生增加所致。研究表明,活性氧损伤和神经变性的表现与包括铜在内的必需金属有关。铜在 PD 中起双重作用:一是游离铜与增加的氧化应激、α-syn 聚集及路易小体有关;铜作为重要抗氧化酶的辅助因子,可以减少氧化应激。血液中铜和铜氧化酶(ceruloplasmin)水平在 PD 中没有改变,故不能代表有效的 PD 诊断指标。

以上,铁、锰、锌、铜或多或少参与了 PD 的发病机制,在其病理生理学中可能发挥关键作用,这些金属在不同脑区出现不同水平的积累,很难分离出它们的特异性毒性,因此维持这些金属的稳态至关重要。除了这四种金属外,铅和汞也是 PD 的潜在危险因素。

(8)溶酶体功能障碍

有研究表明,溶酶体功能障碍是 PD 的主要发病机制。溶酶体蛋白在星形胶质续保中富集,并占据脑组织的 1/3。溶酶体与蛋白质质量控制有关,在 PD 早期解决 α-syn,防止 α-syn 异常聚集产生神经毒性。

（9）其他

人类基因组中存在大小不等的 DNA 大片段的拷贝数目变异（copy number variation，CNVs），与之对应的是功能蛋白量的改变。近年来，CNVs 和神经系统等疾病的关系引起了人们的关注，朱莉亚（Giulia）发现其对 PD 发病机制具有广泛和复杂的遗传作用。

D3R 通过调节运动活动、情绪、记忆和奖励机制在 CNVs 中起重要作用，最近研究表明，D3R 暗中参与 PD 的发病机制。D3R 在 PD 早期增加，增加的 D3R 促进 T 细胞活化并诱导神经炎症，这可能是 D3R 激活在 PD 发病机制中作用的基础，它通过在 T 细胞表面的高密度表达，跨过血脑屏障渗透到黑质中，并诱导小胶质细胞的激活产生更多的炎症因子，进一步诱导神经发炎和神经变性。有研究发现，尼古丁可刺激 D3R，诱导 D3R-nACh 异构体激活，从而减弱 α-syn 的聚集。

非编码 RNA 在 PD 中有重要意义。大量人体和动物实验观察到，PD 患者或动物模型脑组织中存在大量失调的微小 RNA（miRNA），这些 miRNA 与 PD 的发生、发展密切相关，通过对 miRNA 的调控有望为 PD 的治疗提供新策略，同时 miRNA 参与炎症的调节过程，与氧化应激有关。比如小胶质细胞中 miR-7116-5p 的下调会促进 MPTP 小鼠模型中肿瘤坏死因子-α（TNF-α）的产生，导致其他促炎因子的出现，使多巴胺能神经元受损。miR-124 可以通过靶向 p62、p38 和自噬来抑制 PD 发展过程中的神经炎症，也可以通过调节 MEKK3／NF—kB 信号通路来抑制 PD 的神经炎症。研究表明，与年龄相关的 Dicer 酶的下降，再加上多巴胺能神经元细胞应激的增加，也可能会阻碍 miRNA 生物合成，从而导致 PD 相关的神经元变性。参与调节氧化应激的相关 miRNA 可防止 ROS 介导的损伤。

五、PD 症状

首先，PD 患者表现的临床症状分为运动症状和非运动症状。同时，PD 具有隐匿性起病和缓慢性进展的特点，在患者表现出 PD 的典型症状前会有一段时间的前驱症状期。非运动症状是 PD 的重要前驱症状，包括便秘、睡眠紊乱、嗅觉减弱、抑郁和体痛等。

PD 属于 PD 氏病综合征中的一种，PD 氏病综合征分为原发性 PD、血管性 PD（vascular PD，VaP）、多系统萎缩症（multiple system atrophy，MAS）、进行性核上麻痹（progressive supranuclear palsy，PSP）、路易体痴呆症（dementia with lewy body,DLB)、皮质基底节变性(corticobasal degeneration,CBD)、脊髓小脑萎缩症(spinocerebellar ataxia,SCA)和威尔逊氏病(Wilson's disease,WD)。

1. 运动症状

（1）静止性震颤

以震颤为主的 PD,其震颤与特发性震颤(essential tremor,ET)易于混淆。其中 ET 是最常见的运动障碍性疾病,主要为手、头部及身体其他部位的姿位性和运动性震颤,其病因尚不清楚。

（2）肌肉僵直

（3）运动迟缓

运动迟缓表现在两个方面：躯体运动和面部运动。

面部运动迟缓,即常说的"面具脸",表现为眉毛、眼睛、面颊、嘴唇等在运动的速度、弹性和协调性等方面存在不足,严重影响口面部功能,造成语言障碍、流涎等。

2. 非运动症状

（1）感觉症状

① 嗅觉减弱

超过 90%的 PD 患者在疾病早期出现嗅觉障碍,表现为嗅觉减退或缺失,这类症状多早于运动症状 4~6 年,且多为双侧异常。国内一项长期跟踪报告也显示,约 88%的 PD 患者出现嗅觉减退。PD 患者嗅球体积减小,嗅觉功能减退,且嗅觉功能减退程度与嗅球体积减小存在正相关性。嗅觉障碍可能是 PD 的危险因素,可用于评估发生 PD 的风险。最近的证据表明,在运动症状出现前几年,α-syn 在嗅球前嗅核内积累。T.J.斯蒂文森(T.J.Stevenson)关注 PD 嗅球中的非神经细胞类型是否受到 α-syn 影响,结果表明,PD 嗅球中的非神经细胞含有 α-syn 包裹体,说明它们可能在 PD 的进展中发挥重要作用。

② 视觉障碍

视觉障碍可能成为 PD 早期诊断的生物学标志。PD 患者经常伴随着不同程度的视觉障碍,且最常见的表现为视物模糊,复视,光敏感度及空间估计受损及幻觉。研究发现,PD 患者的视网膜内层存在 α-syn 沉积。Ortuno-Lizaran 等对 PD 患者进行尸体解剖,发现磷酸化的 α-syn 在视网膜的累积与大脑的病变保持同步。

③ 疼痛

疼痛是常见的 PD 非运动症状,在 PD 患者中的发生率为 40%~85%,

严重影响患者的生活质量。PD 患者疼痛的表现多样,P.沃克维克(Valkovic P)等统计的 PD 的疼痛包含肌肉骨骼疼痛、肌张力障碍疼痛、中枢神经性疼痛、根性疼痛和其他疼痛(非根性腰痛,关节炎和内脏疼痛)。PD 疼痛以慢性疼痛为主,骨骼肌肉痛是最常见的类型。虽然目前对于 PD 患者疼痛的机制尚不明确,但对 PD 患者皮肤的活检研究发现,α-syn 沉积于皮肤的感觉与自主神经表皮、表皮神经纤维密度下降、神经纤维轴突肿胀有关。

除此之外,还有一些其他感觉障碍,比如听觉障碍。研究发现,在听力丢失和老年性耳聋中,α-syn 沉积于内耳传出神经系统。PD 患者主要表现为高频听力受损。研究者比较 PD 患者组的味觉与嗅觉功能,结果提示 PD 患者组的味觉阈值、嗅觉辨别受损。然而也有研究结果表明,电味觉测量味觉阈值在 PD 患者组与对照组无明显差异。

(2)神经精神

① 焦虑

患者出现情绪障碍尤其是抑郁和焦虑症状,主要就是患者机体的 5-HT 及去甲肾上腺素分泌逐渐减少。

② 冷漠

统计表明,约 40% 的 PD 患者有冷漠表现,并且大部分患者不合并抑郁和痴呆,因此冷漠被视为一项独立的非运动症状。J.Y.洪(J.Y.Hong)等对 PD 患者和对照组进行冷漠评分,结果 PD 患者组高于对照组。推测其原因,可能是 PD 患者的多巴胺神经元缺失导致内侧额叶-基底神经节环路受损,引发情感冷漠。情感冷漠会大大减少患者的日常活动,进而加重患者的失能表现。

③ 疲劳

PD 疲劳的患病率约为 50%。目前研究证据表明,疲劳是与 PD 内在病理机制相关的一种主要临床症状,与睡眠障碍、情绪障碍及药物相关是独立的。

④ 抑郁

PD 患者通常在病发后会出现 50% 的精神障碍病症,抑郁更是 PD 患者最为常见的精神病征之一。张光勇等学者经研究认为,PD 患者均伴随出现抑郁、焦虑病症,但是需要重视的是该种抑郁表现通常会在一定程度上更加促进患者的认知功能下降。

⑤ 认知障碍和痴呆

PD 认知功能障碍是 PD 常见的非运动症状,包括 PD 轻度认知损害(PD-MCI)和 PD 痴呆(PDD)。研究显示,PD 痴呆的 8 年累计患病率高达

78.2%。19%~36%的 PD 患者伴有认知功能障碍,有 10%的患者会演变为 PD 痴呆。痴呆是 PD 的主要症状,给患者生活带来严重影响。当前,临床尚未明确 PD 痴呆的发病机制,但均认为其病理学改变为 α-syn 沉积、皮质路易体形成等。

⑥ 睡眠异常

睡眠障碍是 PD 患者最常见的非运动症状,可能是 PD 中最早出现的临床症状。研究发现,快速眼动睡眠行为障碍可早于其他临床表现 10 年出现。67%~88%的 PD 患者存在不同程度的睡眠障碍,主要临床症状为失眠、白天过度嗜睡、异态睡眠等。其中异态睡眠包括不宁腿(RLS)和快眼睡眠障碍(RBD)。

(3) 自主神经

① 胃肠功能障碍

PD 患者的胃肠功能障碍表现在流涎、吞咽困难、胃排空减少、便秘及排便受损,便秘和排便困难是 PD 患者中最常见的胃肠道症状。2001 年,R.阿伯特(R.Abbott)认为便秘是 PD 发病的危险因素。2004 年,蔡军红通过研究比较得出,PD 患者便秘的发生率高达 88%。

迷走神经背核在肠自主神经中起重要作用,在 PD 中这一区域发生改变。E.吉尔(E.Gelpi)等发现 PD 患者胃肠水平上有 α-syn 沉积,然而在健康人中同样有 α-syn 的沉积,并随着年龄的增长而增加。

美国神经学家迈克·格尔松教授最早提出"肠脑轴"的概念,即肠管+肠道神经系统+肠道微生物形成"第二大脑",随着研究的深入,逐渐扩展为微生物-肠-脑轴,即肠脑轴。其实脑肠轴并非新概念,早在 20 世纪 50 年代就有人描述过微生物、肠、脑轴这三者的关系。有研究表明,肠道微生物是治疗 PD 的靶点。比较 PD 患者组与对照组的粪便菌群,发现柔嫩梭菌、拟杆菌门和普雷沃菌科的数量减少,肠杆菌科的数量增加。其中肠杆菌科的数量与姿态不稳和步调艰难的严重程度成正比。

关于 PD 患者便秘的发病机制目前仍在探索中,在病理生理方面可能和与肠神经系统相关的神经退行性改变有关,也可能与 α-syn 在肠神经系统和迷走神经背核的异常堆积及肠肌间多巴胺神经元的丢失有关。

② 泌尿系统症状

泌尿系统功能障碍是 PD 患者最常见的自主神经功能障碍之一,主要表现为尿频尿急和夜尿增多,可出现在疾病的各个阶段,其中夜间频尿是

PD 患者抱怨的首选,严重影响患者的生活质量。PD 患者中表现出泌尿功能障碍的占 27%~63.9%。虽然泌尿系统功能障碍是非运动症状,但一般在运动症状之后出现。研究发现,泌尿系统功能障碍会加重认知损害程度,尤其是执行功能和视空间功能。

③ 心血管功能

PD 心血管系统自主神经功能障碍的表现为血压调节异常,血压调节异常又分为直立性低血压、仰卧位高血压和餐后低血压。临床上 30% 以上的 PD 患者存在体位性低血压。

六、治疗

1. 中药治疗

中药学将 PD 分为肝肾不足型、气血两虚型、痰热动风型、气滞血瘀型等证型,对症下药。

近年来针灸治疗 PD 取得了明确的临床疗效,常用的方法为针刺结合电针,以督脉、胆经、肝经的腧穴为主,尤其注重特定穴位(如原穴和合穴)。艾灸和中医按摩同样可以达到减轻 PD 症状的效果。

2. 西药治疗

PD 运动症状的药物治疗主要以多巴胺类药物(左旋多巴复方制剂+儿茶酚氧位甲基转移酶)为基础,多巴胺激动剂、单胺酶 B 抑制剂、金刚烷胺和抗胆碱能药对于 PD 初期具有良好的治疗效果。左旋多巴复方制剂是治疗 PD 的金标准,但长期服用会有副作用(如"开关现象"、剂末现象和肌张力运动障碍等)。同时随着其他药物服用时间的加长,也会出现不同的副作用。因此应全面比较各类药物的优劣,选择最佳药物搭配治疗 PD。大多数用于治疗非运动症状的药物都是通过除多巴胺以外的神经递质工作的。

3. 物理治疗

主要是通过物理器械进行运动训练来改善 PD 患者的运动症状,提高 PD 患者的生活质量。比如平衡练习、渐进阻力练习、跑步机练习、力量训练、有氧运动、基于音乐与舞蹈的训练和太极拳等。

4. 手术治疗

神经核损毁术:通过化学手段摧毁底丘脑核和基底节的核心功能,从而达到在 PD 动物模型中去除 PD 的效果。由于 DBS 的开展,此类手术已逐步减少。

深部脑刺激(deep brain stimulation,DBS)：用高频电流靶向刺激底丘脑核或者苍白球,以减轻患者症状。

主要参考文献

［1］DORSEY ER, SHERER T, OKUN MS, et al. The Emerging Evidence of the Parkinson Pandemic［J］. *J Parkinsons Dis*, 2018,8(s1):S3-8.

［2］CRISWELL SR, NIELSEN SS, WARDEN M, et al. [18F]FDOPA Positron Emission Tomography in Manganese-exposed Workers［J］. *Neurotoxicology*, 2018(64):43-49.

［3］CHEN SF, YANG YC, HSU CY. Risk of Parkinson's Disease in Patients with Hypothyroidism: A Nationwide Population-based Cohort Study［J］. *Parkinsonism Relat Disord*, 2020(74):28-32.

［4］OBESO JA, STAMELOU M, GOETZ CG, et al. Past, Present, and Future of Parkinson's Disease: a Special Essay on the 200th Anniversary of the Shaking Palsy［J］. *Mov Disord*, 2017,32(09):1264-1310.

［5］BURBULLA LF, SONG P, MAZZULLI JR, et al. Dopamine Oxidation Mediates Mitochondrial and Lysosomal Dysfunction in Parkinson's Disease［J］. *Science*, 2017,357(6357):1255-1261.

［6］CHANG D, NALLS MA, HALLGRIMSDÓTTIR IB, et al. A Meta-analysis of Genome-wide Association Studies Identifies 17 New Parkinson's Disease Risk Loci［J］. *Nat Genet*, 2017,49(10):1511-1516.

［7］SCHAPANSKY J, KHASNAVIS S, DEANDRADE MP, et al. Familial Knockin Mutation of LRRK2 Causes Lysosomal Dysfunction and Accumulation of Endogenous Insoluble α-synuclein in Neurons［J］. *Neurobiol Dis*, 2018(111):26-35.

［8］ROCHA EM, DE MIRANDA BD, SANDERS LH. Alpha-synuclein: Pathology, Mitochondrial Dysfunction and Neuroinflammation in Parkinson's Disease［J］. *Neurobiol Dis*, 2018,109(PtB): 249-257.

［9］GUSTAFSSON G, LINDSTROM V, ROSTAMI J, et al. Alpha-synuclein Oligomer-selective Antibodies Reduce Intracellular Accumulation and Mitochondrial Impairment in Alpha-synuclein Exposed Astrocytes［J］. *J Neuroinflam-mation*, 2017,14(01):241.

［10］GOLDMAN SM, MAREK K, OTTMAN R, et al. Concordance for Parkinson's Disease in Twins：A 20-year Update［J］. *Ann Neurol*, 2019,85（04）:600-605.

［11］SUN Q, WANG T, JIANG TF, et al. Clinical Profile of Chinese Long-term Parkinson's Disease Survivors With 10 Years of Disease Duration and Beyond［J］. *Aging Dis*, 2018,9(01):8-16.

［12］GALBIATI A, VERGA L, GIORA E, et al. The Risk of Neurodegeneration in REM Sleep Behavior Disorder：a Systematic Reviewand Meta-analysis of Longitudinal Studies［J］. *Sleep Med Rev*, 2019(43):37-46.

［13］FOX SH, KATZENSCHLAGER R, LIM SY, et al. International Parkinson and Movement Disorder Society Evidence-based Medicine Review：Update on Treatments for the Motor Symptoms of Parkinson's Disease［J］. *Mov Disord*, 2018,33(08):1248-1266.

［14］MAK MK, WONG-YU IS, SHEN X, et al. Long-term Effects of Exercise and Physical Therapy in People with Parkinson Disease［J］. *Nat Rev Neurol*, 2017,13(11):689-703.

［15］ZHANG S, LIU D, YE D, et al. Can Music-based Movement Therapy Improve Motor Dysfunction in Patients with Parkinson's Disease? Systematic Review and Meta-analysis［J］. *Neurol Sci*, 2017,38(09):1629-1636.

［16］IRANZO A, STEFANI A, SERRADELL M, et al. Characterization of Patients with Longstanding Idiopathic REM Sleep Behavior Disorder［J］. *Neurology*, 2017,89(03):242-248.

［17］POSTUMA RB, IRANZO A, HU M, et al. Risk and Predictors of Dementia and Parkinsonism in Idiopathic REM Sleep Behavior Disorder：a Multicentre Study［J］. *Brain*, 2019,142(03):744-759.

［18］罗蔚锋,王丽君,王晓君,等.老年男性帕金森病患者血尿酸水平的研究[J].中华老年医学杂志,2009,28(01):60-61.

（秦晓凌　罗蔚锋）

嘌呤代谢

一、尿酸概述

尿酸是一种有机弱酸,其 pKa 值为 5.75,水溶性低,生理条件下主要以钠盐形式即尿酸盐存在。尿酸盐存在于所有体液中,主要存在于血浆和脑脊液中。在人及类人猿体内,尿酸是嘌呤代谢的终产物;而在其他哺乳动物体内,尿酸可被尿酸酶(主要表达于肝脏)进一步分解为水溶性较高的尿囊素而排出体外。随着人类的进化,在人及类人猿中编码尿酸酶的基因突变失活,导致人类和类人猿体内缺乏尿酸酶,尿酸无法进一步分解,成为体内嘌呤代谢的终产物。所以,人体内的血浆尿酸水平(4~6 mg/dL;240~360 μm)高于其他哺乳动物体内的血浆尿酸水平(<1 mg/dL;40~60 μm)。根据达尔文提出的"物竞天择、适者生存"规律,在人类进化过程中尿酸的保留可能具有选择性优势,尿酸因其抗氧化作用在人体内发挥重要功能。当然,物极必反,体内尿酸的过度蓄积也与痛风等多种疾病的发生密切相关。

二、尿酸的合成代谢与转运排泄

尿酸是人体内嘌呤代谢的终产物。首先,细胞中的核苷酸在核苷酸酶的作用下水解成核苷。核苷经核苷磷酸化酶作用解离成碱基和核糖-1-磷酸。嘌呤碱既可以通过补救合成途径参与核苷酸的生成,也可以进一步水解。其中,腺嘌呤核糖核苷酸(Adenosine monophosphate,AMP)首先经不同途径转化为次黄嘌呤,后者在黄嘌呤氧化酶的作用下经两次氧化先后生成黄嘌呤和尿酸。鸟苷酸(guanosine monophosphate,GMP)生成鸟嘌呤,后者经脱氨转化为黄嘌呤,最后也是在黄嘌呤氧化酶的作用下生成尿酸(图 1)。黄嘌呤氧化酶是嘌呤核苷酸分解途径中的关键酶,催化次黄嘌呤氧化生成黄嘌呤,再次催化黄嘌呤进一步氧化生成尿酸。上述嘌呤核苷酸的分解代谢主要在肝、小肠及肾中进行,黄嘌呤氧化酶在这些组织中活性较强。正常人体内血浆尿酸水平约为 4~6 mg/dL(240~360 μm)。其中,80%的尿酸来源于嘌呤核苷酸代谢,约20%来自食物摄入。人体内的尿酸主要经肾脏以尿液形式排出体外(约占 2/3),其余由肠道和皮肤等排泄(约占 1/3)。因此,体内的尿酸水平除了受饮食因素影响之外,还受肾功能调节。

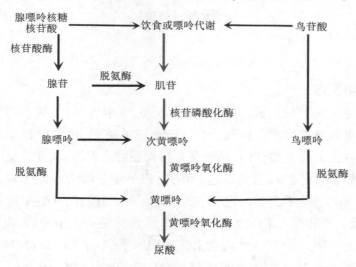

图 1　人体内尿酸生成通路

肾脏是尿酸排泄的主要器官,尿酸经肾脏排泄时主要包括肾小球滤过(几乎达 100%)、近端小管重吸收、分泌及分泌后再吸收等四个过程。总排泄量占滤过的 6%～10%,排出量也与尿酸盐在尿中的溶解度有关,尿液 pH值越大,尿酸在尿液中的溶解度就越大。因此,体内尿酸稳态取决于肾小管中复杂的分泌和再吸收过程,以及肠道排泄的平衡。需要注意的是,在不同的物种之间再吸收和分泌机制的相对重要性是不同的。人类、小鼠和大鼠主要是重新吸收尿酸,而猪、兔、爬行动物和鸟类则有更活跃的分泌机制。

三、血尿酸水平的影响因素

1. 遗传因素

遗传因素对尿酸水平存在一定的影响。尿酸转运体编码基因突变或多态性引起转运体功能变化,影响肾脏等排泄器官对尿酸的重吸收或分泌过程,从而导致血尿酸异常升高或降低。例如,So 等研究发现,尿酸转运蛋白编码基因 Glut9 的等位基因变异对人体血液中的尿酸水平影响较大。

2. 饮食等生活习惯

由于 20% 的尿酸来源于饮食摄入,所以血尿酸水平在很大程度上容易受饮食和生活习惯的影响。譬如,摄入过多的肉类、动物内脏及富含嘌呤的海鲜都会不同程度地提高血浆中的尿酸水平。果糖和麦芽糖会引起腺嘌呤核糖核苷酸分解的增加,促使尿酸生成增多,所以,高尿酸患者也要限制一些软性饮料和含糖量高的水果如西瓜、哈密瓜、榴莲等的摄入。高脂饮食也会引起高尿酸血症。日常生活中,酒类饮料尤其是啤酒的摄入对血尿酸影响非常大,这一点男性尤其要注意。研究提示,血尿酸水平随着啤酒摄入量的增加而升高,但与白酒摄入量不存在类似关系,这可能与啤酒中麦芽糖的含量较高有关。常规牛奶摄入不会增加血尿酸,反而会促进肾小管中尿酸的分泌而降低血尿酸,所以痛风患者可以喝牛奶。还有一些药物如利尿剂、β受体阻断剂、阿司匹林等也会导致血液中尿酸水平的升高。另外,运动等也会影响血尿酸水平。随着机体运动量的增加,排汗量增多,而肾脏血流量减少,尿酸随尿液排出的量相对减少,血尿酸水平也会升高。因此,高尿酸血症患者除了重视基础疾病的治疗与服药影响外,在日常生活中,还应严格限制高嘌呤食物的摄入,戒酒戒烟,控制体重,适度运动,多喝水,多吃新鲜蔬菜,养成良好的生活习惯,这些对控制血尿酸水平都是极其重要的。

四、尿酸转运体

尿酸是弱酸性小分子,具有极性,不能自由通过细胞膜,尿酸排泄主要依赖肾小管上皮细胞刷状缘侧和基底侧膜上的各种尿酸转运蛋白(urate transporter protein,UTP)。因此,转运体功能改变直接影响尿酸在肾脏的转运及排泄。现已发现多种尿酸转运蛋白参与体内尿酸水平的调节,主要包括:(1)尿酸重吸收蛋白,如尿酸盐阴离子转运体1(urate anion transporter 1,URAT1)、有机阴离子转运体4(organic anion transporter 4,OAT4)和葡萄糖转运体9(glucose transporter 9,GLUT9);(2)尿酸分泌蛋白,如有机阴离子转运体1和3(OAT1和OAT3)、尿酸转运蛋白(urate transporter,UAT)、多药耐药蛋白4(mulidrug resistance protein 4,MRP4/ABCC4)、磷酸盐转运蛋白(phosphate transporter,NPT4);(3)其他类型尿酸转运蛋白,如ABC转运蛋白2(ATP-binding cassette subfamily G member 2,ABCG2)、有机阴离子转运体10(organic anion transporters10,OAT10)等。值得注意的是,转运体的表达分布(表1)在不同种属之间存在差异。人体内肾脏近端小管参与尿酸重吸收与分泌。在小鼠中,除了近端小管外,远曲小管也参与了尿酸重吸收与分泌过程。

表 1 尿酸转运体在人体内的分布

尿酸转运体		主要分布
尿酸重吸收蛋白	尿酸盐阴离子转运体 1	位于近端小管顶端(管腔/刷状缘)侧
	有机阴离子转运体 4	主要表达于肾小管上皮的刷状缘侧和基底外侧膜上
	葡萄糖转运体 9	位于近端小管上皮细胞膜的顶端和基底外侧
尿酸分泌蛋白	有机阴离子转运体 1 和 3	主要表达于肾近端小管基底膜
	尿酸转运蛋白	主要表达于肾脏近端小管曲段和升段
	多药耐药蛋白 4	位于管状上皮细胞刷状边缘
	磷酸盐转运蛋白	表达于近端小管上皮细胞的顶膜中
其他类型尿酸转运蛋白	ABC 转运蛋白 2	近端小管上皮细胞膜的顶端和小肠均有表达
	有机阴离子转运体 10	主要表达于肾近端小管上皮细胞顶膜,少量还表达于大脑、心脏及肠道

1. 尿酸重吸收蛋白

顾名思义,尿酸重吸收蛋白主要介导尿酸在肾小管内的重吸收过程,包括尿酸盐阴离子转运体 1、有机阴离子转运体家族中的 OAT4,以及葡萄糖转运体 9。

(1) 尿酸盐阴离子转运体 1

由有机阴离子编码家族 SLC22A 的 SLC22A12 基因编码的一种膜转运蛋白,定位于染色体 llql3,包含 10 个外显子和 9 个内含子,由 555 个氨基酸构成,属于经典的 12 次跨膜转运蛋白,其氨基端和羧基端均位于胞浆内。URAT1 位于近端小管顶端(管腔/刷状缘)侧,不存在于远曲小管。URAT1主要介导尿酸的重吸收,通过与多种单价的有机阴离子和少数无机阴离子交换从而将尿酸从管腔内重吸收至上皮细胞内,重吸收过程依赖于管腔两侧的浓度梯度和电化学梯度,属于电中性的转运体。URAT1 编码基因SLC22A12 突变会影响尿酸重吸收,导致血尿酸水平异常。例如,Guan 等中国学者和 Shima 等日本学者分别在中国和日本的受试者中,证实 SLC22A12基因序列 rs893006 多态性与中国男性高尿酸血症密切相关,而 SLC22A12基因的 G774A 等位基因突变又导致肾性低尿酸血症。实验研究证实,URAT1 功能缺失会导致尿酸排泄分数达 40%~100% 和血清尿酸水平降低。

URAT1 是降低血尿酸水平的主要靶点之一。多种临床药物及内源性分子会影响 URAT1 功能甚至血尿酸水平。例如,苯溴马隆(Benzbromarone)、丙磺舒(Probenecid)、莱西努拉德[Losartan \ Lesinurad,美国食品药品监督管理局(FDA)新批准的治疗痛风药物]抑制 URAT1 功能而降低血尿酸水平;乳酸盐(lactate)、烟酸盐(nicotinate)及抗结核药物吡嗪酰胺(Pyrazinamide)、阿司匹林(Aspirin)促进 URAT1 功能而升高血尿酸水平。

（2）有机阴离子转运体 4

OATs 也是有机阴离子编码家族 SLC22A 编码的一类膜转运蛋白。OATs 表达于体内多种组织器官的细胞膜上,尤其以肝、肾、小肠等排泄器官为主。OATs 家族中的 OAT1、OAT3、OAT4 和 OAT10 均被证明可以通过不同机制参与尿酸在肾脏中的转运。其中,OAT4(由 SLC22A11 基因编码)主要表达于肾小管上皮的刷状缘侧和基底外侧膜上,参与肾脏对尿酸的重吸收。

（3）葡萄糖转运体 9

GLUT9 由 SLC2A9 基因编码,位于 4pl5.3-pl6 染色体上,含有 14 个外显子,其中包括 1 个非编码子和 3 个编码子,有 GLUT9L 和 GLUT9S 两种剪切异构体,分别位于近端小管基底膜和管腔侧,参与肾脏近曲小管顶膜尿酸盐重吸收。除了肾脏之外,肝脏也表达 GLUT9。GLUT9 是尿酸和葡萄糖的双重转运蛋白,所以糖尿病或高血糖都会竞争性地影响血尿酸水平。GLUT9 基因突变与血尿酸水平异常有关。Li 等的研究表明,GLUT9 基因第一外显子起始点上游 1156hp 处的 rsl3137343 多态性与中国汉族男性的高尿酸血症及痛风密切相关。多个研究发现,GLUT9 纯合突变的患者几乎没有尿酸重吸收,其尿酸排泄分数达 100% 或更多。这也提示了 GLUT9 可能是尿酸从近端肾小管内重吸收进入血液的唯一的转运体。

2. 尿酸分泌蛋白

最早的实验证据是在 1950 年,病例对照研究发现低尿酸血症患者存在尿酸盐重吸收障碍,实验结果表明尿酸盐清除率明显高于菊粉,即通过肾脏排出的尿酸盐量高于经肾小球的滤出量,这提示肾小管能分泌尿酸。目前已知的尿酸分泌转运体包括以下几种。

（1）有机阴离子转运体 1 和 3

hOAT1(SLC22A6 基因编码)和 hOAT3(SLC22A8 基因编码)主要表达于肾近端小管基底膜,主要参与将尿酸盐从管周间隙摄取入肾小管上皮细胞这一过程,然后经此分泌至尿液。

（2）尿酸转运蛋白

UAT 广泛表达于各种组织的上皮源性细胞,其中在肾脏表达最丰富,分布于近端小管曲段和升段,主要参与尿酸在肾近曲小管的分泌,进入肾近端小管的尿酸盐大约有 50% 由其介导分泌入管腔,在调节全身尿酸盐稳态中发挥重要作用。UAT 属于电压敏感性离子通道。UAT 与半乳糖凝集素家族尤其是 Galectin9 具有高度同源性。UAT 功能降低或表达减少会导致尿酸排泄降低,引起高尿酸血症。

（3）多药耐药蛋白 4

来源于 ABC（ATP-binding cassette, ABC）家族,由基因 ABCC4 编码,位于染色体 13q32,约 350 kb,由 31 个外显子组成。

（4）磷酸盐转运蛋白（NPT1/4）

3. 其他类型尿酸转运蛋白

例如 ABC 转运蛋白 2,早期研究认为其是一种乳腺癌抗性蛋白,与多种药物的转运相关。后来 Dehghan 等在全基因组相关研究中发现了 ABCG2 与尿酸的相关性,指出 ABCG2 遗传变异与血尿酸异常及痛风发生相关。随后一系列的实验研究表明,近曲小管上皮细胞膜的顶端和小肠中均表达 ABCG2,其在血尿酸稳态调控中发挥重要作用。此外,还有 OAT10,又称"孤对转运蛋白（hoRCTL3）",在近曲小管中依靠尿酸与谷胱甘肽的交换作用来实现尿酸重吸收过程,少量还表达于大脑、心脏及肠道。

4. 尿酸转运体异常与疾病发生

越来越多的研究资料表明,尿酸与多种神经系统疾病的发生有关。然而,关于脑内尿酸的生成与转运调节机制目前了解甚少。有研究报道脑脊液中的尿酸水平仅为血尿酸水平的 1/10,脑脊液内尿酸含量与血浆尿酸水平呈线性相关,脑脊液中的尿酸水平可能还受血脑屏障影响。有研究报道人脑内可以检测到黄嘌呤氧化酶活性,而这正是嘌呤代谢通路中最终催化嘌呤转化生成尿酸的关键酶,这提示我们,除了肝脏及小肠之外,脑内也能产生尿酸。日本有学者运用免疫染色和原位杂交方法研究了尿酸转运体包括 GLUT9、URAT1 和 ABCG2 在小鼠脑内的表达与分布。结果发现,URAT1 定位于室管膜细胞的纤毛和顶端表面;在室管膜细胞、神经元和脑毛细血管中也发现 GLUT9 的阳性染色。在脉络丛上皮和脑毛细血管中同样检测到 ABCG2 阳性染色,而室管膜细胞中没有。另外,其基因突变与 PD 发病延缓相关。以上提示脑内尿酸生成与转运分泌在维持脑内尿酸稳态中起重要作用。然而，诸如脑内尿酸主要是由神经元、神经胶质细胞生成还是二者共同参与生成，其代谢调节的分子机制如何，是否存在脑区分布差异，脑内表达那些尿酸转运蛋白是否受分子机制调控等一系列问题目前尚待进一步研究。

五、尿酸的病理生理功能

1. 促氧化与抗氧化

尿酸是体内重要的抗氧化剂，在人类血浆中，尿酸水平远高于抗坏血酸水平，因此尿酸成为人类主要的内源性抗氧化剂之一。尿酸不仅能抑制过氧化亚硝酸盐介导的硝化反应，还能清除氧自由基和其他一些活性自由基。有研究表明，其抗氧化能力高于抗坏血酸，具有抑制红细胞膜脂质氧化、防止红细胞溶解等作用；还能增加超氧化物歧化酶活性，防止细胞过氧化。此外，尿酸与铁离子具有很强的结合能力，因此还能抑制铁超载引起的过氧化反应，减轻氧化损伤。除了上述直接抗氧化作用外，实验研究还发现尿酸可以通过激活 Nrf2 信号通路，促进谷胱甘肽等抗氧化剂的生成而减轻氧化应激损伤，对神经元发挥保护作用。然而，过高的尿酸，尤其是尿酸晶体沉积会诱发氧化应激损伤。尿酸可以通过氧化应激破坏胰岛 β 细胞和血管内皮细胞，这可能是高尿酸血症患者常伴有糖尿病和心血管病发生的病理生理基础之一。

2. 促进与抑制炎症

既往大量研究认为，高尿酸血症引起的相关病理生理改变与炎症密切相关，这主要与尿酸盐晶体的形成有关。尿酸是一种有机弱酸，水溶性很低，高尿酸血症时，在局部组织如肾小管、骨关节等容易形成结晶沉积。尿酸盐晶体作为一种损伤相关分子模式信号，被巨噬细胞吞噬后可以通过诱导氧自由基大量产生、破坏溶酶体等多重机制激活巨噬细胞等免疫细胞内的 NLRP3 炎症小体，使得 IL-1β 和 IL-18 大量产生，引起局部组织的剧烈炎症反应，这与痛风发作时关节肿胀和疼痛等症状的产生有关。但有趣的是，尿酸对炎症的影响也是一把双刃剑。最近有实验研究表明，尿酸可以抑制小胶质细胞（脑内固有的免疫细胞）活化及其介导的促炎症细胞因子产生，促进抗炎症细胞因子生成，对细菌脂多糖诱导的帕金森病小鼠模型中黑质多巴胺能神经元丢失发挥间接的保护作用。

总之，无论是对氧化应激还是对炎症反应的调节，尿酸都具有两面性。

遗传进化过程保留的尿酸,在适当较低浓度时具有抗氧化和抑制炎症反应的作用,对机体是有益的;持续长期的高尿酸尤其是尿酸盐晶体沉积,则促进氧化损伤和加剧炎症反应,对机体产生不利的影响。

六、尿酸异常与疾病发生

1. 高尿酸血症相关

在正常嘌呤饮食状态下,两次空腹血尿酸水平(非同一日)男性高于420 μmol/L,女性高于360 μmol/L,即称为高尿酸血症(hyperuricemia,HUA)。高尿酸血症可以分为原发性和继发性两大类。原发性高尿酸血症主要是先天性嘌呤代谢障碍所致。常见包括:(1)5-磷酸核苷酸-1-焦磷酸合成酶活性增加,引起5-磷酸核苷酸-1-焦磷酸合成酶合成过多,尿酸产生过多,遗传特征为X连锁。(2)次黄嘌呤-鸟嘌呤磷酸糖转移酶部分缺少,引起5-磷酸核苷酸-1-焦磷酸合成酶浓度增加,尿酸产生过多,遗传特征为X连锁;次黄嘌呤-鸟嘌呤磷酸糖转移酶完全缺乏,见于Lesch-Nyhan综合征。(3)葡萄糖-6-磷酸酶缺乏,嘌呤合成增多引起尿酸产生过多和清除减少,见于糖原积累病Ⅰ型,遗传特征为常染色体隐性遗传。继发性高尿酸血症常见于慢性肾病、药物或长期高嘌呤饮食导致血尿酸生成增加或排泄减少引起的疾病。

高尿酸血症相关的常见疾病包括以下几种。

(1)痛风

高尿酸血症是痛风的发病基础,但短期内尿酸升高并不一定导致痛风,只有当血尿酸持续升高导致尿酸盐在机体组织中沉积并形成结晶时才会促发炎症反应、造成损害而出现痛风。如果高尿酸血症患者不合理控制饮食,酒类尤其是啤酒的摄入很容易诱发痛风的发生。

(2)心血管疾病

血尿酸水平是高血压和冠心病等心血管疾病发病的独立危险因素。

(3)糖脂代谢紊乱综合征

长期高尿酸血症会破坏胰腺β细胞、抑制胰岛素分泌而诱发糖尿病。糖尿病患者在体内糖酵解及游离脂肪酸代谢过程中其血尿酸生成增加,同时肾脏对尿酸的重吸收增加直接导致高尿酸血症。因此,高尿酸血症与糖尿病、肥胖等糖脂代谢紊乱综合征的发病密切相关。

(4)慢性肾脏病

肾脏是尿酸排泄的主要器官,高尿酸血症与慢性肾脏病关系密切。一方面,尿酸结晶沉积可以促发肾小动脉和慢性间质炎症加重肾脏损害;另一方面,尿酸可直接使肾小球入球小动脉发生微血管病变,导致慢性肾脏疾病。反之,慢性肾病的发生又导致尿酸排泄障碍而升高血尿酸。所以,高尿酸血症患者在未出现明显的肾脏病变时要定期监测肾功能变化。

2. 低尿酸血症相关

高尿酸血症可引起痛风和心血管疾病等病理生理改变,临床上血清尿酸水平常作为痛风和肾功能损害的评价指标,中年以上人群也常将血清尿酸检测纳入体检项目。人们常常谈尿酸而色变,降低血尿酸水平被认为有百利而无一害,甚至在临床上血清尿酸降低(低尿酸血症)常常被忽视。

低尿酸血症分为原发性和继发性两大类。继发性低尿酸血症常见于药物或肾功能损伤等。正常经过肾小球滤过、重吸收、分泌和分泌后再吸收等四个过程,最终随尿液排出的尿酸只占 6% ~ 10%。若肾小管功能损伤,近端肾小管对尿酸的重吸收减少和(或)分泌增加,会导致血尿酸降低或低尿酸血症。原发性低尿酸血症主要是尿酸合成减少引起,如 5-磷酸核苷酸-1-焦磷酸合成酶缺陷引起的 Wilson 病。

其实,尿酸作为人体内重要的抗氧化剂,参与了人体内许多重要的氧化还原反应。近年的大量研究发现,低尿酸血症患者帕金森病发病风险增加。尿酸具有神经保护作用,本章节将以 PD 和缺血性脑卒中为例,重点概括性介绍尿酸的神经保护作用。

(1) 低尿酸血症与帕金森病

近年来国内外多项流行病学及临床研究结果表明,尿酸与 PD 发病密切相关。PD 是中老年人常见的以黑质多巴胺能神经元变性缺失为主的神经退行性疾病,临床主要表现为肌强直、静止性震颤、运动减少等运动障碍,常伴有睡眠障碍、嗅觉减退、便秘等非运动症状。病例对照研究发现,PD 患者组的血尿酸水平低于健康对照组;而且,Gao 等的流行病学研究发现,血尿酸水平与 PD 的风险和进展呈负相关,对于男性更为明显。PD 患者脑内的尿酸水平也是明显下降的,尸检结果提示 PD 患者黑质内尿酸水平显著低于对照的健康人群。我们开展的一项动物实验表明,腹腔注射尿酸对 6-羟基多巴胺脑立体定位注射至纹状体诱导的 PD 模型大鼠的中脑多巴胺能神经元起到神经保护作用,能在一定程度上缓解大鼠的运动障碍症状。总之,尿酸对 PD 表现出保护作用,尿酸水平越低,PD 发病风险越高。因此,有学者提出靶向提高脑内尿酸可能是 PD 治疗的新策略。然而,PD 患者血尿酸水平为何降低？二者之间是否存在因果关系？日本学者利用家蚕突变体研究发现，DJ-1（PD 相关蛋白之一）表达降低的家蚕其黄嘌呤氧化酶表达也降低，体内尿酸水平降低，由此提示 DJ-1 可能影响黄嘌呤氧化酶表达，进而减少体内尿酸的生成；然而，临床上 DJ-1 突变的 PD 患者其血尿酸水平是否降低，尚未见相关研究。另外，尿酸对 PD 的临床治疗价值仍待探究，一项以肌苷片（尿酸前体）治疗早期 PD 患者的临床Ⅲ期试验还在进行中。

（2）低尿酸与急性脑缺血

尿酸对缺血性脑卒中具有保护作用。临床研究发现，基线尿酸水平越低，脑梗死体积越大；反之，卒中入院时较高的尿酸水平与较好的预后有关。急性缺血性卒中后 6 h 内尿酸消耗迅速降低，这可能与尿酸发挥抗氧化作用有关。有研究表明，生理条件下尿酸可以清除血液中大约 60% 的氧自由基。在实验性脑缺血模型中，尿酸和溶栓剂阿替普酶联合用药时产生协同的神经保护作用。最近的一项Ⅱ期试验表明，联合静脉注射尿酸和阿替普酶是安全的。哺乳动物的血尿酸水平与其寿命呈正相关。尿酸氧化酶（urate oxidase，UOX）单倍缺失小鼠的尿酸水平升高，且与年龄呈正相关，与野生型小鼠相比寿命显著延长，雌性更为明显。在局灶性缺血性卒中模型中，与野生型小鼠相比，UOX+/-小鼠表现出脑源性神经营养因子水平升高、蛋白硝化和脂质过氧化水平降低、脑水肿减轻。总之，适量补充尿酸对急性缺血性脑卒中表现出令人鼓舞的神经保护作用，但仍需要大样本临床试验进一步验证。

总结与展望

总之，尿酸作为人类进化过程中保留下来的嘌呤代谢终产物，在机体抗氧化和抗炎等过程中发挥重要功能。体内尿酸稳态的维持，对体内多个器官系统功能的发挥具有积极意义。然而，一旦这种平衡被打破，体内持续的高尿酸或低尿酸就会参与甚至导致痛风等多种疾病的发生。尤其是既往常常被忽略的低尿酸与 PD 等多个神经系统疾病的相关性，提示我们不仅要正视高尿酸引起的"害"，更要重视低尿酸的"弊"。对于神经系统而言，探究尿酸的临床疗效依然任重道远，如何找到并维持血尿酸水平在一个合适范围，既能避免心血管疾病和代谢综合征等的发生，又能延缓甚至预防神经退行性疾病的发展，是一项重要而富有挑战性的课题。

主要参考文献

[1] BAO LH, ZHANG YN, ZHANG JN, et al. Urate Inhibits Microglia Activation to Protect Neurons in an LPS-induced Model of Parkinson's Disease [J]. *Neuroinflammation*, 2018, 15(01): 131.

[2] CHOI HK, CURHAN G. Beer, Liquor, and Wine Consumption and Serum Uric Acid Level: the Third National Health and Nutrition Examination Survey[J]. *Arthritis Rheum*, 2004, 51(06): 1023-1029.

[3] CHOI HK, LIU S, CURHAN G. Intake of Purine-rich Foods, Protein, and Dairy Products and Relationship to Serum Levels of Uric Acid: the Third National Health and Nutrition Examination Survey[J]. *Arthritis Rheum*, 2005, 52 (01): 283-289.

[4] CROTTY GF, ASCHERIO A, SCHWARZSCHILD MA. Targeting Urate to Reduce Oxidative Stress in Parkinson Disease[J]. *Exp Neurol*, 2017, 298(PtB): 210-224.

[5] CUTLER RG, CAMANDOLA S, FELDMAN NH, et al. Uric Acid Enhances Longevity and Endurance and Protects the Brain against Ischemia[J]. *Neurobiol Aging*, 2019, 75: 159-168.

[6] DEHGHAN A, KOTTGEN A, YANG Q, et al. Association of Three Genetic Loci with Uric Acid Concentration and Risk of Gout: a Genome-wide Association Study[J]. *Lancet*, 2008, 372(9654): 1953-1961.

[7] GAO X, O'REILLY EJ, SCHWARZSCHILD MA, et al. Prospective Study of Plasma Urate and Risk of Parkinson Disease in Men and Women[J]. *Neurology*, 2016, 86(06): 520-526.

[8] GONG L, ZHANG QL, ZHANG N, et al. Neuroprotection by Urate on 6-OHDA-lesioned Rat Model of Parkinson's Disease: Linking to Akt/GSK3β Signaling Pathway[J]. *J Neurochem*, 2012, 123(05): 876-885.

[9] GUAN M, ZHANG J, CHEN Y, et al. High-resolution Melting Analysis for the Rapid Detection of an Intronic Single Nucleotide Polymorphism in SLC22A12 in Male Patients with Primary Gout in China [J]. *Scand J Rheumatol*, 2009, 38(04): 276-281.

[10] LI C, CHU N, WANG B, et al. Polymorphisms in the Presumptive Promoter Region of the SLC2A9 Gene Are Associated with Gout in a Chinese

Male Population[J].*PLoS One*,2012, 7(02)：e24561.

[11] LLULL L, AMARO S, CHAMORRO A.Administration of Uric Acid in the Emergency Treatment of Acute Ischemic Stroke[J].*Curr Neurol Neurosci Rep*, 2016,16(01)：4.

[12] O'NEILL RD, LOWRY JP.On the Significance of Brain Extracellular Uric Acid Detected with In-vivo Monitoring Techniques：a Review[J].*Behav Brain Res*, 1995,71(1-2)：33-49.

[13] SHIMA Y, NOZU K, NOZU Y, et al.Recurrent EIARF and PRES with Severe Renal Hypouricemia by Compound Heterozygous SLC2A9 Mutation [J].*Pediatrics*, 2011,127(06)：e1621-1625.

[14] SO A, THORENS B.Uric Acid Transport and Disease[J].*J Clin Invest*, 2010,120(06)：1791-1799.

[15] TABUNOKI H, ONO H, ODE H, et al. Identification of Key Uric Acid Synthesis Pathway in a Unique Mutant Silkworm Bombyx Mori Model of Parkinson's Disease[J].*PLoS One*, 2013, 8(07)：e69130.

[16] TOMIOKA NH, TAMURA Y, TAKADA T, et al. Immunohistochemical and in Situ Hybridization Study of Urate Transporters GLUT9/URATv1, ABCG2, and URAT1 in the Murine Brain[J].*Fluids Barriers CNS*, 2016, 13(01)：22.

[17] UEMURA N, MURAKAMI R, CHIBA Y, et al. Immunoreactivity of Urate Transporters, GLUT9 and URAT1, is Located in Epithelial Cells of the Choroid Plexus of Human Brains[J].*Neurosci Lett*, 2017, 659：99-103.

[18] WU XW, MUZNY DM, LEE CC,et al. Two Independent Mutational Events in the Loss of Urate Oxidase during Hominoid Evolution[J].*J Mol Evol*, 1992, 34(01)：78-84.

[19] ZHANG N, SHU HY, HUANG T, et al. Nrf2 Signaling Contributes to the Neuroprotective Effects of Urate against 6-OHDA Toxicity[J].*PLoS One*, 2014, 9(06)：e100286.

（胡丽芳）

帕金森病与嘌呤代谢的基础研究

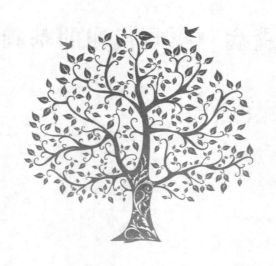

腺苷 A2A 受体和代谢型谷氨酸受体 5 亚型
及其拮抗剂在帕金森病治疗中的作用①

长期应用左旋多巴制剂(5~10 年)会导致约 50%的帕金森病患者出现异动症,称为左旋多巴诱发的异动症(L-DOPA induced dyskinesia,LID),主要表现为舞蹈症和手足徐动症,严重影响 PD 患者的日常生活质量②。LID 的发生与黑质多巴胺能神经元丢失的严重程度、多巴胺波动性刺激引起的直接通路和间接通路的不平衡、突触结构发生可塑性改变及年龄等密切相关③④⑤⑥。腺苷 A2A 受体(adenosine A2A receptor,A2AR)、代谢型谷氨酸受体 5 亚型(metabotropic glutamate receptor 5,mGluR5)及 γ-氨基丁酸(g-aminobutyric acid,GABA)等在其中也起到了重要的作用⑦。

一、腺苷 A2A 受体及其拮抗剂在 PD 和 LID 中的作用

腺苷在中枢神经系统中调节着运动、睡眠、觉醒、疼痛、药物成瘾等重要过程,而这些过程均是由其受体介导的。腺苷受体分为 A1、A2A、A2B、A3 等 4 个亚型,其中 A2A 受体在 PD 治疗方面的作用最为重要⑧。

---

① 本文系江苏省"六大人才高峰"资助项目(项目编号:07-B-005);苏州大学科技创新培育工程重大项目(项目编号:SZ123819)。

② MORISSETTE M, DRIDI M, CALON F, et al. Prevention of Dyskinesia by an NMDA Receptor Antagonist in MPTP Monkeys: Effect On Adenosine A2A Receptors[J].*Synapse*,2006,60(03):239–250.

③ 巴茂文,刘振国,孔敏,等.帕金森病异动症与黑质损伤程度关系的实验研究[J].中华老年医学杂志,2006,25(11):859–862.

④ PAVESE N,EVANS AH,TAI YF,et al.Clinical Correlates of Levodopa-induced Dopamine Release in Parkinson Disease:a PEJ Study[J].*Neurology*,2006,67:1612–1617.

⑤ 曹学兵,孙圣刚,王岚,等.左旋多巴诱发异动症大鼠皮质纹状体突触超微结构与功能的变化[J].中华神经科杂志,2004,37(02):126–130.

⑥ 李先锋,朱武生,陆正齐.帕金森病合并异动症[J].中华老年医学杂志,2009,28(05):438–440.

⑦ MORELLI M,DI PAOLO T,WARDAS J,et al.Role of Adenosine A2A Receptors in Parkinsonian Motor Impairment and 1-DOPA-induced Motor Complications[J].*Prog Neurobiol*,2007,83(05):293–309.

⑧ JENNER P,MORI A,HAUSER R,et al.Adenosine,Adenosine A2A Antagonists,and Parkinson's Disease[J].*Parkinsonism Relat Disord*,2009,15(06):406–413.

1. 腺苷 A2A 受体与 PD 及 LID 的相关性

A2A 受体在脑部主要分布于基底节区,尤其在纹状体的表达最为集中,相对于其他受体其抗 PD 靶点的分布较为局限。A2A 受体选择性地表达于多巴胺 D2 受体和脑啡肽的 γ-氨基丁酸(γ-aminobutyric acid,GABA)能中等棘状神经元(medium spiny neurons,MSNs)上,抗 A2A 受体单克隆抗体超微结构分析显示,A2A 受体主要分布于突触后,少部分分布于突触前,突触后的 A2A 受体通过与 D2 受体及 mGluR5 形成异聚体调节 GABA 的释放①②。

A2A 受体通过与兴奋性 G 蛋白 Gs 相耦联,使腺苷酸环化酶活化,环磷腺苷(cyclic adenosine cyclophosphate,cAMP)合成增加,从而激活依赖 cAMP 的蛋白激酶 A,导致蛋白磷酸化和磷蛋白质如 cAMP 反应元件结合蛋白(cAMP-response element binding protein,CREB)、多巴胺和 cAMP 调节的磷酸化蛋白-32(dopamine and cAMP-regulated phosphoprotein of Mr 32 kD,DARPP-32)等的激活,最终调节 GABA 的释放③。

研究结果显示,多巴胺类药物可以改变 A2A 受体的表达。Zeng 等④对短尾猴进行的研究显示,发生 LID 的猴纹状体 A2A 受体 mRNA 含量要比未发生 LID 的显著增高。Calon 等⑤对死亡后的 PD 患者进行研究,观察到出现 LID 的 PD 患者其脑壳核上 A2A 受体 mRNA 表达水平相对于未出现 LID 的对照组增高,且特异性结合 A2A 受体的放射性配体(H-SCH58261)位点也增多,进一步表明 A2A 受体表达的增加可能与 LID 的发生有关。

2. 腺苷 A2A 受体拮抗剂的动物及临床试验

在动物实验中 A2A 受体拮抗剂能够有效地逆转震颤和肌肉强直⑥。选

① JENNER P,MORI A,HAUSER R,et al.Adenosine,Adenosine A2A Antagonists,and Parkinson's Disease[J].*Parkinsonism Relat Disord*,2009,15(06):406-413.

② SCHWARZSCHILD MA,AGNATI L,FUXE K,et al.Targeting Adenosine A2A Receptors in Parkinson's Disease[J].*Trends Neurosci*,2006,29(11):647-654.

③ MORELLI M,DI PAOLO T,WARDAS J,et al.Role of Adenosine A2A Receptors in Parkinsonian Motor Impairment and 1-DOPA-induced Motor Complications[J].*Prog Neurobiol*,2007,83(05):293-309.

④ ZENG B,PEARCE RK,MACKENZIE GM,et al.Alterations in Preproenkephalin and Adenosine-2A Receptor mRNA,but not Preprotachykinin mRNA Correlate with Occurrence of Dyskinesia in Normal Monkeys Chronically Treated with L-DOPA[J].*Eur J Neurosci*,2000,12(03):1096-1104.

⑤ CALON F,DRIDI M,HORNYKIEWICZ O,et al.Increased Adenosine A2A Receptors in the Brain of Parkinson's Disease Patients with Dyskinesias[J].*Brain*,2004,127(Pt05):1075-1084.

⑥ SALAMONE JD,BETZ AJ,ISHIWARI K,et al.Tremorolytic Effects of Adenosine A2A Antagonists:Implications for Parkinsonism[J].*Front Biosci*,2008,13(10):3594-3605.

择性 A2A 受体拮抗剂(E)-1,3-二丙基-8-(3,4-二甲氧基苯乙烯)-7-甲基-3,7-二氢-1H-嘌呤-2,6-二酮(KW-6002)或 ST1535 与小剂量左旋多巴联合应用时能增强左旋多巴的抗 PD 效应,但并不增加 LID 的发生,表明左旋多巴和 A2A 受体拮抗剂之间存在协同效应①②。此外,研究还显示,KW-6002 和 SCH412348 能够改善 PD 模型大鼠的认知功能③。

多种选择性腺苷 A2A 受体拮抗剂已经进入临床试验,其中 KW-6002 在临床 Ⅱa 和 Ⅱb 试验中均显示能有效改善 PD 症状,且有以下特点:(1)患者对 KW-6002 的耐受性好,不良反应少;(2)KW-6002 能增强小剂量左旋多巴的抗 PD 活性;(3)与左旋多巴相比,KW-6002 使运动障碍的严重程度不变或降低,增加了"开"期时间,减少了"关"期时间④。目前,临床Ⅲ期实验正在进行当中。

3. 腺苷 A2A 受体拮抗剂的神经保护作用

流行病学资料显示,长期饮用咖啡的人群 PD 发病率较低,这可能与咖啡因(非选择性 A2A 受体拮抗剂)拮抗 A2A 受体的神经保护作用有关⑤。研究结果显示,选择性 A2A 受体拮抗剂 KW-6002 及 SCH58261 能够改善 MPTP 诱导的黑质多巴胺能神经元的损伤,MPTP 对 A2A 受体基因敲除动物的多巴胺能神经元毒性显著低于野生型动物⑥⑦,A2A 受体拮抗剂 ST1535 和 ZM241385 能够保护纹状体及对抗鱼藤酮对多巴胺能神经元的神

① ROSE S,JACKSON MJ,SMITH LA,et al. The Novel Adenosine A2A Receptor Antagonist ST1535 Potentiates the Effects of a Threshold Dose of L-DOPA in MPTP Treated Common Marmosets[J]. *Eur J Pharmacol*,2006,546(1−3):82−87.

② MATSUYA T,TAKUMA K,SATO K,et al. Synergistic Effects of Adenosine A2A Antagonist and L-DOPA on Rotational Behaviors in 6-Hydroxydopamine-induced Hemi-Parkinsonian Mouse Model[J]. *J Pharmacol Sci*,2007,103(03):329-332.

③ HIGGINS GA,GRZELAK ME,POND AJ,et al. The Effect of Caffeine to Increase Reaction Time in the Rat during a Test of Attention is Mediated through Antagonism of Adenosine A2A Receptors[J]. *Behav Brain Res*,2007,185(01):32-42.

④ JENNER P,MORI A,HAUSER R,et al. Adenosine,Adenosine A2A Antagonists,and Parkinson's Disease[J].*Parkinsonism Relat Disord*,2009,15(06):406-413.

⑤ SÄÄKSJÄRVI K,KNETKT P,RISSANEN H,et al. Prospective Study of Coffee Consumption and Risk of Parkinson's Disease[J]. *Eur J Clin Nutr*,2008,62(07):908-915.

⑥ JENNER P,MORI A,HAUSER R,et al. Adenosine,Adenosine A2A Antagonists,and Parkinson's Disease[J].*Parkinsonism Relat Disord*,2009,15(06):406-413.

⑦ YACOUBIAN TA,STANDAERT DG. Targets for Neuroprotection in Parkinson's Disease[J]. *Biochim Biophys Acta*,2009,1792(07):676-687.

经毒性作用①。因此,A2AR 拮抗剂可保护黑质多巴胺能神经元,从而延缓疾病的进程。

二、mGluR5 及其拮抗剂在 PD 和 LID 中的作用

谷氨酸作为中枢神经系统重要的兴奋性递质,主要通过兴奋离子型和代谢型谷氨酸受体对神经系统正常功能的维持起重要作用。代谢型谷氨酸受体主要与 G 蛋白相耦联,通过 G 蛋白亚单位作用于离子通道和第二信使,调节神经元和神经胶质细胞的兴奋性。根据其分子结构、药理学特性和信号转导机制的不同,谷氨酸被分为 3 组 8 个亚型,其中第一组包括 mGluRl 和 mGluR5,mGluR5 主要与磷脂酶 C 的磷酸化有关并介导突触后兴奋性效应,同时又与细胞外信号调节激酶(extracellular signal-regulated kinase,GAK)相耦联,最终使 DARPP-32 的 34 位苏氨酸磷酸化②。

1. mGluR5 与 PD 的相关性

多巴胺和谷氨酸均参与正常运动功能的调节,两者介导的神经传导平衡的改变在运动疾病中起关键作用。在 PD 中,由于 D2 受体介导的对纹状体-苍白球神经元抑制作用减弱,间接通路的谷氨酸传导活性明显增强,因此降低间接通路的活性是治疗 PD 的主要目标,可通过增强多巴胺能神经传导或者抑制谷氨酸能神经传导来实现。mGluR5 高度表达于纹状体的投射神经元上,而不存在于自主神经系统的靶器官,克服了传统药物直接作用于多巴胺系统带来的不良反应③。近年来,有报道显示,mGluR5 可能通过调节丘脑底核的谷氨酸释放来改善 PD 的运动障碍孔④。

① BELCASTRO V,TOZZI A,TANTUCCI M,et al. A2A Adenosine Receptor Antagonists Protect the Striatum against Rotenone-induced Neurotoxicity[J]. *Experimental Neurology*,2009,217(01): 231-234.

② MORELLI M,DI PAOLO T,WARDAS J,et al.Role of Adenosine A2A Receptors in Parkinsonian Motor Impairment and 1-DOPA-induced Motor Complications[J].*Prog Neurobiol*,2007,83(05): 293-309.

③ PAQUET M,SMITH Y. Group I Metabotropic Glutamate Receptors in the Monkey Striatum: Subsynaptic Association with Glutamatergic and Dopaminergic Afferents[J]. *J Neurosci*,2003,23(20): 7659-7669.

④ LEVANDIS G,BAZZINI E,ARMENTERO MT. Systemic Administration of an mGlu5 Antagonist,but not Unilateral Subthalamic lesion,Counteracts L-DOPA-induced Dyskinesias in a Rodent Model of Parkinson's Disease[J]. *Neurobiol Dis*,2008,29(01): 161-168.

2. mGluR5 在 LID 时的变化

Samadi 等[①]用 mGluR5 选择性放射配体 2-甲基-6-苯基乙炔基嘧啶〔2 -Methyl－6－(phenylethynyl)pyridine,MPEP)受体结合放射自显影术显示,发生 LID 的 MPTP 毁损的猴纹状体 mGiuR5 结合较对照组明显增多,这为 mGluR5 可能参与 LID 的发生提供了证据。Mela 等[②]的研究显示,选择性 mGluR5 拮抗剂 3-〔(2-甲基-1,3-噻唑-4-)乙炔基〕吡啶｛3 -〔(2－methyl－1,3－thiaol;－4－yl)ethy myl〕－pyridine,MTEP｝可作为左旋多巴治疗 PD 的辅助用药,同时还可以减少 LID 的发生及降低左旋多巴治疗的 PD 小鼠纹状体突触活性。然而,mGluR5 拮抗剂是通过在纹状体水平调节离子型谷氨酸受体 N-甲基 D-门冬氨酸(N－methyl－d－aspartic aci,NMDA)的表达发挥抗异动症效应的[③]。

3. mGluR5 拮抗剂的动物实验

在 LID 大鼠模型中,左旋多巴治疗前 30 mins 予以选择性 mGluR5 拮抗剂 MPEP 腹腔注射,能够明显改善左旋多巴治疗所诱发的异动症症状。有研究报道,mGluR5 拮抗剂 MTEP 不仅能减少左旋多巴治疗诱发异动症的发生,还能改善已经出现的异动症症状[④]。因此应用 mGluR5 拮抗剂将成为改善左旋多巴治疗诱发异动症症状的一种有潜力的治疗手段。

三、腺苷 A2A 受体、mGluR5 及其拮抗剂联合治疗在 PD 和 LID 中的作用

1. 腺苷 A2A 受体、多巴胺 D2 受体和 mGluR5 形成异聚体

突触后 A2A 受体和多巴胺 D2 受体形成异二聚体,A2A 受体和兴奋性

① SAMADI P, GRGOIRE L, MORISSETTE M, et al. mGlu5 Metabotropic Glutamate Receptors and Dyskinesias in MPTP Monkeys[J]. *Neurobiol Aging*,2008,29(07):1040-1051.

② MELA F,MARTI M,DEKUNDY A,et al. Antagonism of Metabotropic Glutamate Receptor Type 5 Attenuates L-DOPA-induced Dyskinesia and its Molecular and Neurochemical Correlates in a Rat Model of Parkinson's Disease[J]. *J Neurochem*,2007,101(02):483-497.

③ LEVANDIS G,BAZZINI E,ARMENTERO MT. Systemic Administration of an mGluR5 Antagonist,but not Unilateral Subthalamic lesion,Counteracts L-DOPA-induced Dyskinesias in a Rodent Model of Parkinson's Disease[J]. *Neurobiol Dis*,2008,29(01):161-168.

④ LEVANDIS G,BAZZINI E,ARMENTERO MT. Systemic Administration of an mGluR5 Antagonist,but not Unilateral Subthalamic lesion,Counteracts L-DOPA-induced Dyskinesias in a Rodent Model of Parkinson's Disease[J]. *Neurobiol Dis*,2008,29(01):161-168.

蛋白 Gs 相耦联，D2 受体和 Gi 相耦联，两受体之间相互拮抗①。而 A2A 受体和 mGluR5 形成的异二聚体则协同发挥作用，一定量的内源性腺苷与 A2A 受体相结合是 mGluR5 和谷氨酸相结合并发挥作用的前提；同时，腺苷 A2A 受体的兴奋亦需要内源性谷氨酸活化 mGluR5，两受体的共同活化可拮抗内源性多巴胺与 D2 受体结合，而单独活化时效应则降低②。A2A 受体在腺苷酸环化酶水平拮抗性地调节 D2 受体兴奋所引起的抑制效应，而 mGluR5 则通过细胞外信号调节激酶增强 A2A 受体的作用。基于 mGluR5 拮抗剂发挥治疗 PD 运动障碍的作用需要 A2A 受体和多巴胺 D2 受体的参与，研究者提出了腺苷 A2A 受体、多巴胺 D2 受体和 mGluR5 异聚体的概念，这一异聚体的存在，使得调节运动功能的多种信号有可能通过纹状体-苍白球 GABA 能神经元发挥作用③④。

2. 腺苷 A2A 受体和 mGluR5 在 LID 时突触可塑性改变中的作用

皮质纹状体突触活性增强是基底节环路失衡改变中的关键环节，与 LID 的发生密切相关，长期非生理性多巴胺替代治疗使纹状体部神经元为适应这一改变而发生异常的可塑性变化⑤。研究显示，A2A 受体与 D2 受体之间不仅存在相互拮抗作用，而且两受体之间的相互作用增强了 A2A 受体信号，因此，LID 可能是由于细胞膜 A2A/D2 异二聚体相对于 A2A 受体平衡性改变而引起。在细胞膜表面由于异常 A2A 受体信号增加使其占主导地位，A2A 受体活化 PKA 和抑制蛋白磷酸酶-1(protein phosphatase-1，PP-1)的活性，使异常的受体嵌合体(特异的异质寡聚物)过度磷酸化形成错误的记

① TOZZI A，TSCHERTER A，BELCASTRO V，et al. Interaction of A2A Adenosine and D2 Dopamine Receptors Modulates Corticostriatal Glutamatergic Transmission[J]. *Neuropharmacol*，2007，53(06)：783-789.

② NISHI A，LIU F，MATSUYAMA S，et al. Metabotropic mGlu5 Receptors Regulate Adenosine A2A Receptor Signaling[J]. *Proc Natl Acad Sci USA*，2003，100(03)：1322-1327.

③ SCHWARZSCHILD MA，AGNATI L，FUXE K，et al. Targeting Adenosine A2A Receptors in Parkinson's Disease[J]. *Trends Neurosci*，2006，29(11)：647-654.

④ FUXE K，MARCELLINO D，RIVERA A，et al. Receptor Interactions within Receptor Mosaics. Impact on Neuropsychopharmacology[J]. *Brain Res Rev*，2008，58(02)：415-452.

⑤ 曹学兵，孙圣刚，王岚，等.左旋多巴诱发异动症大鼠皮质纹状体突触超微结构与功能的变化[J].中华神经科杂志，2004，37(02)：126-130.

忆,从而促使 LID 的发生①。Santini 等②的研究显示,背侧纹状体中等棘状神经元 cAMP/PKA/DARPP-32 途径和细胞外信号调节激酶信号增强可能与 LID 的发生有关。A2A 受体的兴奋激活了 cAMP/PKA/DARPP-32 途径,同时 mGluR5 的兴奋和细胞外信号调节激酶信号增强密不可分,A2A 受体和 mGluR5 可能通过以上两个信号途径促使 LID 的发生和发展。mGluR5 兴奋在膜内和促分裂原活化蛋白激酶(mitogen-activated protein kinase,MAPK)水平通过提高 A2A 受体抑制多巴胺和 D2 受体的结合实现 A2A 受体的效应③。目前对 A2A 受体、mGluR5 在 LID 发生时纹状体中等棘状神经元突触可塑性改变中的机制还不太明确,有待于进一步研究。

3. 腺苷 A2A 受体和 mGluR5 联合治疗 PD 的动物实验

Coccurello 研究组联合应用单独治疗无药效剂量的 A2A 受体拮抗剂和 mGluR5 拮抗剂时可以明显改善由 6-羟多巴胺毁损 PD 大鼠而导致的运动障碍④。Kachroo 等⑤在行为学水平阐明了类似的协同治疗作用,实验显示了 A2A 受体拮抗剂在运动激活中的作用及 mGluR5 拮抗剂在利血平损伤大鼠中的抗 PD 效应。A2A 受体拮抗剂 SCH58261 和 mGluR5 拮抗剂 MTEP 联合治疗 PD 能够发挥协同作用从而减轻肌肉强直及静止性震颤⑥。因此,A2A 受体及 mGluR5 的联合阻断作用为 PD 的治疗提供了一种有潜力的非多巴胺能药物选择。

① ANTONELLI T,FUXE K,AGNATI L,et al. Experimental Studies and Theoretical Aspects on A2A/D2 Receptor Interactions in a Model of Parkinson's Disease. Relevance for L-dopa Induced Dyskinesias[J]. *J Neurol Sci*,2006,248(1-2):16-22.

② SANTINI E,VALJENT E,USIELLO A,et al. Critical Involvement of cAMP/DARPP-32 and Extracellular Signal-regulated Protein Kinase Signaling in L-DOPA-induced Dyskinesia[J].*J Neurosci*,2007,27(26):6995-7005.

③ MORELLI M,DI PAOLO T,WARDAS J,et al.Role of Adenosine A2A Receptors in Parkinsonian Motor Impairment and 1-DOPA-induced Motor Complications[J].*Prog Neurobiol*,2007,83(05):293-309.

④ COCCURELLO R,BREYSSE N,AMALRIC M. Simultaneous Blockade of Adenosine A2A and Metabotropic Glutamate mGlu5 Receptors Increase their Efficacy in Reversing Parkinsonian Deficits in Rats[J]. *Neuropsychopharmacology*,2004,29(08):1451-1461.

⑤ KACHROO A,ORLANDO LR,GRANDY DK,et al. Interactions between Metabotropic Glutamate 5 and Adenosine A2 Receptors in Normal and Parkinsonian Mice[J]. *J Neurosci*,2005,25(45):10414-10419.

⑥ MORELLI M,DI PAOLO T,WARDAS J,et al.Role of Adenosine A2A Receptors in Parkinsonian Motor Impairment and 1-DOPA-induced Motor Complications[J].*Prog Neurobiol*,2007,83(05):293-309.

四、展望

目前,腺苷 A2A 受体及 mGluR5 拮抗剂成为治疗帕金森病十分有前景和可行的非多巴胺类药物,为中晚期出现 LID 等并发症的 PD 患者带来了转机,早期应用可延缓疾病的进展。对腺苷 A2A 受体及 mGluR5 在中枢神经系统神经生物学、病理生理学方面的作用还有待基础及临床的进一步研究。

(黄译腺 李 丹 罗蔚锋)

(本文原载于《中华老年医学杂志》2010 年第 29 卷第 3 期)

尿酸减轻 6-羟基多巴胺对 PC12 细胞的毒性作用①

摘要：6-羟基多巴胺（6-hydroxydopamine,6-OHDA）对 PC12 细胞的毒性作用。

方法：应用 PC12 细胞制作帕金森细胞模型,分为对照组、尿酸组、6-OHDA 组、尿酸+6-OHDA 组。采用 MTT 测定各组 PC12 细胞活性,免疫荧光法观察各组 PC12 细胞 caspase-3 激活情况,流式细胞术检测各组 PC12 细胞凋亡率。尿酸 100～400 μmol/L 不影响 PC12 细胞生存率,尿酸 100～400 μmol/L 可显著提高 6-OHDA 50 μmol/L 作用 6 h、12 h 和 24 h 造成的 PC12 细胞生存率的下降（$P<0.01$）;尿酸能减少 6-OHDA 导致的 PC12 细胞 caspase-3 激活,降低 6-OHDA 导致的凋亡率（$P<0.05$）。

结论：尿酸具有减轻 6-OHDA 对 PC12 细胞毒性的作用。

关键词：尿酸;帕金森病;PC12 细胞,6-羟基多巴胺。

Protective Effect of Uric Acid on the Cell Damage of PC12 Cells Induced by 6-OHDA

Aim：To investigate the protective effect of UA on the injury of PC12 cells induced by 6-OHDA.

Methods：PC12 cells injured by 6-OHDA were used as the Parkinson's disease cell models, which were divided into four groups: control group, UA group, 6-OHDA group and UA+6-OHDA group. The cell viability were assessed by MTT method. The apoptosis of cells were assessed by observing the caspase-3 protein level by using immunocytochemistry, and calculating apoptosis rate using

---

① 本文系苏州市科技计划（社会发展及医药）项目;江苏省高校自然研究计划项目（项目编号:08KJB320012）。

flow cytometry（FCM）technique.

Results：50 μmol/L of 6-OHDA decreased the viability of PC12 cells at 6, 12,24 h. 100~400 μmol/L of UA had no significant effect on the viability of PC12 cells. 100~400 μmol/L of UA reversed the decease of PC12 cells induced by 6-OHDA. The caspase-3 protein level and apoptosis rate of PC12 cell were increased after 6-OHDA（50 μmol/L）treatment for 24 h,which were decreased by UA（200 μmol/L）treatment（$P<0.05$）.

Conclusion：6-OHDA can decrease the viability of PC12 cells and increase the apoptosis of PC12 cells. UA can protect PC12 cells from injury induced by 6-OHDA.

Key words：uric acid；Parkinson's disease；PC12 cell；6-OHDA.

帕金森病是中老年人常见的神经退行性疾病,病理改变主要为中脑黑质多巴胺能神经元进行性减少和路易小体形成,其发生机制与氧化应激反应增强、线粒体功能障碍密切相关。UA 是一种重要的生理性天然抗氧化剂、铁螯合剂、自由基清除剂。近年的流行病学及临床研究发现,PD 发病及进展与 UA 密切相关[1][2][3][4][5]。为提供 UA 保护多巴胺能神经元的直接证据,本实验采用 PC12 细胞和 6-OHDA 建立 PD 细胞模型,评价 UA 减轻 6-OHDA 对 PC12 细胞的毒性作用。

一、材料与方法

1. 主要试剂与细胞株

UA、6-OHDA（Sigma 公司,美国）,DMEM（Dulbecco's modified Eagle's medium）培养基,流式细胞凋亡检测试剂盒（GIBCO Invitrogen 公司,英国）,

① WEISSKOPF MG, O'REILY E, CHEN H, et al.Plasma Urate and Risk of Parkinson's Disease[J]. *Am J Epidemiol*, 2007, 166(05):561-567.

② DE VERA M, RAHMAN MM, RANKIN J, et al.Gout and the Risk of Parkinson's Disease:a Cohort Study[J].*Arthritis Rheum*, 2008, 59(11):1549-1554.

③ ANNANMAKI T, MUURONEN A, MURROS K. Low Plasma Uric Acid Level in Parkinson's Disease [J].*Mov Disord*, 2007, 22(08):1133-1137.

④ 王丽君, 罗蔚锋, 王恒会, 等.帕金森病患者血尿酸水平[J].中华神经科杂志, 2008,41(03):157-158.

⑤ SCHWARZSCHILD MA, SCHWID SR, MAREK K, et al. Serum Urate as a Preditctor of Clinical and Radiographic Progression in Parkinson Disease[J]. *Arch Neurol*, 2008, 65(06):716-723.

羊抗 caspase-3 一抗（Santacruz 公司，美国），cy3 标记兔抗羊二抗、MTT、DMSO（上海碧云天生物技术有限公司）；PC12 细胞株由苏州大学神经变性与衰老疾病实验室秦正红教授赠予。

2. PC12 细胞培养[①]

PC12 细胞用含 10% 小牛血清的 DMEM 进行常规培养，2~3 d 换液。待细胞增长至 80% 融合时，用 0.25% 胰酶消化细胞，加含血清的培养基终止消化，吹打成为单细胞悬液，按 1：4 比例传代分瓶。

3. MTT 检测 PC12 细胞生存率和分组[②]

用含 10% 小牛血清的 DMEM 将 PC12 细胞浓度调整至 7×10^4/mL 接种于 96 孔板中（每孔体积 100 μL），接种细胞的孔板放置于 37 ℃、5%CO_2 培养箱中孵育。首先用 MTT 法检测 UA 对 PC12 细胞生存率的影响，设正常对照组（DMEM 培养基）、UA 100、200、300、400 和 500 μmol/L 组，孵化 24 h。在此基础上，再选取对 PC12 细胞生存率没有影响的 UA 浓度观察其对 6-OHDA 造成的细胞损伤是否具有保护作用。分组为：对照组（DMEM 培养基）、6-OHDA（50 μmol/L）组和 UA（100 μmol/L）+6-OHDA（50 μmol/L）、UA（200 μmol/L）+6-OHDA（50 μmol/L）、UA（300 μmol/L）+6-OHDA（50 μmol/L）、UA（400 μmol/L）+6-OHDA（50 μmol/L）、药物作用时间为 6 h、12 h 和 24 h。

检测前 4 h 每孔加入 MTT（5 mg/mL）10 μL，将孔板放入培养箱中继续孵育 4 h，终止培养。吸出上清液，每孔加入 DMSO100 μL，摇床上振荡 10~15 mins，待紫色甲瓒结晶充分溶解后，应用酶标（BIO-TEK Power Wave XS）选择 570 nm 波长测定各孔吸光度（A）值。每组设 5 个复孔。

$$细胞生存率（\%）=（加药组 A/内对照组 A）\times 100\%$$

4. Caspase-3 免疫荧光染色法[③]

将细胞接种于铺有小玻片的 24 孔板（每孔体积 1 mL）中。分别加 UA、

① FENG L, MENG H, WU F, et al. Olfactory Ensheathing Cells Conditioned Medium Prevented Apoptosis Induced by 6-OHDA in PC12 Cells through Modulation of Intrinsic Apoptotic Pathways[J]. *Int J Dev Neurosci*, 2008, 26(3-4):323-329.

② FENG L, MENG H, WU F, et al. Olfactory Ensheathing Cells Conditioned Medium Prevented Apoptosis Induced by 6-OHDA in PC12 Cells through Modulation of Intrinsic Apoptotic Pathways[J]. *Int J Dev Neurosci*, 2008, 26(3-4):323-329.

③ 邹万新，江悦琴，姜叙诚.Caspase-3 和 bcl-xL 在胃癌中的表达及意义[J].癌症，2001,20(07)：726-729.

6-OHDA 和 UA+6-OHDA 后旋转于 37.0 ℃、5% CO_2 培养箱中孵育 24 h,从 24 孔板取出细胞爬片,PBS 洗涤 3 次,4%多聚甲醛固定 30 mins,PBS 清洗,用 1% triton 打孔 15 mins,PBS 清洗后加抗 caspase-3 一抗(1:1 000)37 ℃ 孵育 2 h,PBS 充分清洗,加 cy3 标记的二抗 (1:500)37 ℃孵育 1 h,PBS 充分漂洗,加入 DAPI(1:10 000)染色 5 mins,PBS 清洗后封片在荧光显微镜下观察。细胞内红色荧光的强弱代表 caspase-3 的激活程度,红色荧光越强,caspase-3 的活性越高。

Caspase-3 免疫荧光染色后选取其中一个保护作用明显、单独对 PC12 细胞生存率没有影响的 UA 浓度(200 μmol/L),观察其对 6-OHDA 造成的 caspase-3 活性影响。分为正常对照组(DMEM 培养基)、6-OHDA(50 μmol/L) 组、UA(200 μmol/L)组和 UA(200 μmol/L)+6-OHDA(50 μmol/L)组。

5. Annexin V/PI 双染法检测细胞凋亡率[①]

分组用 caspase-3 免疫荧光染色。将细胞接种于培养瓶中,待细胞生长融合至 60%~70%时加入药物,作用 24 h 后收集培养瓶中各组细胞,分别制成单细胞悬液,1 000 r/min 离心 5 mins,弃上清,PBS(4 ℃预冷)洗涤细胞 2 次,1 000 r/min 离心,弃上清。用制备好的 annexin blinding buffer 100 μL 将细胞制备成悬液,然后加入 PI(1 μL)和 488 (5 μL),对细胞进行标记,染色 15 mins 后再加入 annexin blinding buffer 400 μL,利用流式细胞仪(EPICS XL)进行双参数分析。流式细胞仪检测时,每个样本检测≥7 000 个细胞,重复 4 次。

细胞凋亡率=被荧光标记的阳性细胞数/所有检测细胞数

6. 统计学方法

所有数据采用"$\bar{x}\pm s$"表示,采用 SSPS 10.0 统计软件进行分析,组间比较用单因素方差分析(One-way ANOVA)检验。

二、结果

1. MTT 测定 UA、6-OHDA 和 UA+6-OHDA 对 PC12 细胞生长的影响

UA 100~500 μmol/L 分别作用 PC12 细胞 24 h,PC12 细胞生存率分别

① CHEN XW, SUN SG, CHENG DB, et al. Overexpression of 14-3-3 Protein Protects Pheochromocytoma Cells against 1-methyl-4-phenylpyridinium Toxicity[J]. *Neurosci Bull*, 2006, 22(05):281-287.

为(93.3±6.0)%、(98.9±6.8)%、(105.0±4.0)%、(106.6±5.0)%和(131.5±16.4)%。其中 UA 100~400 μmol/L 组和对照组（100±3.7)%相比较，差异无统计学意义($P>0.05$)，对 PC12 细胞生存率无明显影响；而 UA 500 μmol/L 组 PC12 细胞生存率与对照组相比有显著提高($P<0.01$)（表1）。

表1　不同浓度尿酸对 PC12 细胞生存率的影响($\bar{x}\pm s$)
Tab.1　Effect of Uric Acid on the Survival Rate of PC12 Cells($\bar{x}\pm s$)

	对照组 Control Group	尿酸组 UA Group				
		100 μmol/L	200 μmol/L	300 μmol/L	400 μmol/L	500 μmol/L
细胞生存率(%) Survival Rate of Cell Viability(%)	100±3.7	93.3±6.0	98.9±6.8	105.0±4.0	106.6±5.0	131.5±16.4
P 值 P Value		0.86	0.83	0.64	0.06	0.002

6-OHDA50 μmol/L 作用 6 h、12 h 和 24 h 后 PC12 细胞生存率进行性下降，分别为(95.5±2.4)%、(88.7±5.1)%和(73.8±10.0)%。其中 12 h 和 24 h 细胞生存率显著下降($P<0.01$)。UA 100~400 μmol/L 6-OHDA 50 μmol/L 作用 6 h、12 h 和 24 h 所造成的 PC12 细胞生存率下降有显著减缓($P<0.01$)（表2）。

表2　不同组 PC12 细胞生存率的比较[($\bar{x}\pm s$)%]
Tab.2　Comparison of Survival Rate of PC12 in Different Groups[($\bar{x}\pm s$)%]

时间 Time	对照组 Control Group	6-OHDA 50 μmol/L 组 6-OHDA 50 μmol/L Group	6-OHDA 50 μmol/L+尿酸组 6-OHDA 50 μmol/LGroup+UA Group			
			UA 100 μmol/L	UA 200 μmol/L	UA 300 μmol/L	UA 400 μmol/L
6 h	100±4.5	95.5±2.4	109.7±5.6[2]	113.9±5.6[2]	118.5±4.6[2]	119.9±3.8[2]
12 h	100±3.6	88.7±5.1[1]	101±6.3[2]	100.9±3.3[2]	114.4±4.4[2]	107.6±7.7[2]
24 h	100±5.3	73.8±10.0[1]	91.6±7.6[2]	104.7±8.3[2]	106.6±16.1[2]	113.7±5.7[2]

注：与对照组比较，[1]$P<0.01$；与 6-OHDA 组比较，[2]$P<0.01$。
Notes：versus the Control Group，[1]$P<0.01$；versus the 6-OHDA Group，[2]$P<0.01$。

2. PC12 细胞 caspase-3 免疫荧光检测

结果显示,对照组和 UA 200 μmol/L 组可见弱的红色荧光;6-OHDA 50 μmol/L 组可见强烈的红色荧光;UA 200 μmol/L+6-OHDA 50 μmol/L 组的红色荧光较 6-OHDA 50 μmol/L 组减弱(图 1)。

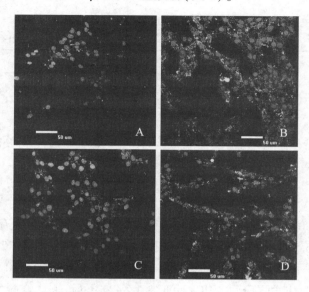

图 1 免疫荧光检测 PC12 细胞内 caspase-3 的活性

Fig.1 Activation of Caspase-3 in PC12 Cells by Immunofluorescence Technology

注:蓝色表示细胞核,红色表示 caspase-3 的活性。A 为对照组;B 为 6-OHDA 50 μmol/L 组;C 为 UA 200 μmol/L 组;D 为 UA200 μmol/L+6-OHDA 50 μmol/L 组。

Notes:Red represents the activation of caspase-3, and blue indicates nuclei. A,cells were control group;B,cells were treated with 6-OHDA 50 μmol/L group;C,cells were treated with UA 200 μmol/L group;D,cells were treated with 6-OHDA 50 μmol/L+UA 200 μmol/L group.

3. Annexin V/PI 双染法检测细胞凋亡率

UA 单独作用于 PC12 细胞 24 h 的凋亡率(3.2±0.8)%和对照组(3.5±1.3)%比较,其差异无统计学意义($P>0.05$)。加入 6-OHDA 50 μmol/L 作用 24 h 后,细胞的凋亡率(9.8±2.3)%和对照组相比显著增高($P<0.05$),而 UA 200 μmol/L+6-OHDA 50 μmol/L 组的细胞凋亡率[(6.0±1.5)%]和 6-OHDA[(9.8±2.3)%]组比较显著降低($P<0.05$)(图 2)。

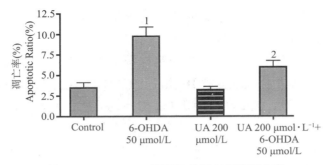

图 2　Annexin V/PI 双染法检测各细胞凋亡率

Fig.2　Apoptotic Ratio of PC12 Cells Assessed by Flow Cytometry(FCM)

注：与对照组比较，[1]$P<0.05$；与 6-OHDA 组比较，[2]$P<0.05$。

Notes：versus the non-treated group，[1]$P<0.05$；versus the 6-OHDA-treated group，[2]$P<0.05$.

讨　论

　　氧化应激在 PD 的发生中起重要作用。生理情况下,黑质纹状系统自由基的生成和清除保持相对动态平衡,当自由基产生过多或机体对自由基的清除能力下降时,就会造成细胞的氧化应激损伤。氧化应激可使饱和、不饱和脂肪酸发生脂质过氧化,从而对蛋白质和 DNA 产生氧化损伤并诱导细胞凋亡,导致黑质多巴胺能神经元的变性死亡、数量减少。多巴胺在 B 型单胺氧化酶(monoamine oxidase,MAO-B)的氧化作用下可以产生自由基和活性半醌,参与氧化应激的形成。6-OHDA DA 是 DA 类似物,其结构与 DA 相类似,常被误作为 DA 神经递质摄入 DA 能神经元,选择性地破坏 DA 能神经元,造成 DA 能神经元死亡,在 PD 患者脑内和尿样中检测到 6-OHDA。6-OHDA DA 在氧化时可以产生 H_2O_2 和半醌,前者通过产生氧化应激作用于线粒体引起细胞色素 C 释放,激活 caspase-3/7 而导致细胞凋亡[1],后者是通过氧化应激以外的途径造成对细胞的操作,它通过 caspase-8、caspase-12 激活 caspase-3 启动细胞凋亡[2]。超氧化物歧化酶(superoxide dismutase,SOD)

　　① HANROTT K, GUDMUMSEN L, WONNACOTT S. 6-hydroxydopamine-induced Apoptosis is Mediated via Extracellular Auto-oxidation and Caspase 3-dependent Activation of Protein Kinase Cδ[J]. *J Biol Chem*, 2006, 281(09):5373-5382.

　　② SAITO Y, NISHIO K, OGAWA Y, et al. Molecular Mechanisms of 6-hydroxydopamine-induced Cytotoxicity in PC12 Cells:Involvement of Hydrogen Peroxide-dependent and Independent Action[J]. *Free Radic Biol Med*, 2007, 42(05):675-685.

可以完全阻止 H_2O_2 对细胞造成的损害,却不能完全阻止 6-OHDA 对细胞造成的损伤。Caspase-3 是半胱氨酸蛋白酶家族中的一个,它可以参与重要底物的剪切,诱导细胞凋亡①。PC12 细胞株源于大鼠肾上腺嗜铬细胞瘤,细胞质富含 DA 受体并合成或分解 DA 所需的各种酶,生理及生化功能等方面接近于 DA 能神经元,被广泛应用于 DA 能神经元死亡方式及毒性损害的研究,本实验以 PC12 细胞和 6-OHDA 建立 PD 细胞模型为研究对象。

UA 是嘌呤代谢产物,具有清除自由基、增加 SOD 活性及螯合铁离子的作用②③④,能降低 PD 的氧化速度,减少 H_2O_2 产生的速度,减轻氧化应激⑤。流行病学及临床研究发现,在血 UA 水平相对低的人群中 PD 的发生率较高⑥⑦,PD 患者的 UA 水平显著低于正常人⑧⑨。在 PD 病例中,UA 水平高的患者比 UA 水平低的患者病情进展缓慢⑩。本研究结果提示:在 UA 浓度为 100~400 μmol/L 不影响细胞活性的情况下,对 6-OHDA 作用 12 h 和 24 h 所造成的 PC12 细胞生存率下降有显著的提高;UA 能减少 6-OHDA 导致的 PC12 细胞 caspase-3 激活,降低 6-OHDA 导致的凋亡率增高。UA 减轻 6-OHDA 对 PC12 细胞毒性的作用机制还不完全清楚,考虑与 UA 清除自

① 谭玉燕,周海燕,陈生弟. 帕金森病的细胞凋亡[J].中华老年医学杂志,2007,26(09):709-712.

② AMES BN, CATHCART R, SCHWIERS E, et al. Uric Acid Provides an Antioxidant Defense in Humans against Oxidant-and radical-caused Aging and Cancer: a Hypothesis[J]. *Proc Natl Acad Sci USA*, 1981, 78(11):6858-6862.

③ HINK HU, SANTANAM N, DIKALOV S, et al. Peroxidase Properties of Extracellular Superoxide Dismutase:Role of Uric Acid in Modulating in Vivo Activity[J]. *Arterioscler Thromb Vasc Biol*, 2002, 22(09):1402-1408.

④ YU ZF, BRUCE-KELLER AJ, GOODMAN Y, et al. Uric Acid Protects Neurons against Excitotoxic and Metabolic Insults in Cell Culture, and against Focal Ischemic Brain Injury in Vivo[J]. *J Neurosci Res*, 1998, 53(05):613-625.

⑤ 罗蔚锋,刘春风.尿酸水平与帕金森病[J].中华神经科杂志,2008,41(08):552-553.

⑥ WEISSKOPF MG, O'REILY E, CHEN H, et al.Plasma Urate and Risk of Parkinson's Disease[J]. *Am J Epidemiol*, 2007, 166(05):561-567.

⑦ DE VERA M, RAHMAN MM, RANKIN J, et al.Gout and the Risk of Parkinson's Disease:a Cohort Study[J].*Arthritis Rheum*, 2008, 59(11):1549-1554.

⑧ ANNANMAKI T, MUURONEN A, MURROS K. Low Plasma Uric Acid Level in Parkinson's Disease [J].*Mov Disord*, 2007, 22(08):1133-1137.

⑨ 王丽君,罗蔚锋,王恒会,等.帕金森病患者血尿酸水平[J].中华神经科杂志,2008,41(03):157-158.

⑩ SCHWARZSCHILD MA, SCHWID SR, MAREK K, et al. Serum Urate as a Predictor of Clinical and Radiographic Progression in Parkinson Disease[J]. *Arch Neurol*, 2008, 65(06):716-723.

由基、增加 SOD 活性、螯合铁离子的作用,减轻氧化应激压力密切相关。临床研究提示,UA 处于高 1/5 水平的男性 PD 患者疾病的进展速度显著慢于 UA 处于低 1/5 水平的男性 PD 患者,而在女性 PD 患者中尽管有类似的趋势,但未达到差异有统计学意义的程度①。流行病学调查同样发现,咖啡因也可以减少 PD 的发生②,而咖啡因不具有清除自由基螯合铁等作用,UA 和咖啡因具有相似的结构。Guerreiro 等③报道,UA 对 DA 能神经元的保护作用可能与其碳八结构相关。UA 对 DA 能神经元的保护作用可能还存在其他机制,尚待进一步研究证实。

本研究应用体外 PC12 细胞培养的方法,为 UA 保护 DA 能神经元作用提供了直接的证据。本实验证实,UA 100~400 μmol/L 在不影响细胞生存率的情况下,对 6-OHDA 造成损伤的细胞有保护作用。为了进一步证明 UA 的保护作用,本研究选取 6-OHDA 作用于细胞后 caspase-3 明显激活的时间段④观察 UA 是否减少其激活,选择其中一个对 PC12 细胞生存率无影响,同时对 6-OHDA 造成损伤有保护作用的 UA(200 μmol/L)进行实验,由免疫荧光结果可以观察到 UA 作用于 PC12 细胞 24 h 后 caspase-3 激活和对照组比较无显著差别,UA 200 μmol/L 能减少 6-OHDA 导致的 caspase-3 激活;流式细胞检测证实相同浓度的 UA 能降低 6-OHDA 导致的凋亡($P<0.05$)。本实验为进一步提高 PD 保护性治疗效果的研究奠定了基础。

(叶　艳　罗蔚锋　朱婷鸽　杨亚萍　周旭平　刘春风　包仕尧)
(本文原载于《中国临床神经科学》2010 年第 18 卷第 2 期)

———————————

①　GAO X, CHEN H, CHOI HK, et al. Diet, Urate, and Parkinson's Disease Risk in Men[J].*Am J Epidemiol*, 2008, 167(07):831-838.

②　ASCHERIO A, ZHANG SM, HERNAN MA, et al. Prospective Study of Caffeine Consumption and Risk of Parkinson's Disease in Men and Woman[J].*Ann Neruol*, 2001, 50(01):56-63.

③　GUERREIRO S, PONCEAU A, TOULORGE D, et al. Protection of Mibrain Dopaminergic Neurons by the End Product of Purine Metabolism Uric Acid:Potentiation by-low Level Depolarization[J]. *J Neurochem*, 2009, 109(04):1118-1128.

④　AMES BN, CATHCART R, SCHWIERS E, et al. Uric Acid Provides an Antioxidant Defense in Humans against Oxidant-andradical-caused Aging and Cancer:a Hypothesis[J]. *Proc Natl Acad Sci USA*, 1981, 78(11):6858-6862.

尿酸减轻 6-OHDA 介导 PC12 细胞 SOD 活性下降和损伤的实验研究①

目的：探讨尿酸对 6-OHDA 介导的 PC12 细胞氧化损伤的作用。

方法：采用高分化 PC12 细胞制作帕金森病细胞模型，实验分为对照组、6-OHDA 组、UA 组和 6-OHDA+UA 组。药物作用 6 h、12 h 和 24 h，采用比色法检测细胞 SOD 的活性和乳酸脱氢酶（lactic dehydrogenase，LDH）活力，硫代巴比妥酸法测定细胞内脂质过氧化产物丙二醛（malondialdehyde，MDA）的含量。

结果：100 μmol/L 6-OHDA 作用于 PC12 细胞 12 h、24 h 后，与对照组相比，SOD 活性降低，LDH 释放增加，MDA 生成增多（$P<0.05$）；UA 组与对照组相比各项指标均无统计学差异（$P>0.05$）；6-OHDA+UA 组与 6-OHDA 组相比，SOD 活性升高，LDH 释放显著降低、MDA 的生成减少（$P<0.05$）。

结论：尿酸具有减轻 6-OHDA 介导的 PC12 细胞损伤的作用，其作用机制可能与提高 SOD 活性有关。

关键词：尿酸；帕金森病；PC12 细胞；6-羟基多巴胺。

The Protective Role of Uric Acid in 6-hydroxydopamine-induced Injury of PC12 Cells

Abstract：Objective to investigate the protective role of UA in oxidative injury induced by 6-OHDA in PC12 cells.

Methods：The highly differentiated PC12 cells were divided into 4 groups：the control，6-OHDA，UA and 6-OHDA+UA. Each group was subdivided into 3 subgroups and cultured for 6，12 and 24 hours in vitro，respectively. The content of Lactate dehydrogenase（LDH），SOD in the culture medium，and intracellular

---

① 本文系江苏省自然科学基金（项目编号：BK2010229）；江苏省高校自然研究计划项目（项目编号：08KJB320012）；苏州市科技发展计划（社会发展及医药）项目（项目编号：200815404）。

malondialdehyde（MDA）were detected.

Results：The release of LDH and content of MDA in the group treated with 100 μmol/L 6-OHDA for 12 h and 24 h were significantly increased compared with the control group，while the activity of SOD was decreased，which were reversed by 200 μmol/L UA treatment.

Conclusion：These results suggest that UA treatment can prevent PC12 cell from oxidative stress-mediated injury，which may associated with the increased activity of SOD.

Key words： uric acid；Parkinson's disease；PC12 cells；6-hydroxydopamine.

帕金森病是中老年人常见的神经系统退行性疾病之一，其主要病理特征为中脑黑质致密部多巴胺能神经元的进行性变性减少，导致黑质纹状体系统多巴胺水平降低。尽管 PD 的确切发病机制仍不十分清楚，但研究资料显示与以下因素密切相关：鱼藤酮，1-甲基-4-苯基-1，2，3，6-四氢吡啶等物质的毒性作用；含有抗氧化剂食物的摄入减少，以及体内尤其是黑质纹状体内产生和清除自由基平衡系统障碍所导致的氧化应激反应增强；线粒体功能障碍等①②③。尿酸是嘌呤代谢的终产物，流行病学及临床研究提示，高水平的血尿酸可以显著降低发生 PD 的危险性，PD 患者的血尿酸水平显著降低④⑤⑥，伴有认知功能损害患者的血尿酸水平更低⑦。我们之前的实验结果提示，适当提高体内的 UA 水平能够减轻 6-OHDA 对 SD（Sprague

① SANTIAGO RM，BARBIEIRO J，LIMA MM，et al. Depressive-like Behaviors Alterations Induced by Intranigral MPTP，6-OHDA，LPS and Rotenone Models of Parkinson's Disease are Predominantly Associated with Serotonin and Dopamine［J］. *Prog Neuropsychopharmacol Biol Psychiatry*，2010，34（06）：1104-14.

② LOGROSCINO G，GAO X，CHEN H，et al. Dietary Iron Intake and Risk of Parkinson's Disease［J］. *Am J Epidemiol*，2008，168（12）：1381-1388.

③ JENNER P，OLANOW CW. The Pathogenesis of Cell Death in Parkinson's Disease［J］. *Neurology*，2006，66（10 Suppl 4）：S24-S36.

④ WEISSKOPF MG，O'REILLY E，CHEN H，et al. Plasma Urate and Risk of Parkinson's Disease［J］. *Am Epidemiol*，2007，166（05）：561-567.

⑤ 王丽君，罗蔚锋，王恒会，等. 帕金森病患者血尿酸水平［J］. 中华神经科杂志，2008，41（03）：157-158.

⑥ HUANG YX，LUO WF. Potential Role of Uric Acid as a Biomarker for Parkinson's Disease［J］. *Med Hypotheses*，2010，75（02）：273.

⑦ 王晓君，罗蔚锋，王丽君，等. 帕金森病患者认知功能与尿酸及相关因素分析［J］. 中华医学杂志，2009，89（23）：1633-1635.

Dawley)大鼠黑质纹状体系统多巴胺能神经元的毒性作用,但其机制还不甚清楚①。本实验采用 PC12 细胞和 6-OHDA 制作 PD 细胞模型,从细胞水平上探讨 UA 对 6-OHDA 介导的 PC12 细胞氧化损伤的作用及其机制。

一、材料与方法

1. 材料

PC12 细胞株由苏州大学神经变性与衰老疾病实验室秦正红教授赠予。UA、6-OHDA(Sigma 公司,美国),高糖 DMEM 培养基(GIBCO Invitrogen 公司,英国),LDH、SOD 试剂盒(南京建成生物工程研究所有限公司);IP 细胞裂解液、MDA、BCA 蛋白质定量测定试剂盒均购于上海碧云天生物技术有限公司。

2. 方法

（1）细胞培养及药物处理

PC12 细胞置于含 10% 胎牛血清、高糖 DMEM 的培养基中培养,每 48 h 换培养液,细胞融合至 80%~90% 后,以 1∶3 分瓶传代,选取对数生长期的细胞用于实验。实验分为 4 组:① 对照组[PBS(phosphate buffered saline)组];② 6-OHDA(100 μmol/L)组;③ UA(200 μmol/L)组;④ 6-OHDA(100 μmol/L)+UA(200 μmol/L)组。

（2）乳酸脱氢酶释放的测定

LDH 能催化乳酸生成丙酮酸,丙酮酸与 2,4-二硝基苯肼反应生成丙酮酸二硝基苯腙,在碱性溶液中呈棕红色,通过比色可求出酶活力。药物处理后,每组样品收集培养上清液 80 μL,加入基质缓冲液 250 μL、辅酶 I 50 μL,混匀,37 ℃水浴 15 mins;再加入 2,4-二硝基苯肼 250 μL,混匀,37 ℃水浴,15 mins;最后加入 0.4 mol/L NaOH 2.5 mL 混匀,室温放置 3 mins,酶标仪取波长 440 nm,每组样品设 3 个平行样,检测 OD 值,并重复该实验 3 次。

（3）超氧化物歧化酶的测定

黄嘌呤及黄嘌呤氧化酶反应系统产生超氧阴离子自由基(O_2^-),后者氧化羟胺形成亚硝酸盐,在显色剂的作用下呈现紫红色,在 550 nm 处有最大吸收峰。药物处理后,取细胞上清液 100 μL,按试剂盒说明书操作,比色法

---

① 王丽君,罗蔚锋,王恒会,等.尿酸对 6-羟基多巴胺致大鼠黑质纹状体系统毒性的影响[J].中华医学杂志,2010,90(19):1362-1365.

测定细胞上清液中 SOD 的 OD 值并计算其活性,其活性单位以 U/mL 计,重复测定 3 次。

（4）PC12 细胞内丙二醛含量的测定

药物处理 6 h、12 h、24 h 后,吸去培养液,用冷 PBS 洗涤细胞 3 次,用塑料细胞刮子刮下细胞,加入裂解液进行细胞裂解提取蛋白,按试剂盒说明书具体操作,每组样品设 3 个平行检测样品在 535 nm 的吸光度,并重复该实验 3 次。依标准曲线测出样品 MDA 的浓度。另根据 BCA 蛋白定量检测试剂盒说明计算出最初样品中 MDA 的含量。

（5）统计学处理

所有数据采用均数±标准差"$\bar{x}\pm s$"表示,采用 SPSS17.0 统计软件进行分析,组间比较用单因素方差分析（One-way ANOVA）检验。

二、结果

1. 尿酸减轻 6-OHDA 对 PC12 细胞 LDH 释放的作用

100 μmol/L 6-OHDA 作用于 PC12 细胞 6 h、12 h、24 h 后,12 h 及 24 h LDH 释放量较对照组显著增加,表明 6-OHDA 可以使 PC12 细胞膜受损,LDH 释放至胞外。200 μmol/L UA 可以降低 6-OHDA 所致 LDH 释放量增加,而单纯 UA 组与对照组 LDH 释放量的差异无统计学意义。

2. 6-OHDA 导致 PC12 细胞 SOD 含量的变化

100 μmol/L 6-OHDA 分别作用于 PC12 细胞 6 h、12 h、24 h 后,12 h、24 h 细胞内 SOD 的含量显著减少（图 1）,而 6-OHDA 所致的 SOD 含量减少可以被 200 μmol/L UA 所抑制。

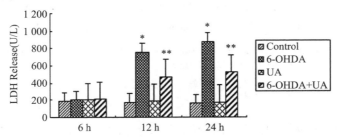

图 1　UA 对 6-OHDA 介导的 PC12 细胞 LDH 释放量的影响

Fig.1　Effects of UA on the Production of LDH Release in 6-OHDA-induced PC12 Cells

注: 6-OHDA 100 μmol/L,UA 200 μmol/L,$\bar{x}\pm s$,N=3; ＊对照组 versus 6-OHDA 组; ＊＊6-OHDA 组 versus 6-OHDA+UA 组,$P<0.05$。

3. PC12 细胞内 MDA 含量的变化

细胞传代 24 h 后,按照对照组、6-OHDA 组（100 μmol/L）、UA 组（200 μmol/L）和 UA（200 μmol/L）+6-OHDA 组（100 μmol/L）,进行加药处理,将细胞继续放入培养箱中孵育 6 h、12 h、24 h（图 2）。作用 12 h、24 h 时细胞内 6-OHDA 组 MDA 的生成量显著增加（与对照组相比,$P<0.05$）,而 UA+6-OHDA 组较 6-OHDA 组 MDA 的生成量显著减少（$P<0.05$）。

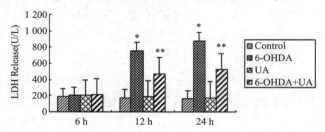

图 2　不同时间点 UA 对 6-OHDA 介导 PC12 细胞 SOD 活力的影响

Fig.2　the Activity of SOD in 6-OHDA Induced PC12 Cells at Different Times

注:6-OHDA 100 μmol/L,UA 200 μmol/L,$\bar{x}\pm s$,$N=3$;＊对照组 versus 6-OHDA 组;＊＊6-OHDA 组 versus 6-OHDA+UA 组,$P<0.05$。

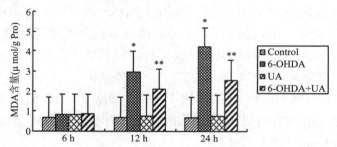

图 3　UA 对 6-OHDA 介导 PC12 细胞的 MDA 含量的变化

Fig.3　Effects of UA on Intracellular Content of MDA in PC12 Cells Induced by 6-OHDA

注:6-OHDA 100 μmol/L,UA 200 μmol/L,$\bar{x}\pm s$,N＝3;＊对照组 versus 6-OHDA 组;＊＊6-OHDA组 versus 6-OHDA+UA 组,$P<0.05$。

三、讨论

PD 发病的确切原因目前仍不十分清楚,氧化应激和线粒体功能障碍与 PD 发病密切相关[1],其中氧化应激在 PD 的发病机制中有重要作用,它可使

---

[1]　ZHOU C,HUANG Y,PRZEDBORSKI S. Oxidative Stress in Parkinson's Disease:a Mechanism of Pathogenic and Therapeutic Significance[J]. *Ann N Y Acad Sci*,2008,1147:93-104.

蛋白质和 DNA 产生氧化损伤,饱和、不饱和脂肪酸发生脂质过氧化,诱导细胞凋亡,导致细胞变性死亡。DA 能神经元对超氧化物尤其敏感,很容易引起线粒体、DNA 及蛋白质氧化损伤,从而导致细胞功能障碍和死亡。正常生理情况下,自由基的生成和清除保持动态平衡,自由基产生过多或机体对自由基的清除能力下降,易造成细胞的氧化损伤。

在 PD 患者的脑内和尿液中可检测到 6-OHDA,6-OHDA 是一种神经毒素,通过多巴胺能神经元上的多巴胺转运体摄取并积聚到细胞内,在单胺氧化酶-B(MAO-B)的作用下降解,一方面产生 H_2O_2 超氧阴离子生成 OH-和·OH 两种自由基,作用于线粒体导致细胞色素 c 释放,从而激活 caspase-3、caspase-7 导致细胞凋亡[1];另一方面产生半醌,通过 caspase-8、caspase-12 激活 caspase3 启动细胞凋亡[2]。PC12 细胞富含多巴胺受体及合成、分解多巴胺所需的各种酶,本实验用 6-OHDA 作用的 PC12 细胞建立 PD 的细胞模型。我们之前的实验结果发现,100~400 μmol/L UA 对 PC12 细胞存活率无影响,同时对 6-OHDA 所致的 PC12 细胞损伤具有保护作用[3],因此,本次实验 UA 的浓度采用 200 μmol/L。

LDH 为完全的胞浆酶,细胞释放 LDH 增加,通常表明细胞出现不可逆损伤、细胞膜通透性增加。本实验中 100 μmol/L 6-OHDA 分别作用于 PC12 细胞 12 h、24 h 后,与对照组相比,LDH 释放显著增加,6-OHDA+UA 组与 6-OHDA 组相比,LDH 释放显著降低,提示 UA 对 6-OHDA 介导的 PC12 细胞损伤具有保护作用。

SOD 是重要的抗氧化剂,可通过一系列化学反应缓冲及清除自由基引发连锁反应的起始基-超氧阴离子,它的活性大小反映了细胞抗氧化能力的高低;MDA 是不饱和脂肪酸降解的中间产物,其含量可反映细胞代谢过程中脂质的过氧化强度并间接反映氧自由基对细胞的损伤程度。本实验结果表明,6-OHDA 组与对照组相比,12 h、24 h 后,SOD 活力显著下降,具有统计

① HANROTT K,GUDMUMSEN L,O'Neill MI,et al. 6-hydroxydopamine-induced Apoptosis is Mediated via Extracellular Auto-Oxida-Tion and Caspase3-dependent Activation of Protein Kinase C Delta [J]. *Biol Chem*,2006,281(09):5373-5382.

② SAITO Y, NISHIO K, OGAWA Y, et al. Molecular Mechanisms of 6-hydroxydopmine-induced Cytotoxicity in PC12 Cells:Involvement of Hydrogen Peroxide-dependent and-Independent action [J]. *Free Radic Biol Med*,2007,42(05):675-685.

③ 叶艳,罗蔚锋,朱婷鸽,等. 尿酸减轻 6-羟基多巴胺对 PC12 细胞的毒性作用[J]. 中国临床神经科学,2010,18(02):135-139.

学意义($P<0.05$),MDA 含量显著增加,具有统计学意义($P<0.05$),提示 6-OHDA 导致 PC12 细胞损伤,与 SOD 水平下降,缓冲或清除超氧阴离子能力降低,超氧阴离子与生物膜中的多不饱和脂肪酸过氧化反应增强有关。另外,超氧阴离子能直接与 DNA 分子反应,导致 DNA 链断裂、DNA 蛋白交联等氧化性 DNA 损伤。

朱红灿等通过培养孕 SD 大鼠中脑原代细胞,利用 6-OHDA 制作 PD 模型,通过 TH 免疫组化染色观察到 6-OHDA,则 TH+细胞明显减少,而预先加入 UA 后再加入 6-OHDA,TH+细胞明显多于单纯 6-OHDA 组($P<0.05$),表明 UA 能减轻由 6-OHDA 所致的多巴胺能神经元损伤[①]。本实验 6-OHDA+UA 组与 6-OHDA 组相比,12 h、24 h 后 SOD 含量显著增加,具有统计学意义($P<0.05$),MDA 含量和 LDH 释放显著降低,具有统计学意义($P<0.05$),提示 UA 对 6-OHDA 介导的 PC12 细胞损伤发挥保护作用,与其提高 SOD 水平密切相关。

UA 对神经元的保护作用可能还存在其他机制,如 UA 具有中和过氧化亚硝酸盐和螯合金属铁离子的作用[②③]。黄嘌呤是 UA 的直接前体物质,只有八位碳取代基不同,却无神经保护作用,故推测 UA 的保护作用可能与八位碳结构具有相关性[④]。另有研究表明,UA 在星形胶质细胞存在下才能减轻谷氨酸对脊髓神经元的毒性作用,提示 UA 还可能通过星形胶质细胞传导机制来保护神经元[⑤]。UA 对多巴胺能神经元保护作用的确切机制还有待进一步研究。

（朱婷鸽　张琪林　黄婷婷　周旭平　罗蔚锋　刘春风）
（本文原载于《分子诊断与治疗杂志》2011 年第 3 卷第 2 期）

---

① 朱红灿,蔡春生,耿利娇,等.尿酸对帕金森病模型大鼠多巴胺能神经元氧化应激的影响[J].中华老年医学杂志,2010,29(04):319-323.

② KELLER JN,KINDY MS,HOLTSBERG FW,et al. Mitochondrial Manganese Superoxide Dismu-tase Prevents Neural Apoptosis and Reduces Ischemic Brain Injury：Suppression of Peroxynitrite Production,Lipid Peroxidation and Mitochondrial Dysfunction[J]. *Neurosci*,1998,18(02)：687-697.

③ SIAN J,DEXTER DT,LEES AJ,et al. Alterations in Glutathione Levels in Parkinson's Disease and Other Neurodegenerative Disorders Affecting Basal Ganglia[J]. *Ann Neurol*,1994,36(03)：348-355.

④ GUERREIRO S,PONCEAU A,TOULORGE D,et al. Protection of Midbrain Dopaminergic Neurons by the End-Product of Purine Metabolism Uric Acid：Potentiation by Low-Level Depolarization[J]. *Neurochem*, 2009,109(04)：1118-1128.

⑤ DLUY,CHEN CP,TSENG CY,et al. Astmglia-mediated Effects of Uric Acid to Protect Spinal Cord Neuron from Glutamate Toxicity[J]. *Glia*,2007,55(05)：463-472.

Neuroprotection by Urate on 6-OHDA-lesioned Rat Model of Parkinson's Disease: Linking to Akt/GSK3β Signaling Pathway

Abstract: Higher plasma urate level is reported to be associated with a reduced risk and slower progression of Parkinson's disease. In this study, we explored the effects of urate on dopaminergic neurons in nigrostriatal pathway in the 6-hydroxydopamine unilaterally lesioned rats. Uric acid, when given twice daily at 200 mg/kg intraperitoneally for 10 consecutive days, elevated urate (the anionic form of UA) in plasma and striatum by 55% and 36.8%, respectively, as compared with the vehicle group. This regimen of UA was found to ameliorate the behavioral deficits, dopaminergic neuron loss as well as dopamine depletion in the nigrostriatal system. Moreover, UA administration was capable of increasing glutathione level and superoxide dismutase activity while decreasing malondialdehyde accumulation in striatum. In addition, the phosphorylation of both protein kinase B (Akt) and glycogen synthase kinase 3 beta (GSK3β) in the lesioned striata of 6-OHDA-lesioned rats was dramatically reduced as compared with sham-operated rats. This reduction was attenuated in the Parkinsonian rats receiving UA treatment. Similarly, Vitro findings showed that UA alleviated the decrease in Akt activation and the increase in GSK3β activity caused by 6-OHDA. Furthermore, neuroprotection by urate and its regulation on GSK3β phosphorylation at Ser 9 was found to be abolished in the presence of PI3K inhibitor. Therefore, our findings demonstrated that urate was able to protect dopaminergic neurons in rat nigrostriatal pathway against the neurotoxicity of 6-OHDA, and showed that its beneficial effects may be related to its regulation on Akt/GSK3β signaling.

Keywords: 6-OHDA; neuroprotection; oxidative stress; Parkinson's disease; urate.

Parkinson's disease is a neurodegenerative disorder characterized by a progressive loss of dopaminergic neurons in substantia nigra and depletion of the neurotransmitter dopamine in striatum. Although it has been extensively investigated for many decades, the exact pathogenic factors responsible for dopaminergic neuron degeneration remain to be illuminated. Accumulating evidence suggests that oxidative stress and mitochondrial dysfunction are major contributing factors in the pathogenesis of PD. In fact, these two pathogenic factors interact with each other. An increase in oxidative stress causes damage to mitochondria, resulting in more accumulation of reactive oxygen species (ROS), mitochondrial membrane permeabilization, energy depletion, and eventually cell death. Hence, strategies that aim to limit or clear reactive oxygen/nitrogen species have been proposed to relieve dopaminergic neuron degeneration in PD.

Urate is the anionic form of uric acid and an endogenous antioxidant in humans. Its antioxidant property is mainly attributed to its capacity to react with ROS, such as peroxynitrite, peroxides, hypochlorous acid, and to chelate transition metal ions. On the other hand, urate acts as a pro-oxidant under some circumstances. For instance, urate may enhance the copper-induced low-density lipoprotein oxidation. In fact, altered serum urate concentrations have been linked to a number of disease conditions. An abnormally high urate level has been associated with gout, hypertension, cardiovascular disease, and renal disease; whereas reduced urate concentration has been linked to PD, Alzheimer's disease, multiple sclerosis, and optic neuritis. In 1994, Church WH and Ward VL reported that urate was significantly lower by 54% in the SN of PD patients compared with age-matched controls. Consistently, other groups further demonstrated that besides SN, plasma urate levels were also lower in PD patients. In the meantime, several prospective and cohort studies have shown that higher plasma urate levels are associated with a lower risk of PD. The clinical findings further raised the possibility that the higher the urate level in serum, the slower the PD clinical progression. Thus, urate was postulated to be a neuroprotective agent. However, this assumption has not yet been verified in animal models and clinical trials, although several *in vitro* studies including our previous work have shown that urate could protect against 6-hydroxydopamine (6-OHDA)-induced cell injury via antioxidant mechanisms in PC12 cells. Here, we further tested this assumption in the 6-OHDA unilaterally lesioned rat model of PD with histochemical, behavioral, neurochemical, and also molecular techniques, by intraperitoneal (i.p.) injection of UA for 10 consecutive days to enhance plasma urate levels.

1. Material and Methods

(1) Drugs and Chemicals

UA, 6-OHDA, mouse anti-tyrosine hydroxylase (TH) monoclonal antibody were purchased from Sigma (St Louis, MO, USA). Antibodies against Akt, phospho-Akt(Ser473), GSK3β, and phospho-GSK3β(Ser9) were obtained from Cell Signaling Technology (Beverly, MA, USA). The antibody against phospho-GSK3β(Tyr216) was purchased from Santa Cruz Biotechnology(Santa Cruz, CA, USA).

(2) Experimental Procedure and Animal Surgery

Sprague-Dawley(SD) male rats (180~220 g), 130 in total, were purchased from the Center for Experimental Animals, Soochow University (certificate No. 20020008, Grade Ⅱ). Animals were housed at a 12-h light/dark cycle with free access to food and water. NIH Guidelines for the Care and Use of Laboratory Animals were followed in all animal procedures.

The overall experimental procedure was illustrated as Fig. 1. Our study comprised two parts of work. In the first part, the effects of UA injection via i.p. on both plasma and brain urate levels in rats were assessed. In brief, 70 male SD rats were used and randomly divided into five treatment groups, and subject to injection for five and 10 consecutive days, respectively. Rats were injected(i.p.) with UA at doses of 50, 100, 200, 400 mg/kg, or its vehicle twice daily 2 h apart ($N=7$ for each treatment at one time point). On the 5th and 10th day, 1h after last injection, blood was sampled via caudal vein and put into an anticoagulant tube. After centrifugation at 835 g for 10 mins, plasma was transferred into Eppendorf tubes and stored at -80 ℃ for urate measurement later. Rats were killed and brain tissues(striatum) were then harvested.

Part I

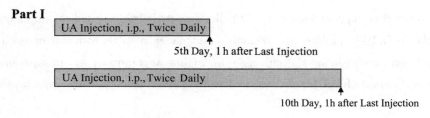

Part II

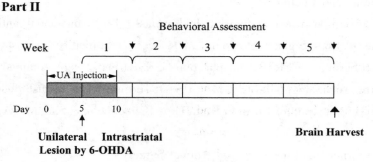

Fig.1   Experimental Procedure

In the second part, the potential protection by urate at an appropriate dose, which was chosen in accordance with the results obtained from part one, in 6-OHDA-induced Parkinsonian rats were further investigated. In total, 60 rats were randomly divided into four groups ($N = 15$ for each group. Among these, 10 rats were used for behavioral test, histology study, and DA assay. The others were used for measuring oxidative parameters and the western blot analysis of protein expression in striatum): sham-operated group, UA treatment plus sham-operated group, 6-OHDA-injected group, and UA treatment plus 6-OHDA-injected group. Briefly, rats were injected (i. p.) with UA or its vehicle twice daily for five consecutive days before and after stereotaxic surgery. On the 5th day between the two injections, all rats received a unilateral stereotaxic injection of 6-OHDA or saline into the right striatum. The injection was performed on anesthetized rats (3.6% chloral hydrate, 0.18 g/kg, i. p.) via a 10 μL Hamilton syringe using stereotaxic apparatus (David Kopf Instruments, Tujunga, CA, USA) according to rat brain atlas. The lesions were made by injection of 6-OHDA into the right striatum at two sites (10 μg 6-OHDA hydrochloride in 5 μL of 0.02% ascorbic acid saline solution, 5 μg 6-OHDA each site) with the coordinates: (ⅰ) AP,

-0.7；L，-3.0；DV，-4.5 mm；(ⅱ)AP，-0.2；L，-2.6；DV，-6.0 mm from bregma at the rate of 0.5 μL/min. At the end of injection，the needle was left in place for an additional 5 mins and then withdrawn at a rate of 1 mm/min. Sham-lesioned rats were infused with 5 μL saline containing 0.02% ascorbic acid. After surgery，the rats were kept in cages with constant temperature(25 ℃) and humidity，and were exposed to a 12：12-h light/dark cycle with unrestricted access to tap water and food.

(3) Plasma and Striatum Urate Level Determination in Normal Rats

Striatum tissues were homogenized and sonicated in normal saline (1：5,mg/uL) for 1 min and then centrifuged at 20 000 g for 15 mins at 4 ℃. Protein concentrations were determined using the BCA kit(Pierce Chemical，Rockford，IL，USA). The urate levels in plasma and striatum were assessed using the Uric Acid Assay Kit from Bio Vision，according to the manufacturer's instructions. The urate levels in plasma and striatum were expressed as μmol/L and nmol per mg wet tissue，respectively.

(4) Behavioral Assessment

Deficits in forepaw adjusting steps in PD rat model provide a simple and consistent behavioral phenomenon similar to akinesia in PD. Forepaw adjusting step was measured once a week after 6-OHDA lesion as previously described. The rat was held by the rear part of torso and placed on treadmill surface so that its weight was on one forepaw. The treadmill was set to move at a rate of 90 cm/5 s in the direction opposite to the weightbearing forepaw，resulting in the outward lateral shifting of the torso relative to the weight-bearing forepaw. The number of forepaw adjusting steps，defined as the movement of weight-bearing forepaw toward torso to compensate for the outward lateral movement of body，was counted. Each stepping test consisted of five trials for each forepaw，alternating between forepaws，and each trial lasted 5 s. The average of five trials for each forepaw was used for analysis.

(5) Immunohistochemistry Staining

Formalin-fixed and paraffin-embedded sections(5 μm in thickness)received deparaffinization and rehydration treatments. Endogenous peroxidase activity was inactivated with 0.3% H_2O_2 for 30 mins. The sections were then blocked with 5%

normal goat serum in 1% bovine serum albumin for 30 mins and incubated with a mouse monoclonal TH antibody (1 : 5 000) at 4 ℃ overnight. The slides were incubated with biotin-conjugated anti-mouse IgG and thereafter, streptavidin-horseradish peroxidase(1 : 1 000) for another 1 h. Immunoreactivities were finally developed with diaminobenzidine solution and sections were counter-stained with Mayer's Hematoxylin, dehydrated, and mounted. The sections were observed and photographed using a Zeiss microscope(Axio Scope A1; Zeiss Corp, Goettingen, Germany). The number of TH^+ neurons in SN was manually counted using a superimposed grid to facilitate the procedure. At least five sections for each rat were examined and counting was performed by researchers blind to the treatments received.

(6) Determination of DA and its Metabolites in Striatum

The levels of DA and its metabolites 3, 4-dihydroxyphenylacetic acid (DOPAC), and homovanilic acid(HVA) in striatum were determined by high-performance liquid chromatography-tandem mass spectrometry(HPLC-MS/MS). HPLC was carried out on an Agilent 1100 system(Agilent Technologies, Palo Alto, CA, USA) consisting of a vacuum degasser, a quaternary pump, and an autosampler. An API 4000 triple-quadrupole mass spectrometer (Applied Biosystems Sciex, Ontario, Canada) equipped with a Turbo Ion Spray ionization (ESI) source was used for mass analysis and detection. Data acquisition and integration were controlled using Applied Biosystems Analyst Software(Applied Biosystems/MDS Sciex, version 1. 4. 2). The tissue was homogenized and sonicated in a mixture of normal saline and methanol(1 : 1, v/v, 10 μL mixture per mg brain tissue) for 1 min and then centrifuged at 18 000 g for 5 mins at 4 ℃. After that, the supernatant was mixed with internal standard at the same volume, and was filtered (0.2 μm, Millipore, Billerica, MA, USA). A volume of 20 μL final solution was injected into HPLC-MS/MS system for analysis. The mobile phase was a mixture of water containing 0.015% formic acid and methanol (92 : 8, v/v), and was pumped at a flow rate of 0.3 mL/ min under gradient elution. The precursor to product-ion transitions m/z 152.1→122.1, m/z 138.1→122.0, and m/z 180.9→137.0 were used to quantify DA, DOPAC, and HVA, respectively. The concentrations were expressed as ng/mg tissue.

（7）Malondialdehyde, Glutathione（GSH）, and Superoxide Dismutase Activity Measurement

The striatal contents of MDA—a compound produced during lipid peroxidation, and SOD—an important antioxidant enzyme that plays a pivotal role in clearing ROS, as well as GSH were measured using commercially available detection kits（Nanjing Jiancheng Biochemical Reagent Co. Nanjing, China）according to the manufacturers' instructions.

（8）Western Blot Analysis

Striatal tissues were homogenized in lysis buffer and centrifuged at 12 000 g for 30 mins. Protein samples were heated at 97 ℃ for 5 mins before loading. Equal amounts of protein were electrophoresed on 10% sodium dodecyl sulfate-polyacrylamide gel and transferred onto a polyvinylidene difluoride membrane（PALL, East Hills, NY, USA）. The resulting blots were blocked with 5% milk in Tris Buffer Saline Tween20 buffer（10 mmol/L Tris, 150 mmol/L NaCl, 0.1% Tween-20, pH 8.0）for 1 h and then incubated at 4 ℃ overnight with primary antibodies that recognize proteins of interest. Bound antibodies were detected by a secondary antibody conjugated to horseradish peroxidase and visualized by ECL chemiluminescence（GE healthcare, Buckinghamshire, UK）.

（9）Cell Viability Determination

Cell viability was measured using 3-（4, 5-Dimethylthiazol-2-yl）-2, 5-diphenyltetrazolium bromide（MTT）reduction assay. In brief, regular medium was replaced, and MTT at the final concentration of 0.5 mg/mL was added at the end of treatment. Cells were further incubated at 37 ℃ for 4 h. After that the insoluble formazan was dissolved with dimethyl sulphoxide. The absorbance was finally measured at 570 nm with a reference wavelength at 630 nm using a microplate reader（Tecan M200; TECAN, GmbH, Austria）.

（10）Statistical analysis

All data were presented as mean±SEM. Statistical significance was assessed with one-way analysis of variance followed by Dunnett's test for multiple group comparison. In addition, we further analyzed the time-and dose-dependent effects of the behavioral test results jointly by using a two-way ANOVA followed by a several *post hoc* paired *t*-tests. Differences with *p*-values of less than 0.05 were considered statistically significant.

2. Results

（1）Intraperitoneal Injection of UA Raises Urate Levels in Plasma and Striatum

The temporal changes of plasma and striatal urate levels were determined and monitored before exploring the potential of urate neuroprotection. UA, at various doses of 0, 50, 100, 200, and 400 mg/kg was administered i.p. twice daily at 2h intervals for five and 10 consecutive days, respectively. On the 5th and 10th day, the plasma and striatum urate levels were determined at 1h after last injection. It was found that at doses above 200 mg/kg, UA administration was able to enhance the urate level both in plasma and striatum in a dose-dependent manner, as shown in Fig.2.A and Fig.2.B. Specifically, on the 5th and 10th day

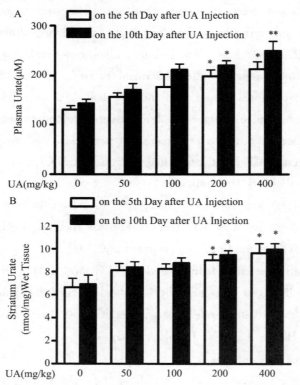

Fig.2　Effect of UA treatment on plasma and striatum urate level in normal SD rats. UA (50, 100, 200, 400 mg/kg) or its vehicle was intraperitoneally given twice a day at a 2 h interval for five and 10 consecutive days, respectively. Urate levels in plasma (A) and striatum (B) on the 5th and 10th day after injection were measured using a kit from Bio Vision. Data are expressed as mean ± SEM, $N = 7$. $^{*}p < 0.05$, $^{**}p < 0.01$ versus vehicle-treated group.

after injection with UA at 200 mg/kg twice daily, the plasma urate level increased by 52.9% (from 130.1±0.46 μmol/L to 198.9±0.71 μmol/L) and 55% (from 142.5±0.49 μmol/L to 220.8±0.58 μmol/L), whereas the urate level in striatum increased by 32.3% (from 6.8±0.17 nmol/mg to 9.0±0.18 nmol/mg) and 36.8% (from 6.9±0.13 nmol/mg to 9.5±0.12 nmol/mg) respectively.

(2) UA Treatment Improves Behavioral Deficits in 6-OHDA-lesioned Rats

To evaluate the effects of UA treatment on motor performance, the rats that received different treatments were subjected to forepaw adjusting step test for five times at 1 week interval after surgery. Sham-operated rats (S) served as controls and data were shown in Fig.3. As anticipated, unilateral 6-OHDA injection caused a significant reduction in forepaw adjusting steps at the 4th and 5th week after surgery compared with controls. Post hoc analysis revealed that UA treatment (200 mg/kg twice daily for five consecutive days before and after surgery) to 6-OHDA-lesioned rats significantly improved stepping in the forepaws when compared with saline-treated rats. Of note, UA treatment at the same regimen to the sham-operated rats did not affect the forepaw adjusting steps.

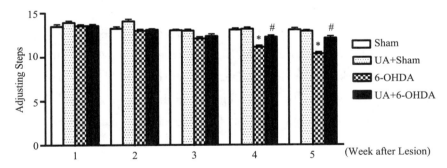

Fig.3 Effect of UA treatment on behavioral deficits in 6-OHDA-induced Parkinsonian rats. UA (200 mg/kg, i.p. twice daily) or its vehicle was injected 5 days before and after stereotaxic injection of 6-OHDA or saline (sham-operated). The movement deficits were evaluated by forepaw adjusting steps (90 cm in 5 s) at different time points (1st, 2nd, 3rd, 4th, 5th week) after unilateral 6-OHDA or saline lesion. Data are expressed as mean± SEM, N=10. *p<0.05 versus sham group; #p<0.05 versus 6-OHDA-lesioned group.

（3）UA Treatment Alleviates Dopaminergic Neuron Loss in the Nigrostriatal Pathway in 6-OHDA-lesioned Rats

We continued to examine the effect of UA on dopaminergic neuron degeneration in the nigrostriatal pathway in intrastriatal 6-OHDA unilaterally lesioned rats with immunohistochemistry study and western blot analysis as well. As shown in the representative pictures in Fig.4.A and Fig.4.C, unilateral 6-OHDA lesion induced a dramatic loss of TH^+ neurons in both SN pars compacta (SNc, Fig.4.A) and striatum (Fig.4.C) in the lesioned side. However, there was no significant reduction of TH^+ staining in the intact hemisphere and in sham-lesioned rats. UA, when given twice daily at 200 mg/kg intraperitoneally, markedly attenuated the loss of TH^+ neurons in SN and fibers in striatum caused by 6-OHDA injection. The observation was verified by counting the number of TH^+ neurons in SN(Fig.4.B), and by western blot analysis of protein lysates from striatum(Fig.4.D). As can be seen from Fig.4.B, the number of TH^+ neurons in the 6-OHDA-lesioned side was reduced by 45.4% as compared with sham-lesioned side, while it merely reduced by 28.2% in the 6-OHDA-lesioned side of rats receiving UA treatment. Western blot analysis also showed that TH expression in the lesioned striata of 6-OHDA-treated group decreased by 72.8%, as compared with sham-lesioned side. This decrease was obviously attenuated in the UA-treated Parkinsonian rats, which reduced only by 46.2%. The findings indicate that UA treatment, by enhancing plasma urate level, was able to protect against dopaminergic neuron loss in the nigrostriatal pathway of 6-OHDA unilaterally lesioned rats.

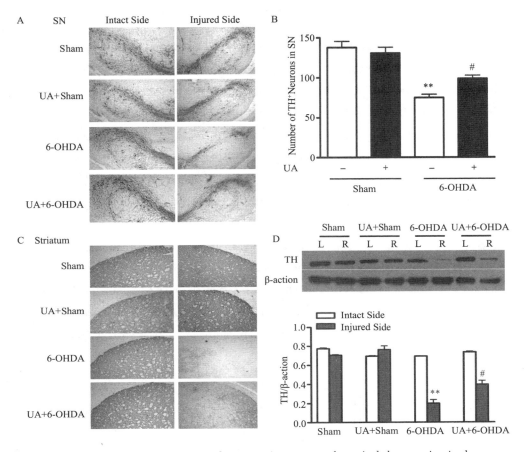

Fig.4　Effect of UA treatment on dopaminergic neuron and terminal degeneration in the nigrostriatal pathway. A and C, representative pictures showing UA (200 mg/kg, twice daily,i.p.) treatment alleviated tyrosine hydroxylase (TH⁺) neuron (A) and terminal (C) loss in substantia nigra (SN) and striatum in 6-OHDA-lesioned Parkinsonian rats, determined by immunostaining. B, group data showing the number of TH⁺ neurons in the right side of SNc at 5 weeks after surgery.Data of each group were obtained by calculating the mean value of TH⁺ neuron number from four rats. Five sections were included for counting and analysis for each rat.Photos were taken at ×50 magnification. D, western blots showing UA treatment attenuated the down-regulation of TH expression in striata of Parkinsonian rats. Data are expressed as mean ± SEM, $N = 3$. ** $p < 0.01$ versus the corresponding value in the sham group;#$p<0.05$ versus the injured side in the 6-OHDA-lesioned rat.L, left(intact side) ;R, right(injured side).

（4）UA Attenuates Dopamine Reduction in Striatum

Next, the contents of DA and its metabolites in striatum were determined by HPLC to confirm the neuroprotection on dopaminergic neurons by urate. The effects of both saline and UA treatment on the levels of DA, DOPAC, and HVA in the intact(left) versus lesioned(right) striata of 6-OHDA unilaterally lesioned rats were shown in Fig.5. It was observed that in the saline-treated Parkinsonian rats, the DA content in the lesioned striata was significantly reduced by 64.9% compared with intact side. Likewise, the DA metabolites, DOPAC and HVA levels also dramatically dropped in the lesioned side. These observations indicate that 6-OHDA administration induces a significant DA depletion in striatum, consistent with our findings on dopaminergic neuron loss in SN as shown in Fig.4.A and Fig.4.B. These data also suggest the successful establishment of Parkinsonian rat model in this study. The levels of DA, HVA, as well as DOPAC in the lesioned side of UA-treated group were about 69.1%, 70.2%, and 69.0% of those in intact striatum, significantly higher than those in saline-treated group, as shown in Fig.5.

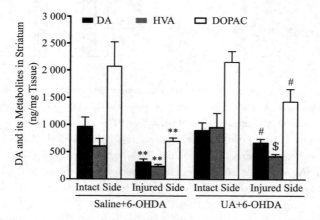

Fig.5　Effect of UA treatment on DA reduction in striatum. The contents of DA(column in black) and its metabolites DOPAC(column in hollow) and HVA(column in shaded line) in striata of 6-OHDA-lesioned rats with saline or UA treatment were determined by HPLC. The results were expressed as ng/mg tissue. Data are expressed as mean±SEM, $N=$ 5. $^*p<0.05$, $^{**}p<0.01$ versus the intact striatum in saline-treated group; $^\#p<0.05$ versus the injured striatum in saline-treated group; $^\$ p<0.05$ versus the intact side in UA-treated group.

（5）UA Treatment Ameliorates Oxidative Damage in Striatum

As urate is a natural antioxidant, the effect of UA treatment on oxidative damage in the striata of 6-OHDA-lesioned rats was also determined by measuring the levels of MDA, total GSH, and the activities of SOD as well. As shown in Fig.6, there was no significant difference of the striatal MDA levels in the intact side between saline and UA-treated Parkinsonian rats. Similar trends were observed for SOD activity and GSH content between the two groups. Of note, the MDA level in the injured side of saline-treated group was significantly higher than that of the intact side and also higher than the injured side of UA-treated

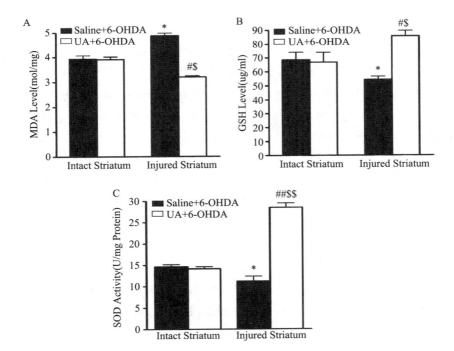

Fig.6 Effect of UA treatment on the oxidative damage in striatum. The oxidative level was evaluated by measuring the levels or activities of malondialdehyde (MDA) (A), glutathione(GSH) (B), and superoxide dismutase (SOD) (C) in both intact and injured striata of 6-OHDA unilaterally lesioned rats receiving saline or UA treatment, using commercially available kits as indicated in methods. Data are expressed as mean±SEM, $N = 5$. $^*p < 0.05$ versus the intact striatum in saline-treated group; $^#p < 0.05$, $^{##}p < 0.01$ versus the intact striatum in UA-treated group; $^\$ p < 0.05$, $^{\$\$}p < 0.01$ versus the injured side in saline-treated group.

71

rats lesioned by 6-OHDA intrastriatal injection (Fig. 6. A), implying that 6-OHDA lesion caused the increase of lipid peroxidation, which was relieved by UA administration. Furthermore, it was observed that in the saline-treated group, the GSH level and SOD activity in the injured side were markedly lower than those in intact side, indicating GSH depletion and SOD activity reduction as a result of 6-OHDA lesion. UA treatment significantly enhanced the GSH contents and SOD activity in the injured striata compared to those of saline-treated group(Fig.6.B and Fig.6.C). Interestingly, it was found that in the UA treated group, the SOD activity in the injured side was remarkably higher than that of the intact side.

(6) AKT/GSK3β Signaling Contributes to the Neuroprotection by Urate

To explore the possible signaling pathways mediating the neuroprotection by urate, the phosphorylation levels of Akt at Ser473 and GSK3β at Ser9 and Tyr216 sites in the striatum were examined by western blot analysis as the changes in Akt and GSK3β activity have been reported in *in vivo* and *in vitro* PD models. As shown in Fig.7. A and Fig.7. B, the phosphorylation levels of Akt(Ser473) and GSK3β (Ser9) were obviously reduced in the injured side (right) of 6-OHDA-injected rats, as compared with either the intact side (left) of 6-OHDA-injected rats or the lesioned side of sham-operated rats. This reduction was markedly alleviated in the 6-OHDA-injected rats receiving UA treatment(200 mg/kg, i.p.twice daily). However, no significant change of phosphorylated GSK3β at Tyr216 was observed in the injured striata of 6-OHDA-injected rats compared with sham-operated group (data not shown). UA administration did not affect the phosphorylation of Akt or GSK3β in sham-operated rats.

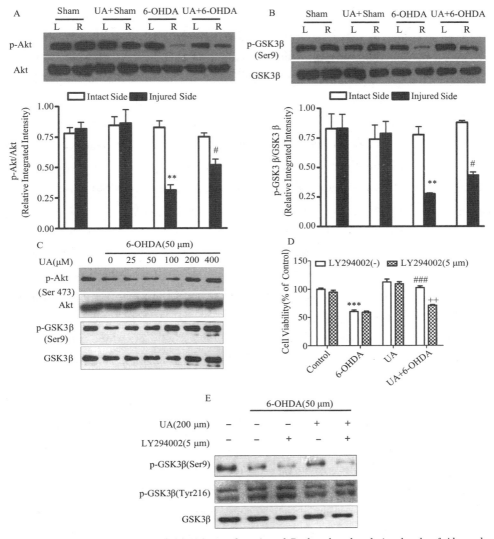

Fig.7　Effect of UA on Akt and GSK3β signaling. A and B, the phosphorylation levels of Akt and GSK3β in striatum at 5 weeks after surgery, determined by western blot analysis. L, left (intact side), indicated as hollow column; R, right (injured side), indicated as black column. Mean±SEM, $N = 3$ for each group. $^{**}p < 0.01$ versus the corresponding value in sham group; $^{#}p < 0.05$ versus the injured side of striatum in 6-OHDA-lesioned rats. C-E, SHSY5Y cells were pretreated with UA at indicated concentration for 30 mins, in the presence or absence of LY294002 (5 μm), and then exposed to 6-OHDA treatment. C and E, western blot results show the representatives of at least three independent experimental results. D, cell viability determined by MTT method. $N = 6$ for each group and the experiment was repeated four times. $^{***}p < 0.001$ versus control; $^{###}p < 0.001$ versus 6-OHDA-treated group without LY294002; $^{++}p < 0.01$ versus UA + 6-OHDA-treated group without LY294002.

To establish the role of Akt/GSK3β signaling pathway in the neuroprotection by urate against 6-OHDA-induced neurotoxicity, we further assessed its beneficial effects in the presence and absence of a phosphoinositide 3-kinase (PI3K) inhibitor LY294002 with *in vitro* study using human neuroblastoma cell line SH-SY5Y. Western blot analysis displayed that consistent with our *in vivo* results, 6-OHDA markedly inhibited the phosphorylation of Akt at Ser473, implying an inhibitory effect on Akt activity. Pretreatment with UA for 30 min, at concentrations from 25 μm to 400 μm, appeared to alleviate the inhibition on Akt activation caused by 6-OHDA in a concentration-dependent manner, as shown in the upper two panels in Fig. 7. C. The cell viability measurement showed that UA(200 μm) pretreatment was able to protect against 6-OHDA(50 μm, 14 h)-induced toxicity to SH-SY5Y cells. But, this beneficial effect was abolished in the presence of LY294002(5 μm), which inhibits Akt activation, as shown in Fig. 7. D. Furthermore, western blot analyses demonstrated that 6-OHDA markedly dephosphorylated GSK3β at Ser9 (Fig. 7. C), but hyperphosphorylated that at Tyr216 (Fig. 7. E), both of which indicated a stimulatory effect by 6-OHDA on GSK3β activity. LY294002 was observed to enhance the inhibition by 6-OHDA on GSK3β phosphorylation at Ser9, whereas it failed to affect that at Tyr216, implying that GSK3β activation was secondary to Akt inhibition by LY294002. Of interest, UA was able to attenuate the alterations in GSK3β phosphorylation at both Ser9 and Tyr216 caused by 6-OHDA, which indicates a dual inhibition by urate on GSK3β activity. Similarly, LY294002 was found to abolish the effect by urate on GSK3β phosphorylation at Ser9, but not that at Tyr216. These results clearly suggest that the neuroprotective effects by urate on 6-OHDA-induced Parkinsonian rats may be mediated, at least in part, by Akt/GSK3β signaling.

3. Discussion

Urate has emerged as a promising candidate therapeutic target for neuroprotection in PD based on a remarkable convergence of biological, epidemiological, and clinical data. However, this still lacks consolidated experimental evidence both *in vivo* and *in vitro*. Our previous study demonstrated that UA pre-treatment was capable of protecting PC12 cells against 6-OHDA-induced injury *in vitro*. In this study, intraperitoneal injection of UA was found to elevate plasma and brain urate levels. This elevation was particularly obvious when the dose of UA was above 200 mg/kg. Therefore, treatment with UA, at a dose of 200 mg/kg twice daily was chosen to explore the effects and underlying mechanisms of UA administration on 6-OHDA-induced Parkinsonian rats. Our data showed that UA treatment alleviated the impairment of motor performance, loss of dopaminergic neurons in SN, reduction of DA and its metabolites in striatum, accumulation of lipid oxidation, as well as depletion of GSH and SOD activity in striatum caused by 6-OHDA unilaterally injected into striatum (right side). These findings clearly demonstrate that UA treatment at this regimen could protect dopaminergic neurons in SN against 6-OHDA-induced degeneration, in agreement with our previous findings. In addition, western blot analysis showed that 6-OHDA lesion remarkably reduced the phosphorylation of Akt (activation) and induced the dephosphorylation of GSK3β (activation) in the lesioned striatum, which was significantly alleviated in the UA-treated Parkinsonian rats. This indicates that Akt activation and GSK3β inactivation may, at least in part, be involved in the beneficial effects of UA treatment.

6-OHDA is toxic in both central and peripheral nervous system. However, this neurotoxin is incapable of crossing the blood-brain barrier; thus, its toxicity to the central nervous system is achieved only when directly injected into brain by means of stereotaxic surgery. Therefore, it is generally accepted that the intact side could serve as a good internal control without the interference of individual variability. In addition, the infusion of 6-OHDA into striatum was reported to alter the redox homeostasis in rat brain. The chronic and persistent imbalance between ROS formation generation and antioxidant defenses characterizes many pathological processes and disease conditions including PD. Several studies demonstrated the oxidation products of lipid, protein, and nuclei acid were significantly enhanced in urine, serum, and substantia nigra of 6-OHDA-lesioned animal models of PD. This implies that antioxidant agents are capable of relieving 6-OHDA-induced neurotoxicity.

Urate was found to reduce 6-OHDA-induced oxidative products such as

MDA and 8-hydroxy-deoxyguanosine (8-OHdG), but increase the SOD activity and GSH levels in an *in vitro* model of PD. Likewise, the increase in SOD activity and GSH level exerted by UA treatment was observed in this *in vivo* study. More importantly, we found that the SOD activity and GSH level in the injured striata of UA-treatment group were even higher than those in intact side. This may be explained by the mechanism that the locally accumulated urate in striatum resulted in an overshoot in enhancing SOD activity and GSH level to defend against the excessive ROS generation in striatum caused by 6-OHDA local injection. It is supported by our findings that i. p. injection of UA yielded an increase of urate in plasma and striatum by 52.9% and 32.3%, respectively, on the 5th day after injection. This also indicates a tight correlation between blood and brain urate, although detailed information on urate modulation in periphery and brain remains to be determined. In short, the data in this study provided evidence that UA treatment could elevate plasma urate level and enhance the resistance to oxidative injury *in vivo*.

However, it is still debatable whether urate is accumulated into neurons or not. Guerreiro *et al.* reported that urate is not significantly accumulated into neurons, which indicates that its antioxidant effect occurs extracellularly. But, Cipriani *et al.* recently demonstrated that exogenous application of urate raises intracellular urate level about four folds 24 h later. This discrepancy was explained by the different sensitivity of the analytical methods applied. Although this discrepancy exists, researchers consistently agree that urate, at appropriate levels, may produce antioxidant action in cells, which could be mediated by some undefined receptor (s) even if urate does not enter cells. In fact, our recent findings showed that urate could produce antioxidant effect intracellularly by promoting nuclear factor erythroid-related factor Nrf 2 nuclear translocation and the up-regulation of antioxidant enzymes such as γ-glutamate cysteine ligase (unpublished data). Therefore, UA treatment, at the regimen employed in this work, could provide neuroprotection against oxidative stress and thus rescue the loss of dopaminergic neurons and terminals in the nigrostriatal pathway in 6-OHDA-lesioned rats. Because of the selective dopaminergic neuron degeneration induced by 6-OHDA, we believed that an appropriate elevation of plasma urate level could exert specific neuro protective effects on dopaminergic neurons in PD models. Although the whole picture is yet to be uncovered, the dysregulation of urate homeostasis should play a crucial role in dopaminergic neuron degeneration in PD.

Growing evidence shows that Akt/GSK3β signaling takes a dominant role in preventing cellular degeneration. Decreased Akt signaling, associated with increase in GSK3β activity, has been reported in the *in vitro* and *in vivo* PD models. Akt is a serine/threonine protein kinase and its signaling depends on its phosphorylation by PI3K. GSK3β activity is differently regulated by the phosphorylation level of two critical sites Ser9 and Tyr216. Specifically, Ser9 phosphorylation reduces GSK3β activity, whereas Tyr216 phosphorylation increases its activity. Physiologically, Akt activation inhibits GSK3β activity by enhancing its phosphorylation at Ser9. Our *in vivo and in vitro* observations consistently showed that 6-OHDA treatment markedly dephosphorylated Akt at Ser473 and GSK3β at Ser9, implying the inactivation of Akt but activation of GSK3β by 6-OHDA. We found that 6-OHDA also enhanced the GSK3β activity by hyper-phosphorylating it at Tyr216 *in vitro*, which was not observed in *in vivo* study. These led us to postulate that there are other mechanisms involved in modulating GSK3β phosphorylation at Tyr216 *in vivo*. Nevertheless, our present observations clearly show that UA treatment could attenuate the decrease in Akt phosphorylation at Ser473 and GSK3β phosphorylation at Ser9, as well as the increase in GSK3β phosphorylation at Tyr216 caused by 6-OHDA. The differentially regulatory effects by urate on GSK3β phosphorylation at Ser9 and Tyr216 consistently imply the inhibition on GSK3β activation exerted by urate. More importantly, our results showed that the PI3K inhibitor LY294002 was able to abolish the protective effects of urate on cell survival and its regulation on GSK3β phosphorylation at Ser9 in 6-OHDA-treated SH-SY5Y cells. Herein, we proposed that Akt/GSK3β signaling pathway may play a critical role in the neuroprotection by urate on dopaminergic neurons in SN of 6-OHDA-lesioned parkinsonian rats.

In addition to PD, the neuroprotection by urate have been reported in *in vitro* and *in vivo* models of other neurological disorders. In an experimental allergic encephalomyelitis model of multiple sclerosis, urate and its precursor inosine were found to delay the onset and improve the behavioral deficits in mice. Urate has also been shown to protect embryonic rat spinal cord neuron cultures against glutamate toxicity, and it protected against secondary damage and improved functional recovery after spinal cord injury *in vivo*. Studies also proved that in Alzheimer's disease, there is defective tubular urate transport and a plasma natriuretic factor. Of note, among these neurodegenerative diseases, PD is most closely related to urate. This may be because of a possible link between the antioxidant action of urate and the vulnerability of dopaminergic neurons to oxidative damage. To this end, further investigation is warranted to enhance our understanding of urate biology and to translate it into improved PD treatments.

In conclusion, our present data demonstrated a significantly neuroprotective effect by urate on dopaminergic neurons in SN, supported by the evidence that UA treatment enhanced DA and its metabolite DOPAC content in striatum and improved the behavioral activities. Apart from these, UA treatment alleviated oxidative stress and induced an increase in phosphorylation of Akt(Ser473) and GSK3β(Ser9), both *in vivo* and *in vitro*. The *in vitro* findings further show that PI3K inhibitor LY294002 abolished the neuroprotection by urate and its regulation on GSK3β phosphorylation at Ser9. Thus, the findings clearly demonstrate that the *in vivo* neuroprotection by urate was possibly mediated by Akt/ GSK3β signaling. These findings offered an experimental basis for the clinical usage of urate, and also provided promising approaches or drug combinations for PD therapy.

4. Acknowledgements

We would like to thank Ms. Wang Fen for technical support. In our study, Dr Luo gave contributions to conception and design. Dr Hu made critical reading of the manuscript and gave helpful discussion and revision of our manuscript. Qi-Lin Zhang and Wen-Yan Hua focused on HPLC-MS/MS determination while Li Gong, Yi-Xian Huang, and Ping-Wei Di performed all other experiments in this study. This work was supported by grants from The Suzhou Foundation for Development of Science and Technology (200815404), Suzhou Technology

Support Project（SS201112）, Jiangsu Ordinary University Science Research Project（08KJB320012）, and also Natural Science Foundation of Jiangsu Province, China（BK2010229）. There is no conflict of interest to be disclosed.

References

［1］ANNANMAKI T, MUURONEN A, Murros K. Low Plasma Uric Acid Level in Parkinson's Disease［J］.*Mov Disord*,2007,22(08):1133−1137.

［2］BECKER BF. Towards the Physiological Function of Uric Acid［J］. *Free Radic Biol Med*,1993,14(06):615−631.

［3］CHANG LW, CHIEN PY, LEE CT. Measurement of Absolute Displacement by a Double-modulation Technique Based on a Michelson Interferometer［J］.*Appl Opt*,1999,38(13):2843−2847.

［4］CHEN G, BOWER KA, MA C, et al. Glycogen Synthase Kinase 3β（GSK3β）Mediates 6-hydroxydopamine-induced Neuronal Death［J］.*FASEB J*, 2004,18(10):1162−1164.

［5］CHUNG CY, KOPRICH JB, Endo S, et al. An Endogenous Serine/Threonine Protein Phosphatase Inhibitor, G-substrate, Reduces Vulnerability in Models of Parkinson's Disease［J］.*J Neurosci*,2007,27(31):8314−8323.

［6］CHURCH WH, Ward VL. Uric Acid is Reduced in the Substantia Nigra in Parkinson's Disease：Effect on Dopamine Oxidation［J］.*Brain Res Bull*, 1994,33(04):419−425.

［7］CIPRIANI S, Desjardins CA, Burdett T C. Urate and its Transgenic Depletion Modulate Neuronal Vulnerability in a Cellular Model of Parkinson's Disease［J］.*PLoS One*,2012, 7(05):0037331.

［8］DAVIES KJ, SEVANIAN A, MUAKKASSAH-KELLY SF, et al. Uric Acid-iron Ion Complexes. A new Aspect of the Antioxidant Functions of Uric Acid［J］. *J Biochem*,1986,235(03):747−754.

［9］DU Y, CHEN CP, TSENG CY, et al. Astroglia-mediated Effects of Uric Acid to Protect Spinal Cord Neurons from Glutamate Toxicity［J］.*Glia*,2007, 55(05):463−472.

［10］FITZMAURICE PS, ANG L, GUTTMAN M, et al. Nigral Glutathione Deficiency is not Specific for Idiopathic Parkinson's Disease［J］.*Mov Disord*,

2003,18(09):969-976.

[11] FRANKE TF,KAPLAN DR, CANTLEY LC.PI3K: Downstream AKT Ion Blocks Apoptosis[J].*Cell*,1997, 88(04):435-437.

[12] GUERREIRO S,PONCEAU A,TOULORGE D, et al. Protection of Midbrain Dopaminergic Neurons by the End-product of Purine Metabolism Uric Acid: Potentiation by Low-level Depolarization [J]. *J Neurochem*, 2009, 109 (04):1118-1128.

[13] HOOPER DC, BAGASRA O, Marini J. C. et al. Prevention of Experimental Allergic Encephalomyelitis by Targeting Nitric Oxide and Peroxynitrite: Implications for the Treatment of Multiple Sclerosis[J].*Proc Natl Acad Sci USA*,1997, 94(06):2528-2533.

[14] JENNER P, OIANOW C. W. Understanding Cell Death in Parkinson's Disease[J].*Ann Neurol*,1998,44(3 suppl 1):S72-84.

[15] JOHNSON RJ,KANG DH,FEIG D,et al.Is there a Pathogenetic Role for Uric Acid in Hypertension and Cardiovascular and Renal Disease? [J]. *Hypertension*,2003, 41(06):1183-1190.

[16] KIKUCHI Y, YASUHARA T, AGARI T, et al. Urinary 8-OHdG Elevations in a Partial Lesion Rat Model of Parkinson's Disease Correlate with Behavioral Symptoms and Nigrostriatal Dopaminergic Depletion [J]. *J Cell Physiol*,2011,226(05):1390-1398.

[17] KUTZING M.K., FIRESTEIN B.L. Altered Uric Acid Levels and Disease States[J].*J Pharmacol Exp Ther*,2008,324(01),1-7.

[18] DE LAU LM,KOUDSTAAL PJ,HOFMAN A,et al.Serum Uric Acid Levels and the Risk of Parkinson Disease[J].*Ann Neurol*,2005,58(05):797-800.

[19] MAESAKA JK, WOLF-KLEIN G, PICCIONE JM, et al. Hypouricemia,Abnormal Renal Tubular Urate Transport,and Plasma Natriuretic Factor(s)in Patients with Alzheimer's Disease[J]. *J Am Geriatr Soc*,1993,41 (05):501-506.

[20] PATTERSON RA, HORSLEY ET, Leake DS. Prooxidant and Antioxidant Properties of Human Serum Ultrafiltrates toward LDL: Important Role of Uric Acid[J].*J Lipid Res*,2003,44(03):512-521.

［21］SCHWARZSCHILD MA,SCHWID SR,MAREK K,et al.Serum Urate as a Predictor of Clinical and Radiographic Progression in Parkinson Disease ［J］.*Arch Neurol*,2008,65(06):716-723.

［22］SCOTT GS,SPITSIN SV,KEAN RB,et al.Therapeutic Intervention in Experimental Allergic Encephalomyelitis by Administration of Uric Acid Precursors［J］.*Proc Natl Acad Sci USA*,2002, 99(25):16303-16308.

［23］SCOTT GS,CUZZOCREA S,GENOVESE T,et al. Uric Acid Protects against Secondary Damage after Spinal Cord Injury［J］.*Proc Natl Acad Sci USA*, 2005,102(09):3483-3488.

［24］SIMOLA N,MORELLI M, Carta AR.The 6-hydroxydopamine Model of Parkinson's Disease［J］.*Neurotox Res*,2007,11(3-4):151-167.

［25］WANG LJ, LUO WF, WANG HH, et al. Protective Effects of Uric Acid on Nigrostriatal System Injury Induced by 6-hydroxydopamine in Rats［J］. *Zhonghua Yi Xue Za Zhi*,2010, 90(09):1362-1365.

［26］WEISSKOPF MG, O'REILLY E, CHEN H,et al. Plasma Urate and Risk of Parkinson's Disease［J］.*Am.J.Epidemiol*,2007,166(05):561-567.

［27］ZHU TG, WANG XX, LUO WF, et al. Protective Effects of Urate Against 6-OHDA-induced Cell Injury in PC12 Cells through Antioxidant Action ［J］.*Neurosci Lett*,2012,506(02):175-179.

(Li Gong, Qi-Lin Zhang, Ning Zhang, Wen-Yan Hua, Yi-Xian Huang, Ping-Wei Di, Tingting Huang, Xing-Shun Xu,Chun-Feng Liu, Li-Fang Hu and Wei-Feng Luo)

(本文原载于 *Journal of Neurochemistry* 2012 年第 123 卷第 5 期)

Protective Effects of Urate against 6-OHDA-induced Cell Injury in PC12 Cells through Antioxidant Action

Abstract: There is evidence to support that oxidative stress is increased in Parkinson's disease and contributes to the degeneration of dopaminergic neurons. Recent research has shown that higher blood urate concentrations have now been linked to decreased risks and progression rates of PD. However, the mechanisms about urate to protect dopaminergic neurons are less clear. Our study investigated the effect of urate on oxidative stress induced by 6-Hydroxydopamine in neuronal differentiated PC12 cells. We found that urate significantly reduced 6-OHDA-induced lactate dehydrogenase (LDH), malondialdehyde (MDA), and 8-OHdG generation but increased the superoxide dismutase activity and glutathione (GSH) levels in the PC12 cells. These results suggested that urate can prevent PC12 cells from oxidative injury induced by 6-OHDA, which may play an important role in the mechanisms underlying the association of high plasma levels of urate with reduced risk and slower progression of PD. Urate treatment could be a potential therapeutic strategy for PD.

Keywords: 6-Hydroxydopamine; urate; oxidative stress; Parkinson's disease.

1. Introduction

Parkinson's disease is a common neurodegenerative disorder characterized by progressive loss of dopaminergic neurons in substantia nigra pars compacta. The exact mechanisms underlying neuronal death are incompletely understood, but oxidative stress, lipid peroxidation and mitochondrial dysfunction are generally thought to play a prominent role[1]. Different epidemiological studies

---

① JENNER P.Oxidative Stress in Parkinson's Disease [J]. *Ann Neurol*, 2003, 53 (Suppl 3) : S26 – 36 (discussion S36–38).

indicate that reductions in dietary or endogenous antioxidants decrease the capacity to suppress oxidative stress and consequently increase the risk and progression of PD①②.

Urate, the end-product of purine nucleoside catabolism, is a strong natural antioxidant in blood and brain tissue, scavenging superoxide, peroxynitrite and hydroxyl radical③. Several epidemiological studies have found that higher blood urate concentrations are associated with a decreased risk and delayed progression of PD④⑤. Moreover, recent studies also demonstrated that individuals with gout, a rheumatic disease resulting from hyperuricemia, had a significantly reduced occurrence of PD⑥⑦.Consistent with thesefindings, urate levels were significantly lower in the substantia nigra, striatum and serum of PD patients compared to those of controls subjects⑧⑨.As an antioxidant, urate might be a protective factor against this neurodegenerative disorder. Indeed, our previous study shown that urate can protect dopaminergic neurons in nigrostriatal system of rats from the toxic effects of 6-Hydroxydopamine⑩. Furthermore, protection by urate in cell

① DRECHSEL DA, PATEL M. Role of Reactive Oxygen Species in the Neurotoxicity of Environmental Agents Implicated in Parkinson's Disease[J].*Free Radic Biol Med*,2008,44(11):1873−1886.

② GAO X,CHEN H,CHOI HK, et al.Schwarzschild, A. Ascherio, Diet, Urate, and Parkinson's Disease Risk in Men[J].*Am J Epidemiol*,2008,167(07):831−838.

③ DAVIES KJ,SEVANIAN A,MUAKKASSAH-KELLY SF, et al.Uric Acid-iron Ion Complexes:A new Aspect of the Antioxidant Functions of Uric Acid[J].*Biochem J*,1986,235(03):747−754.

④ MG WEISSKOPF, O'REILLY E, CHEN H, et al.Plasma Urate and Risk of Parkinson's Disease[J].*Am J Epidemiol*,2007, 166(05):561−567.

⑤ WINQUIST A, STEENLAND K, SHANKAR A. Higher Serum Uric Acid Associated with Decreased Parkinson's Disease Prevalence in a Large Community-based Survey[J].*Mov Disord*,2010, 25(07):920−945.

⑥ AIONSO A, RODRIGUEZ LA, LOGROSCINO G, et al. Gout and Risk of Parkinson Disease: a Prospective Study[J].*Neurology*,2007,69(17):1696−1700.

⑦ ALONSO A,SOVELL KA.Gout,Hyperuricemia and Parkinson's Disease: a Protective Effect[J]. *Curr Rheumatol Rep* 2010, 12(02):149−155.

⑧ ANNANMAKI T,MUURONEN A,MURROS K.Low Plasma Uric Acid Level in Parkinson's Disease [J]. *Mov Disord*,2007,22(08):1133−1137.

⑨ CHURCH WH, WARD VL. Uric Acid is Reduced in the Substantia Nigra in Parkinson's Disease: Effect on Dopamine Oxidation[J]. *Brain Res Bull*,1994,33(04):419−425.

⑩ WANG LJ,LUO WF,WANG HH, et al.Protective Effects of Uric Acid on Nigrostriatal System Injury Induced by 6-Hydroxydopamine in Rats[J]. *Zhonghua Yi Xue Za Zhi*,2010, 90(19):1362−1365.

culture models of PD has strengthened this possibility[1][2]. However, the mechanisms about urate to protect dopaminergic neurons are less clear.

In the present study, we used 6-Hydroxydopamine a neurotoxin commonly used to lesion dopaminergic pathways, to generate experimental models of PD, investigated the effect of urate on oxidative stress, and explored the protection of urate in vitro in 6-OHDA induced PC12 cells.

2. Materials and Methods

（1）Materials

A PC12 cell line, which spontaneously differentiates into neuron-like cells, was a gift from the Institute of Neuroscience, Soochow University. Urate, 6-OHDA were purchased from Sigma-Aldrich (USA), and Dulbecco's modified Eagle's medium was purchased from GIBCO Inc. (USA). The lactate dehydrogenase and superoxide dismutase assay kit were purchased from Nanjing Jiancheng Biological Technology Company (Nanjing, China); IP cell lysate, malondialdehyde, glutathione kit and BCA-200 Quantitative protein assay kit were purchased from Beyotime Institute of Biotechnology (Shanghai, China). ELISA assay of 8-OHdG was purchased from U.S.R & D companies.

（2）Methods

① Cell Culture

The neuronal differentiated PC12 cells were cultured in Dulbecco's modified Eagle's medium, supplemented with 10% fetal calf serum at 37 ℃ in a humidified atmosphere containing 5% CO_2. The medium was replaced every 2 days as the cells were grown to $80\% \sim 90\%$ confluent. Then the cells were lifted by incubation with 0.25% trypsin and replaced in 75 cm^2 culture flasks. The logarithmic growing cells were used as indicated for all experiments, and every experiment was repeated three times. All cells were divided into 8 experimental

---

① GUERREIRO S, PONCEAU A, TOULORGE D, et al. Protection of Midbrain Dopaminergic Neurons by the End-product of Purine Metabolism Uric Acid: Potentiation by Low Level Depolarization[J]. *J Neurochem*, 2009,109(04):1118−1128.

② HABERMAN F, TANG SC, ARUMUGAM TV, et al. Soluble Neuroprotective Antioxidant Uric Acid Analogs Ameliorate Ischemic Brain Injury in Mice[J]. *Neuromolecular Med*, 2007,9(04):315−323.

groups: the control group, urate (100, 200 or 400 μmol/L) groups, 6-OHDA (100 μmol/L) group, 6-OHDA (100 μmol/L) +urate (100, 200 or 400 μmol/L) groups. Cells were incubated urate and/or 6-OHDA for 6 h, 12 h or 24 h.

② Lactate Dehydrogenase Assay

Cells were treated for 6 h, 12 h, and 24 h, and then 80 μL culture medium was collected to detect the LDH according to the manufacturer's instructions. The plasma membrane damage of the PC12 cells was assessed by measuring the release of LDH into culture medium.

③ Measurement of Glutathione and Malondialdehyde

After treatment for 6 h, 12 h and 24 h, cells were rinsed with PBS for three times, then scraped from the flask. Lysis buffer was added into cells and homogenized for 40 mins on ices. The lysates were then centrifuged at 4 ℃ at 12 000 rpm for 10 mins. After that, the supernatant was collected for analysis according to the manufacturer's instructions. GSH and MDA concentration was determined by a commercial colorimetric GSH and MDA assay kit (Beyotime Institute of Biotechnology, Shanghai, China). In the end, BCA protein assay kit was used to measure the protein concentration to calculate the content of GSH and MDA per gram proteins.

④ SOD Activity Assay

SOD is an important anti-oxidant enzyme that plays a pivotal role in the clearance of reactive oxygen species. After treatment for 6 h, 12 h or 24 h, 100 μL supernatant was used to measure the SOD activity with a spectrophotometry by using a commercially available detection kit (Nanjing Jiancheng Biochemical Reagent Co. Nanjing, China) according to the manufacturer's instructions.

⑤ Analysis of 8-hydroxydeoxyguanosine by ELISA

8-OHdG is one of the predominant forms of free radical-induced oxidative lesions, therefore, cellular 8-OHdG, urinary 8-OHdG, or 8-OHdG level in the culture medium has been widely used as a biomarker of oxidative stress①②③. In our study, we examined 8-OHdG level in the culture medium according to the method used by Arimoto and his colleague④. We have used the enzyme-linked immunosorbent assay (ELISA) to detect the content of 8-OHdG in the PC12 cells. After treatment for various time intervals, 50 μL culture medium was collected for analysis according to the manufacturer's instructions.

⑥ Statistical Analysis

Data were expressed as mean±SD. We analyzed the data by using ANOVA followed by Scheffe multiple-comparison test to compare the difference if there was a significant difference between groups. A value of $P<0.05$ was considered statistically significant.

3. Results

(1) LDH Release in Differentiated PC12 Cells

Following treatment with 6-OHDA (100 μmol/L), cells were incubated for up to 24 h, and toxicity was assessed as an index of membrane integrity (release of LDH). According to the results as shown in Fig. 1, urate alone at concentrations of 100, 200 or 400μmol/L, did not affect the release of LDH in the neuronal differentiated PC12 cells. There was no significant effect of 6-OHDA to the PC12 cells after 6 h incubation, however, compared with control group, 12 h and 24 h treatment of 6-OHDA caused a significant increase of LDH release ($P<0.05$). While cells were incubated with 6-OHDA and urate, the increased LDH release was dramatically reduced by urate at the dose of 200 and 400 μmol/L

① ARIMOTO T, YOSHIKAWA T, TAKANO H, et al. Generation of Reactive Oxygen Species and 8-hydroxy-2'-deoxyguanosine Formation from Diesel Exhaust Particle Components in L1210 Cells [J]. *Jpn J Pharmacol*, 1999, 80(01):49-54.

② KIKUCHI Y, YASUHARA T, AGARI T, et al. Urinary 8-OHdG Elevations in a Partial Lesion Rat Model of Parkinson's Disease Correlate with Behavioral Symptoms and Nigrostriatal Dopaminergic Depletion[J]. *J Cell Physiol*, 2011, 226(05):1390-1398.

③ YASUHARA T, HARA K, SETHI KD, et al. Increased 8-OHdG Levels in the Urine, Serum, and Substantia Nigra of Hemiparkinsonian Rats[J]. *Brain Res*, 2007, 1133(01):49-52.

④ ARIMOTO T, YOSHIKAWA T, TAKANO H, et al. Generation of Reactive Oxygen Species and 8-hydroxy-2'-deoxyguanosine Formation from Diesel Exhaust Particle Components in L1210 Cells [J]. *Jpn J Pharmacol*, 1999, 80(01):49-54.

（ P <0.05），but not at the dose of 100μmol/L（ P >0.05）.

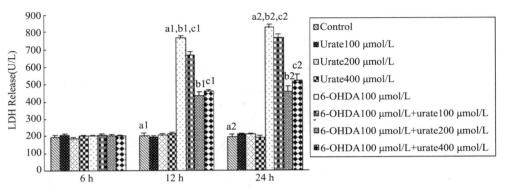

Fig.1　Effects of urate on the release of LDH in the medium of differentiated PC12 cells after 6-OHDA treatment. After treatment of 6-OHDA for 12 h and 24 h, there was a significant increase in LDH release, and it was reversed by urate（200,400 μmol/L）. Data were expressed as mean±S.D. N =3, a1, a2, P <0.05 versus control group, b1, b2, c1, c2, P <0.05 versus 6-OHDA group.

（2）Changes of Oxidation Products MDA and 8-OHdG after 6-OHDA treatment in Differentiated PC12 Cells

We continued to examine the underlying mechanisms for the beneficial effects of urate against 6-OHDA-induced cell injury in the PC12 cells. In vitro studies have suggested that oxidative stress is the main mediator in 6-OHDA-mediated cell death. Moreover, oxidative damage to lipids, proteins, and DNA occurs in PD. To this end, we measured the levels of MDA, a biomarker of lipid oxidation and 8-OHdG, a principal stable marker of hydroxyl radical damage to DNA to test whether the protective effects of urate observed in this study is related to its anti-oxidant action. As shown in Fig.2.A and Fig.2.B, there was no striking difference between 6-OHDA and control group after treatment for 6 h, moreover, 24 h after treatment, urate alone（100,200 or 400μmol/L）was not significantly change the production of MDA and 8-OHdG compared with control group. The levels of MDA and 8-OHdG dramatically increased following incubation with 6-OHDA for 12 h or 24 h and attenuated by urate at the concentrations of 200 or 400 μmol/L. This indicated that urate prevented 6-OHDA-induced oxidative stress in the PC12 cells.

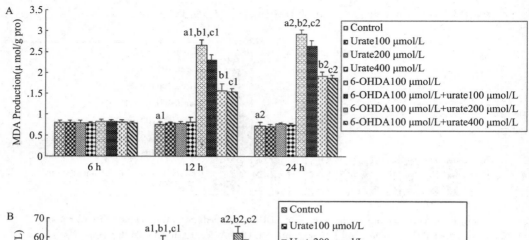

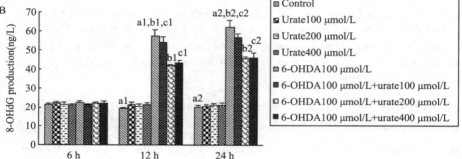

Fig.2   A, change of MDA in differentiated PC12 cells after treatment. PC12 cells were treated with 6-OHDA（100 μmol/L）and urate（100,200,400 μmol/L）for 6 h,12 h and 24 h.The content of MDA was significant increased post 6-OHDA treated for 12 h and 24 h, and urate（200, 400 μmol/L）attenuated the generation of MDA. Data were expressed as mean ± S.D. $N=3$, a1, a2, $P<0.05$ versus control group, b1, b2, c1, c2, $P<0.05$ versus 6-OHDA group. B, change of 8-OHdG in differentiated PC12 cells after treatment. ELISA method was used to detected the content of 8-OHdG in PC12 cells. After treatment of 6-OHDA for 12h and 24h, the levels of 8-OHdG was dramatically increased, and it was reversed by urate（200, 400 μmol/L）. Data were expressed as mean±S.D.$N=3$, a1, a2, $P<0.05$ versus control group, b1, b2, c1, c2, $P<0.05$ versus 6-OHDA group.

（3）Changes of GSH and SOD in differentiated PC12 cells

To clarify whether the protection of urate against 6-OHDA in the PC12 cells is involved in its anti-oxidant action. We further measured the most abundant anti-oxidant reagents SOD and GSH in cells. From the results shown in Fig.3.A and Fig.3.B, we found that there was no significant difference between the groups after 6 h incubation. In addition, the incubation with urate for 6 h, 12 h or 24 h, no significant difference was detected compared with the control group. However, after treatment with 6-OHDA for 12 h or 24 h, intracellular content of GSH and SOD significantly reduced. Because urate at the concentration of 200 or 400 μmol/L can decrease the levels of MDA and 8-OHdG, so we determined the effect of urate at the concentration of 200 or 400 μmol/L on cellular levels of GSH and SOD. We found that 6-OHDA-induced decrease of GSH and SOD was partially reversed by urate (200 or 400μmol/L, $P<0.05$). All results suggested that urate protected against 6-OHDA-induced cell injury in the PC12 cells, probably associated with its anti-oxidant activity.

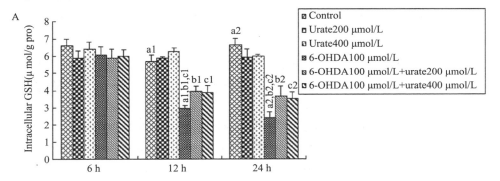

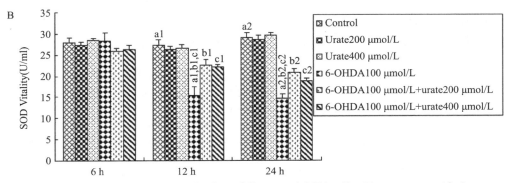

Fig.3 A, measurement of GSH levels in differentiated PC12 cells. After treatment with 6-OHDA for 12 h and 24 h, intracellular content of GSH significantly reduced, although the 6-OHDA-induced decrease of GSH could be partly reversed by urate (200,400 μmol/L), it was obvious lower than the control group. Data were expressed as mean±S.D. $N=3$, a1, a2, $P<0.05$ versus control group, b1, b2, c1, c2, $P<0.05$ vs 6-OHDA group. B, measurement of SOD levels in differentiated PC12 cells. Similarly, post incubation with 6-OHDA for 12 h and 24 h, intracellular content of SOD significantly reduced, and it was improved following treatment with urate (200,400 μmol/L). Data were expressed as mean±S.D. $N=3$, a1, a2, $P<0.05$ versus control group, b1, b2, c1, c2, $P<0.05$ versus 6-OHDA group.

4. Discussion

There is long-standing evidence that oxidative stress contributes to the neuronal cell death across neurodegenerative disease, such as Parkinson disease[1][2].PD occurs as a result of free radicals and scavenging of the normal balance has been severely damaged, leading to the death of dopamine neurons. Urate is an important natural antioxidant, iron chelator, and free radical scavenger in blood and brain tissue. Several evidence from clinical and epidemiological researches suggested that higher blood urate concentrations has now been linked to decreased risks and progression rates of PD[3][4][5][6]. However, the underlying mechanisms were not identified. In the present study, we investigated the influence of urate in 6-OHDA-induced neuronal differentiated PC12 cells, which have been proved to be a useful cell model to study neurodegenerative disease, such as PD.

6-OHDA-induced cell death is widely used as an experimental model of PD both in vivo and in vitro since this neurotoxin induces cell death of such neurons, as well as symptoms of the disease[7][8]. In the present study, 6-OHDA, which shares some structural similarities with dopamine, exhibiting a high affinity for dopamine transporters (DAT), was applied to the neuronal differentiated PC12 cells to generate cell models for PD.In vitro, 6-OHDA incubation for up to 12 h

① JENNER P.Oxidative Damage in Neurodegenerative Disease[J].*Lancet*,1994, 344(8925):796-798.

② MILLER RL, JAMES-KRACKE M, SUN GY, et al. Oxidative and Inflammatory Pathways in Parkinson's Disease[J].*Neurochem* Res,2009,34(01):55-65.

③ ANDREADOU E, NIKOLAOU C, GOURNARAS F, et al. Serum Uric Acid Levels in Patients with Parkinson's Disease: their Relationship to Treatment and Disease Duration[J].*Clin Neurol Neurosurg*,2009,111(09):724-728.

④ DE LAU LM, KOUDSTAAL PJ, HOFMAN A, et al.Serum Uric Acid Levels and the Risk of Parkinson Disease[J].*Ann Neurol*,2005,58(05):797-800.

⑤ WEISSKOPF MG, O'REILLY E, CHEN H, et al.Plasma Urate and Risk of Parkinson's Disease[J].*Am J Epidemiol*,2007, 166(05):561-567.

⑥ WINQUIST A, STEENLAND K, SHANKAR A. Higher Serum Uric Acid Associated with Decreased Parkinson's Disease Prevalence in a Large Community-based Survey[J].*Mov Disord*,2010, 25(07):932-936.

⑦ HANROTT K, GUDMUNSEN L, O'NEILL MJ, et al. 6-Hydroxydopamine-induced Apoptosis is Mediated via Extracellular Auto-oxidation and Caspase 3-dependent Activation of Protein Kinase C δ[J].*J Biol Chem*,2006,281(09):5373-5382.

⑧ WANG LJ, LUO WF, WANG HH, et al.Protective Effects of Uric Acid on Nigrostriatal System Injury Induced by 6-Hydroxydopamine in Rats[J].*Zhonghua Yi Xue Za Zhi*,2010, 90(19):1362-1365.

induced cellular membranes damaged and LDH released①②. These findings are consistent with our results, indicating 6-OHDA could induce cells injury in neuronal differentiated PC12 cells. However, it could be partly reversed by urate, a natural antioxidant that may reduce oxidative stress. Based on this, a mechanism, its anti-oxidant action, thought to play a role in this experimental model of PD.

It has been demonstrated that oxidative DNA damage is played a prominent role in the pathogenesis of PD. Several studies demonstrated that 8-OHdG, the oxidation product most frequently measured as an indicator of oxidative DNA damage, was significantly elevated in urine, serum, and substantia nigra of 6-OHDA-lesioned animal models of PD③④. In our study, we used ELISA methods to assay the content of 8-OHdG⑤, which may serve as indicator of oxidative stress. We demonstrated 6-OHDA marked increased the levels of 8-OHdG compared with the control group in the PC12 cells. Similarly, the levels of MDA, a biomarker of lipid oxidation was significant increased after incubation with 6-OHDA. However, it could be in part reversed by urate, a natural antioxidant. This results suggested that 6-OHDA initiated the neurotoxicity in the PC12 cells, moreover, oxidative stress showed to mediate neuron damage of 6-OHDA, for the increases of oxidation products. Urate exerted protective effects, decreased the production of oxidative injury in these in vitro models of Parkinson disease.

To our best knowledge, a chronic imbalance between formation of ROS and

① HANROTT K, GUDMUNSEN L, O'NEILL MJ, et al. 6-Hydroxydopamine-induced Apoptosis is Mediated via Extracellular Auto-oxidation and Caspase 3-dependent Activation of Protein Kinase C δ[J]. *J Biol Chem*, 2006, 281(09): 5373−5382.

② RODRIGUEZ-BLANCO J, MARTIN V, HERRERA F, et al. Intracellular Signaling Pathways Involved in Post-mitotic Dopaminergic PC12 Cell Death Induced by 6-Hydroxydopamine [J]. *J Neurochem*, 2008, 107(01): 127−140.

③ KIKUCHI Y, YASUHARA T, AGARI T, et al. Urinary 8-OHdG Elevations in a Partial Lesion Rat Model of Parkinson's Disease Correlate with Behavioral Symptoms and Nigrostriatal Dopaminergic Depletion[J]. *J Cell Physiol*, 2011, 226(05): 1390−1398.

④ YASUHARA T, HARA K, SETHI KD, et al. Increased 8-OHdG Levels in the Urine, Serum, and Substantia Nigra of Hemiparkinsonian Rats[J]. *Brain Res*, 2007, 1133(01): 49−52.

⑤ ARIMOTO T, YOSHIKAWA T, TAKANO H, et al. Generation of Reactive Oxygen Species and 8-hydroxy-2'-deoxyguanosine Formation from Diesel Exhaust Particle Components in L1210 Cells [J]. *Jpn J Pharmacol*, 1999, 80(01): 49−54.

antioxidant defenses characterizes many pathological processes and disease conditions including PD[①]. In addition, free radicals are neutralized by an elaborate antioxidant defense system consisting of enzymes such as SOD and non-enzymatic antioxidants such as GSH. To verify the anti-oxidation mechanism of urate against 6-OHDA, furthermore, we measured the contents of GSH and SOD to assay antioxidant defense system status. The results showed that urate increased the contents of antioxidants after incubation of 6-OHDA, which indicated that urate played antioxidant effect and reduced consumption of other antioxidants, such as GSH and SOD. In short, urate could improve the ability of scavenging the free radicals and anti-oxidant action in PD cell models induced by 6-OHDA.

Urate protected differentiated PC12 cells against 6-OHDA induced cell injury, at least in part via an anti-oxidation mechanism. First of all, it has been demonstrated that oxidative stress, lipid peroxidation, mitochondrial dysfunction and oxidative DNA damage are generally thought to play an important role in the pathogenesis of PD, and their oxidation products, MDA, carbonyl group and 8-OHdG also can damage mesencephalon dopaminergic neurons. Secondly, urate, the iron chelating agent, can neutralize reactive species such as peroxynitrites, hydroxyl radicals[②] via a Fentontype chemical reaction and to inhibit free radical-mediated chain reactions that result in lipid peroxidation[③][④]. All of above illustrated that urate can protect neurons through an antioxidant mechanism. However, other molecular protection mechanisms of urate could be considered. Several studies have suggested that nitric oxide promoted oxidative stress and the apoptosis of cells. Nitric oxide may react with superoxide to generate peroxynitrite, which as a strong oxidant can elevate the contents of 3-nitrotyrosine

① ALLEN RG, TRESINI M. Oxidative Stress and Gene Regulation[J]. *Free Radic Biol Med*, 2000, 28(03):463-499.

② DAVIES KJ, SEVANIAN A, MUAKKASSAH-KELLY SF, et al. Uric Acid-iron Ion Complexes: A new Aspect of the Antioxidant Functions of Uric Acid[J]. *Biochem J*, 1986, 235(03):747-754.

③ ALVAREZ-FISCHER D, GUERREIRO S, HUNOT S, et al. Modelling Parkinson-like Neurodegeneration via Osmotic Minipump Delivery of MPTP and Probenecid[J]. *J Neurochem*, 2008, 107(03):701-711.

④ MURAOKA S, MIURA T. Inhibition by Uric Acid of Free Radicals that Damage Biological Molecules[J]. *Pharmacol Toxicol*, 2003, 93(06):284-289.

(3-NT)[1] and inhibition of electron transfer in mitochondria, induce depletion of ATP and cell injury[2][3]. Urate, a specific scavenger of peroxynitrite, can prevent the formation of 3-NT and reduce the levels of oxidative stress. In addition, xanthine, the precursor of urate is different from it only at 8-one moiety, which is failed to afford neuroprotection. So we surmised that this chemical group greatly contributed to the protection of urate.

5. Conclusion

In present study, we have provided evidence that urate exerted protective effects, at least in part via an anti-oxidation mechanism, in an in vitro model of Parkinson disease, which suggests that increased levels of urate could offer a new neuroprotective approach to decrease incidence of PD or slow the progression of PD.

6. Acknowledgement

The work was supported by the Suzhou Foundation for Development of Science, Technology(200815404), Jiangsu Ordinary University Science Research Project(08KJB320012) and Natural Science Foundation of Jiangsu Province, China(BK2010229).

(Ting-Ge Zhu, Xiao-Xia Wang, Wei-Feng Luo, Qi-Lin Zhang, Ting-Ting Huang, Xing-Shun Xu, Chun-Feng Liu)

(本文原载于 *Journal of Neurochemistry* 2012 年第 123 卷第 5 期)

① SCHULZ JB, MATTHEWS RT, MUQIT MM, et al. Inhibition of Neuronal Nitric Oxide Synthase by 7-nitroindazole Protects against MPTP-induced Neurotoxicity in Mice[J]. *J Neurochem*, 1995, 64(02):936-939.

② INOUE S, KAWANISHI S. Oxidative DNA Damage Induced by Simultaneous Generation of Nitric Oxide and Superoxide[J]. *FEBS Lett*, 1995, 371(01):86-88.

③ PACHER P, BECKMAN JS, LIAUDET L. Nitric Oxide and Peroxynitrite in Health and Disease[J]. *Physiol Rev*, 2007, 87(01):315-424.

Nrf2 Signaling Contributes to the Neuroprotective Effects of Urate against 6-OHDA Toxicity[①]

Background: Mounting evidence shows that urate may become a biomarker of Parkinson's disease diagnosis and prognosis and a neuroprotectant candidate for PD therapy. However, the cellular and molecular mechanisms underlying its neuroprotective actions remain poorly understood.

Results: In this study, we showed that urate pretreatment protected dopaminergic cell line(SH-SY5Y and MES23.5) against 6-hydroxydopamine and hydrogen peroxide-induced cell damage. Urate was found to be accumulated into SHSY5Y cells after 30 mins treatment. Moreover, urate induced NF-E2-related factor 2 (Nrf2) accumulation by inhibiting its ubiquitination and degradation, and also promoted its nuclear translocation; however, it did not modulate Nrf2 mRNA level or Kelch-like ECH-associated protein 1 (Keap1) expression. In addition, urate markedly up-regulated the transcription and protein expression of γ-glutamate-cysteine ligase catalytic subunit (γ-GCLC) and heme oxygenase-1 (HO-1), both of which are controlled by Nrf2 activity. Furthermore, Nrf2 knockdown by siRNA abolished the intracellular glutathione augmentation and the protection exerted by urate pretreatment.

Conclusion: Our findings demonstrated that urate treatment may result in Nrf2-targeted anti-oxidant genes transcription and expression by reducing Nrf2 ubiquitination and degradation and promoting its nuclear translocation, and thus offer neuroprotection on dopaminergic cells against oxidative stresses.

1. Introduction

Parkinson's disease is the second most common neurodegenerative disorder.

① This work was supported by grants from National Natural Science Foundation of China(81171212), Natural Science Foundation of Jiangsu Province, China(BK2010229, BK2010228) and also Suzhou Technology Support Program(SS201112).

It is pathologically featured by dopaminergic neuron losses in substantia nigra and the formation of cytoplasmic inclusion bodies, although its etiology remains elusive. Dopamine replacement therapy remains the first line strategy in PD treatment; however, its effectiveness fades with disease progression. Therefore, more potential targets are needed to be identified to expand the therapeutic strategies.

1/LUrate constitutes the end product of purine metabolism in primates due to the lack of urate oxidase, which catalyzes the conversion of urate to allantoin. Relatively higher levels of urate exist in human plasma. The reference ranges of urate in clinical practices are typically 3.4~7.2 mg/dL (200~430 μmol/L) for men and 2.4~6.1 mg/dL for women (140~360 μmol/L)[1]. However, its concentration in human brain (30 μmol/L) is much lower than in blood. In 1994, a post-mortem study revealed that urate was lower in the nigrostriatal tissue of PD patients compared with age matched controls[2]. Subsequently, several epidemiological studies consistently showed that higher but still normal level of plasma urate was associated with lower risk and slower progression of PD.[3] Urate also favored the outcomes of non-motor symptoms of PD and other neurodegenerative disorders[4]. All these lines of evidence suggest a beneficial role of urate in PD. In recent years, our and other groups' work in both *in vitro* and *in*

① ENOMOTO A, KIMURA H, CHAIROUNGDUA A, et al. Molecular Identification of a Renal Urate Anion Exchanger that Regulates Blood Urate Levels[J]. *Nature*, 2002, 417(6887): 447–452.

② CHURCH WH, WARD VL. Uric Acid is Reduced in the Substantia Nigrain Parkinson's Disease: Effect on Dopamine Oxidation[J]. *Brain Res Bull*, 1994, 33(04): 419–425.

③ SCHWARZSCHILD MA, SCHWID SR, MAREK K, et al. (2008) Serum Urate as a Predictor of Clinical and Radiographic Progression in Parkinson Disease[J]. *Arch Neurol*, 2008, 65(06): 716–723.

④ ANNANMAKI T, PESSALA-DRIVER A, HOKKANEN L, et al. Uric Acid Associates with Cognition in Parkinson's Disease[J]. *Parkinsonism Relat Disord*, 2008, 14(07): 576–578.

vivo PD models substantiated the neuroprotective actions of urate①②③. However, the cellular and molecular mechanisms were poorly understood.

Recent studies identified that nuclear factor E2-related factor 2(Nrf2) was strongly induced in nucleus of PD nigral neurons④.Nrf2 is a transcription factor regulating the expression of antioxidant response elements(ARE) contained genes such as heme oxygenase-1 (HO-1), NAD (P) H quinone oxidoreductase-1, glutathione-S-transferases and other glutathione synthesizing enzymes⑤. Alterations in Nrf2 signaling were linked to abnormal redox homeostasis.Loss of Nrf2-mediated transcription exacerbated the vulnerability of dopaminergic neurons to oxidative stresses⑥. Nrf2 knockout mice showed a greater loss of dopaminergic neurons compared with wild type mice when exposure to 1-methyl-4-phenyl-1,2,3,6-tetrahydropyridine ⑦.Therefore, Nrf2 may serve as a critical signaling molecule in the neuroprotective strategies against PD pathogenesis. In the present study, we sought to examine whether Nrf2 signaling is involved in the protective effect of urate on dopaminergic cells. Our findings demonstrated that urate could activate Nrf2 transactivity by inhibiting its ubiquitination and degradation without disrupting Nrf2 association with Kelch-like ECH-associated protein 1, and thus protected dopaminergic cells (SH-SY5Y and MES23. 5)

① GONG L,ZHANG QL,ZHANG N.et al.Neuroprotection by Urate on 6-OHDA-lesioned Rat Model of Parkinson's Disease: Linking to Akt/GSK3 beta Signaling Pathway[J]. *J Neurochem*,2012, 123(05): 876-885.

② GUERREIRO S,PONCEAU A,TOULORGE D.et al. Protection of Midbrain Dopaminergic Neurons by the End-product of Purine Metabolism Uric Acid: Potentiation by Low-level Depolarization[J]. *J Neurochem*, 2009, 109(04): 1118-1128.

③ ZHU TG,WANG XX,LUO WF.et al.Protective Effects of Urate against 6-OHDA-induced Cell Injury in PC12 Cells through Antioxidant Action[J]. *Neurosci Lett*,2012, 506(02): 175-179.

④ RAMSEY CP, GLASS CA, MONTGOMERY MB. et al. Expression of Nrf2 in Neurodegenerative Diseases[J]. *J Neuropathol Exp Neurol*,2007, 66(01): 75-85.

⑤ ANSARI N, KHODAGHOLI F, AMINI M. 2-Ethoxy-4, 5-diphenyl-1, 3-oxazine-6-one Activates the Nrf2/HO-1 Axis and Protects against Oxidative Stress-induced Neuronal Death[J]. *Eur J Pharmacol*,2011, 658 (2-3): 84-90.

⑥ JAKEL RJ,TOWNSEND JA,KRAFT AD, et al.Nrf2-mediated Protection against 6-hydroxydopamine [J]. *Brain Res*,2007,1144: 192-201.

⑦ CHEN PC,VARGAS MR,PANI AK.et al. Nrf2-mediated Neuroprotection in the MPTP Mouse Model of Parkinson's Disease: Critical Role for the Astrocyte[J]. *Proc Natl Acad Sci USA*,2009, 106(08): 2933-2938.

against oxidative insults.

2. Materials and Methods

（1）Reagents and Antibodies

Uric acid and 6-OHDA were purchased from Sigma-Aldrich（St Louis, MO, USA）. Cycloheximide（CHX）was obtained from Beyotime（Nantong, China）and lipofectin amine 2000 from Invitrogen（Carlsbad, CA, USA）. The antibodies against γ-glutamate-cysteine ligase catalytic subunit, γ-glutamate-cysteine ligase modifier（γ-GCLM）, HO-1 and Nrf2, Keap1, ubiquitin were purchased from Abcam（New Territories, Hong Kong, china）and Santa Cruz（California, USA）, respectively. Other primary antibodies were obtained from Cell Signaling Technology（Boston, MA, USA）. All reagents for cell culture were obtained from Life technologies（Van Allen Way, Carlsbad, USA）.

（2）Cell Culture and Treatment

Undifferentiated SH-SY5Y cells were purchase from ATCC and cultured in Dulbecco's modified Eagle's Medium supplemented with 10% fetal bovine serum and 1% penicillin/streptomycin in a 5% CO_2 atmosphere at 37 ℃. MES23.5 cells（kindly provided by Prof. Wei-dong Le, Institute of Health Science, Shanghai Institutes For Biological Sciences, CAS）were cultured in DMEM/F12 growth medium supplemented with 5% fetal bovine serum, 2 μmol/L glutamine and Sato's chemically defined medium to a final concentration of 5 mg/mL insulin, 5 mg/mL transferrin, 48.6 mg/mL pyruvic acid, 6.3 ng/mL progesterone, 5 ng/mL sodium selenite and 4 mg/mL putrescine[①].

（3）Cell Viability Measurement

Cell viability was determined as previously described[②]. In brief, at the end of treatment, culture medium was replaced with the medium containing MTT at a

① CRAWFORD GD, JR, LE WD, et al. A Novel N18TG2 x Mesencephalon Cell Hybrid Expresses Properties that Suggest a Dopaminergic Cell Line of Substantia Nigra Origin[J]. *J Neurosci*, 1992, 12（09）: 3392-3398.

② GONG L, ZHANG QL, ZHANG N, et al. Neuroprotection by Urate on 6-OHDA-lesioned Rat Model of Parkinson's Disease: Linking to Akt/GSK3beta Signaling Pathway[J]. *J Neurochem*, 2012, 123（05）: 876-885.

final concentration of 0.5 mg/mL and cells were incubated at 37 ℃ for 4 h. After that, culture supernatant was carefully removed. The insoluble formazan was then dissolved in dimethyl sulphoxide. The absorbance was determined at 570 nm with the reference wavelength at 630 nm using a microplate reader (TECAN M200 Pro, Grodig, Austria).

(4) Urate Measurement

Urate was assessed with an assay kit from Cayman Chemical (Ann Arbpr, MI, USA) according to the manufacturer's instructions. In brief, SH-SY5Y cells were treated with 200 μmol/L urate. After incubation for indicated time periods, the culture supernatants were collected for extracellular urate assay. Cells were then washed twice with phosphate-buffered saline (PBS) and harvested in a solution of 150 μmol/L phosphoric acid. After centrifugation at 15 000 g for 15 mins at 4 ℃, the resulting supernatants were used for intracellular urate determination. For urate assay, 20 μL samples were mixed with 30 μL assay buffer in a 96-well plate, followed by the addition of 50 μL reaction mixture that contains the probe and enzyme mix. The mixtures were then incubated at 37 ℃ for 30 mins. Fluorescence was measured at Ex/Em = 535/590 nm in a microplate reader (TECAN, GmbH, Austria). The intracellular urate level was normalized by the protein level and expressed as μmol/g protein. The protein concentrations were determined using the BCA kit (Pierce Chemical, Rockford, IL, USA).

(5) Protein Carbonyl Determination

For protein carbonyl assay, SH-SY5Y cells were cultured in 100 mm dishes until they reached confluence. Cells were harvested by centrifugation at 12 000 rpm for 5 mins. The pellets were resuspended in 300 μL ice-cold PBS and sonicated. The supernatants were then collected for protein carbonyls assay using a commercial ELISA kit (BioCell Corp, New Zealand). The carbonyl level was normalized by the protein concentration and expressed as nmol/mg protein.

(6) Immunoblotting and Immunoprecipitation

Whole lysates were prepared by washing cells twice with chilled PBS and homogenized in lysis buffer [150 μm NaCl, 25 μm Tris (pH7.5), 5 μm EDTA, 1% Nonidet P-40] and protease inhibitor cocktail tablets (Roche Diagnostics, Penzberg, Germany). Protein samples were boiled for 5 mins prior to separation on 10% sodium dodecyl sulfate-polyacrylamide gel and transferred onto polyvinylidene fluoride membranes (Millipore, Bedford, MA, USA). Membranes were then blocked and incubated with primary antibodies against proteins of interest at 4 ℃ overnight with gentle shaking. Afterwards, membranes were briefly washed and incubated with HRP-conjugated second antibodies (Jackson Laboratory, USA). The results were visualized by ECL chemiluminescence (GE healthcare, Buckinghamshire, UK). The band densities were quantified by Image J software (National Institute of Health, USA).

For immunoprecipitation(IP), cells were lysed in lysis buffer as mentioned above. Cell lysates were precleared with protein A/G Plus-agarose beads (Santa Cruz, California, USA) and incubated with 5 μg of the affinity-purified antibody overnight at 4 ℃. The lysates were then precipitated by incubation with protein A/G-agarose beads at 4 ℃ for 2 h. After washing with RIPA buffer three times, immunoprecipitation complexes were eluted in sample buffer by boiling for 5 mins and subjected to immunoblotting as described above. When measuring ubiquitinated Nrf2, proteins extracts were denatured first to disrupt the potential association of Nrf2 with other proteins before IP.

（7）Confocal Imaging

Cells were fixed in 4% paraformaldehyde and permeabilized in PBS with 0.1% Triton X-100 for 5 mins. Next, coverslips were blocked in 3% bovine serum albumin/PBS for 1 h. After that, coverslips were incubated with anti-Nrf2 antibodies at 4 ℃ overnight, followed by incubation with Alexa Fluor 488 chicken anti-rabbit IgG (Molecular Probes, Eugene, OR, USA) for another 1 h. Subsequently, coverslips were mounted onto slides with mounting medium containing DAPI. Cells were observed and scanned under a confocal microscope (LSM 700, Zeiss, Germany).

（8）Cytosolic and Nuclear Fraction Lysate Preparation

The cytosolic and nuclear fractions were separated with a kit (Beyotime institute of Biotechnology, China) according to the manufacturer's instructions. In brief, cells were harvested and lysed with 100 μL cytosolic extract A reagent containing 1 μm PMSF and vortexed for 5 seconds. The lysates were then added with 5 μL cytosolic extract B reagent and violently vortexed for another

5 seconds. After that, the lysates were centrifuged at 13 000 g at 4 ℃ for 5 mins and the supernatants were collected and designated as the cytosolic fractions. The resulting pellets were added with 30 μL nuclear extract reagent containing 1 μm PMSF and vortexed for 15~30 seconds every 2 mins interval during a period of 30 mins, and centrifuged again at 13 000 g at 4 ℃ for 10 mins. The resulting supernatants were extracted as nuclear proteins.

(9) Reverse Transcription PCR

RNA was extracted using TRIzol reagent (Invitrogen, Carlsbad, CA, USA). Equal amounts of RNA (1μg) were reversely transcribed into cDNA using cDNA synthesis kit (Fermentas). An equal volume of cDNA product was amplified using PCR Master Mix kit (Fermentas) with primers (Genscript, Nanjing, China) as listed: human GCLC [NM_001498.3] (forward 5′-TGA GAT TTA AGC CCC CTC CT-3′ and reverse 5′-TTG GGA TCA GTC CAG GAA AC-3′); GCLM [NM_002061.2] (forward 5′-TTT GGT CAG GGA GTT TCC AG-3′ and reverse 5′-ACA CAG CAG GAG GCA AGA TT-3′); HO-1 [NM_002133.2] (forward 5′-CCT AAA CTT CAG AGG GGG CG-3′ and reverse 5′-ATG GCT CAA AAA CCA CCC CA-3′); Nrf2 [NM_006164.4] (forward 5′-TTC AAA GCG TCC GAA CTC CA-3′ and reverse 5′-AAT GTC TGC GCC AAA AGC TG-3′) and β-actin [NM_001101.3] (forward 5′-AAG AGA GGC ATC CTC ACC CT-3′ and reverse 5′-TAC ATG GCT GGG GTG TTG AA-3′). PCR products were separated in a 2% agarose gel and stained with Gel view. The band densities were analyzed with Image J software.

(10) Transient Transfection with siRNA Targeting Nrf2

The small interfering RNA (siRNA) oligonucleotides targeting human Nrf2 (si-Nrf2-1: sense 5′-CCC GUU UGU AGA UGA CAA UTT-3′; antisense 5′-AUU GUC AUC UAC AAA CGG GTT-3′; si-Nrf2-2: sense 5′-GCC CAU UGA UGU UUC UGA UTT-3′; antisense 5′-AUC AGA AAC AUC AAU GGG CTT-3′) and nonspecific oligonucleotides were ordered from GenePharma (Shanghai, China). SH-SY5Y cells were transiently transfected with siRNAs using Lipofectamine 2000 (Invitrogen, Carlsbad, CA, USA) when reaching 70% ~ 80% confluence. The Nrf2 knockdown efficiency was determined at 24 h post-transfection with immunoblotting.

（11）Intracellular Glutathione Measurement

Glutathione assays were performed with a kit according to the manufacturer's instructions（Nanjing Jiancheng Biochemical Reagent Co. Nanjing, China）. Briefly, cultures were washed with ice-cold PBS and deproteinated with 10% trichloroacetic acid. After centrifugation, the supernatants were mixed with working buffer containing glutathione reductase, DTNB and total glutathione amortization buffer and incubated for 5 mins, followed by the addition with 0.16 mg/mL NADPH and incubation for 25 mins. Subsequently, the absorbance was measured at 450 nm using a microplate reader as described above. Total glutathione content was determined with a standard curve obtained from the defined concentrations of reduced glutathione.

（12）Statistical Analysis

All data were presented as mean±SEM. Statistical differences were assessed with one-way analysis of variance followed by a post hoc（Tukey）test for multiple group comparison. Differences with $P < 0.05$ were considered statistically significant.

2. Results

（1）Urate Pretreatment Alleviated the 6-OHDA-induced Injury to Dopaminergic Cells

6-OHDA is a commonly used toxin for inducing PD-like models in both *in vivo* and *in vitro* studies. In this study, we observed that 6-OHDA treatment resulted in a significant decrease of cell viability in human dopaminergic neuroblastoma cell line（SH-SY5Y）in concentration and time-dependent manners（Fig.1.A, Fig.1.C）. 50 μmol/L 6-OHDA treatment for 14 h reduced the cell viability by 47.3% as compared to controls. We then evaluated the effect of urate（25, 50, 100, 200 and 400 μmol/L）on 6-OHDA-induced damage in SH-SY5Y cells. It was found that urate pretreatment for 30 mins appeared to attenuate the 6-OHDA-induced toxicity in a concentration-dependent manner. Specifically, at 200 μmol/L and 400 μmol/L, urate increased the cell viability by 37.4% and 43.5% as compared to 6-OHDA-treated group（Fig. 1. B）. Moreover, 200 μmol/L urate pretreatment was still able to protect against the

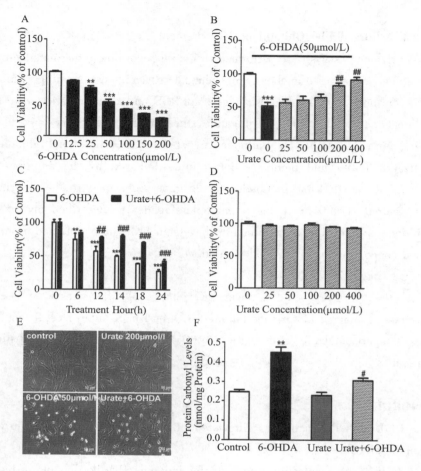

Fig. 1　Effect of urate pretreatment on 6-OHDA-induced injury in SH-SY5Y cells. A, concentration-dependent toxicity of 6-OHDA in SH-SY5Y cells. Cells were treated with various concentrations of 6-OHDA for 14 h. Cell viability was then determined by MTT method. B, effect of urate on 6-OHDA-induced cytotoxicity. Cells were pre-treated with urate (25,50,100,200 and 400 μmol/L) for 30 mins, followed by 50 μmol/L 6-OHDA treatment for 14 h. C, effect of 200 μmol/L urate pretreatment on cell survival when cells were exposed to 50 μmol/L 6-OHDA for different time periods. D, effect of urate treatment for 24 h on SH-SY5Y cell viability at indicated concentrations. E, morphological changes of SH-SY5Y cells when cells were treated with 50 μmol/L 6-OHDA or 200 μmol/L urate, or in combination with both for 14 h. F, cells were pretreated with 200 μmol/L urate for 30 mins followed by 50 μmol/L 6-OHDA for 14 h. The protein carbonyl levels were determined as described in methods. Data were presented as Mean± SEM. $N = 6$ for each group in cell viability assay and the results were repeated three times independently. $^{**}P < 0.01$, $^{***}P < 0.001$ versus controls; $^{\#}P < 0.05$, $^{\#\#}P < 0.01$, $^{\#\#\#}P < 0.001$ versus 6-OHDA group.

cytotoxicity when cells were exposed to 50 μmol/L 6-OHDA for up to 24 h, although the protective effect became less significant than that at earlier time points (Fig.1.C). To preclude the possibility that urate caused any toxicity to SH-SY5Y cells after 24 h incubation, cells were treated with urate alone and the cell viability was determined at 24 h later. The results showed that urate, at tested concentrations (25,50,100,200 and 400 μmol/L), did not produce any toxic effect on SH-SY5Y cells (Fig.1.D). In addition, we observed that SH-SY5Y cells exhibited short spiny neurite-like processes in vehicle-treated group. After exposure to 50 μmol/L 6-OHDA for 14 h, most cells shrank and cell processes disappeared. The morphological changes were markedly alleviated in urate-pretreated group (Fig. 1. E). Considering that 200 μmol/L urate, which was within its physiological range, produced obvious protection against 6-OHDA-induced toxicity, 200 μmol/L urate was then applied in the studies herein reported.

(2) Urate Could be Accumulated into Dopaminergic Cells

Interestingly, we observed urate's protection remained even if urate was washed out before 6-OHDA exposure (Fig. 2. A). It is less likely that this protection was a false positive observation resulted from the direct interaction between urate and 6-OHDA in the extracellular milieu. Next, we assessed whether urate could be transported into SH-SY5Y cells. To achieve this, cells were treated with 200 μmol/L urate for 0.5, 6 and 24 hours. The urate levels in culture supernatant and cell lysates at these time points were then determined and defined as extracellular and intracellular urate content, respectively. It was observed that intracellular urate level increased in a time-dependent manner whilst the extracellular counterpart decreased (Fig.2.B). At 0.5 h after urate addition, the extracellular urate level decreased to 186.75 μmol/L while the intracellular urate reached 0.3±0.01 μmol/g protein, which was about 15 folds over the basal level (0.02±0.01 μmol/g protein). Furthermore, no significant amount of urate was detected in the culture supernatant at another 24 h later when extracellular urate was removed after 24 h incubation (data not shown), implying reverse transportation of urate may not exist in this cell line.

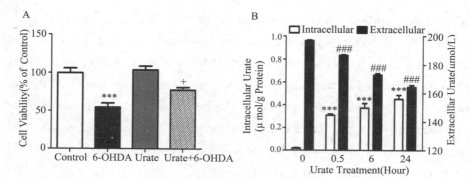

Fig.2　Urate was accumulated into SH-SY5Y cells and exerted protection intracellularly. A,effect of urate pre-treatment on cell viability. Urate was removed by washout after 30 mins pre-incubation,followed by 6-OHDA treatment for 14 h. B,accumulation of urate into SH-SY5Y cells as incubation time increased. Cells were treated with 200 μmol/L urate for different time periods as indicated. The extracellular and intracellular urate content was determined as described in"material and methods". The intracellular urate level was normalized by the protein concentration. Results were shown as Mean±SEM,$N=3$. +$P<$ 0.05 versus 6-OHDA group; *** $P<0.001$ versus controls or intracellular value of controls (0 h);### $P<0.001$ versus extracellular value of controls (0 h).

（3）Urate Protected against H_2O_2-induced Cell Damage to Dopaminergic Cells

As urate was previously reported to act as a pro-oxidant under some conditions[①],we also studied the effect of urate on oxidative stress by determining the protein oxidation product carbonyl levels. We found that 50 μmol/L 6-OHDA treatment enhanced the cellular protein carbonyl levels,which was obviously attenuated in the presence of 200 μmol/L urate pretreatment. Furthermore,urate treatment alone did not affect the protein carbonyl levels,as shown in Fig.1.F.

To determine whether urate was protective against other oxidative insults, SH-SY5Y cells and another dopaminergic cell line（MES23.5）were subjected to H_2O_2 treatment（100,200,400 and 800 μmol/L）for 12 h. As can be seen from Fig.3.A,Fig.3.C,H_2O_2 resulted in a differential toxicity to SH-SY5Y（Fig.3.A）and MES 23.5（Fig.3.C）cells. Specifically,800 μmol/L H_2O_2 treatment reduced the cell viability by 49.3% in SH-SY5Y whilst merely 100μmol/L H_2O_2

① MAHAJAN M,KAUR S,MAHAJAN S,et al. Uric Acid a Better Scavenger of Free Radicals than Vitamin C in Rheumatoid Arthritis[J]. Indian J Clin Biochem,2009, 24(02): 205-207.

decreased it by 49.8% in MES23.5 cell line.Pretreatment with urate at 200 μmol/L and 400 μmol/L for 24 h markedly increased the cell viability as compared to H_2O_2-treated group in SH-SY5Y cells (Fig.3.B).Similar trend was observed in MES23.5 cells (Fig.3.D).

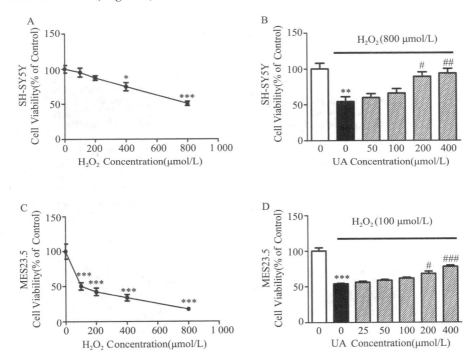

Fig.3   Effect of urate on H_2O_2-induced cell damage in SH-SY5Y and MES23.5 cells. A, B,C,concentration-dependent toxicity of H_2O_2 treatment for 12 h to SH-SY5Y (A) and MES23.5 cells (C).B and D,cells were pretreated with urate (25,50,100,200 and 400μmol/L)for 24 h,followed by H_2O_2 treatment at the indicated concentration in SH-SY5Y(B) and MES23.5(D) cells.The results were repeated three times. $^*P<0.05$, $^{**}P< 0.01$, $^{***}P<0.001$ versus controls; $^\#P<0.05$, $^{\#\#}P<0.01$, $^{\#\#\#}P<0.001$ versus H_2O_2 group.

(4) Urate Suppressed Nrf2 Ubiquitination and Degradation

We then explored the signaling mechanisms that contributed to the protection of urate. Nrf2 is a master regulator against oxidative stress and it controls the transcription of several anti-oxidant genes. We observed that 200 μmol/L urate treatment markedly elevated the protein levels of Nrf2 and its control genes including γ-GCLC and HO-1. The elevation,detected as early as

0.5 h after treatment, lasted at least 6 h and came to decline at 14 h later (Fig.4.A). Notably, the Nrf2 transcription was not altered by urate (Fig.4.B). Moreover, we observed in the presence of CHX, a protein translation inhibitor, Nrf2 protein level decreased rapidly. About 50% of the total Nrf2 was decreased at 10 mins after CHX addition. However, this decrease appeared much slower in the presence of urate (Fig.4.C), implying urate may delay Nrf2 degradation.

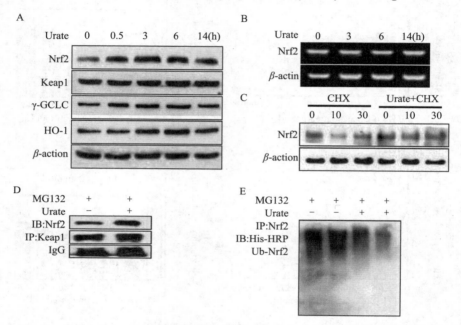

Fig.4　Effect of urate on Nrf2 activation in SH-SY5Y cells. A and B, immunoblotting and reserve transcription PCR analysis showing the protein and mRNA levels of Nrf2, Keap1, γ-GCLC and HO-1. Cells were treated with 200 μmol/L urate for 0.5, 3, 6 and 14 hours. β-actin served as loading controls. C, effect of urate on Nrf2 protein level in the presence of 1 μg/mL CHX. Cells were harvested and lysed at 0, 10 and 30 mins after CHX addition with or without urate treatment. D, urate did not disrupt Keap1-Nrf2 complex. Cells were treated with 200 μmol/L urate for 6 h. The association of this complex was assessed using IP with anti-Keap1, followed by immunoblotting with anti-Nrf2. E, urate inhibited Nrf2 ubiquitination. Cells were treated with or without urate for 6 h in the presence of MG132 (25 μm). For detecting ubiquitinated Nrf2, samples were subjected to IP with anti-Nrf2, followed by IB with an anti-His-HRP-conjugated antibody. The results were independently repeated at least three times.

Nrf2 protein is rapidly degraded by the 26S proteasome with its half-life at approximately 15 mins①②. Keap1, known as Nrf2 repressor, is crucial for its rapid turnover and functions as an adaptor for Nrf2 ubiquitination③④. Therefore, we processed to study the protein level of Keap1 and its interaction with Nrf2 via immunoprecipitation. We observed no significant change in Keap1 expression after urate treatment for up to 14 h. Of interest, we detected a significant increase in Nrf2 level in Keap1 immunoprecipitates from urate-treated cells in the presence of proteasome inhibitor MG132 (Fig.4.D). Furthermore, urate markedly reduced the ubiquitination of Nrf2, as shown in Fig.4.E.

(5) Urate Induced Nrf2 Accumulation and its Nuclear Translocation in Dopaminergic Cells

Nrf2 controls and initiates the transcription of oxidation-related genes such as γ-GCLC and ho-1 once it accumulates and translocates into the nucleus⑤. Therefore, the subcellular distribution of Nrf2 was also studied by confocal scanning in combination with immunoblotting. We observed Nrf2 was mostly distributed in cytoplasm in both control and 6-OHDA (50 μmol/L, 6 h)-treated cells. However, it was mainly localized to the nucleus with urate pretreatment (Fig.5.A). This redistribution was most prominent in urate alone treated cells. To verify these observations, cytosolic and nuclear compartments of SH-SY5Y cells were fractioned and subjected to immunoblotting (Fig.5.B). The results showed Nrf2 protein was present at higher levels in the nuclear fraction than that in the cytosolic after urate treatment (Fig.5.C), implying urate may promote Nrf2 nuclear translocation. The phenomenon was validated in another dopaminergic cell line MES23.5. Similarly, the pictures showed that Nrf2 was predominantly located

① STEWART D, KILLEEN E, NAQUIN R, et al. Degradation of Transcription Factor Nrf2 via the Ubiquitin-proteasome Pathway and Stabilization by Cadmium[J]. *J Biol Chem*,2003, 278(04): 2396–2402.

② ITOH K,WAKABAYASHI N,KATOH Y,et al. Keap1 Regulates both Cytoplasmic-nuclear Shuttling and Degradation of Nrf2 in Response to Electrophiles[J]. *Genes Cells*,2003, 8(04): 379–391.

③ KOBAYASHI A,KANG MI,OKAWA H,et al. Oxidative Stress Sensor Keap1 Functions as an Adaptor for Cul3-based E3 Ligase to Regulate Proteasomal Degradation of Nrf2[J]. *Mol Cell Biol*, 2004, 24(16): 7130–7139.

④ ZHANG DD. Mechanistic Studies of the Nrf2-Keap1 Signaling Pathway[J]. *Drug Metab Rev*,2006, 38(04): 769–789.

⑤ YU J, ZHAO Y, LI B, et al. 17β-estradiol Regulates the Expression of Antioxidant Enzymes in Myocardial Cells by Increasing Nrf2 Translocation[J]. *J Biochem Mol Toxicol*,2012, 26(07): 264–269.

in the cytoplasm of control and 6-OHDA (50 μmol/L, 6 h)-treated cells. There was an obvious Nrf2 accumulation in the nuclei of uratetreated cells, which was more prominent in the cells without 6-OHDA treatment. We also extended our study to 14 h after 50 μmol/L 6-OHDA treatment. The results showed that similar trends of Nrf2 re-distribution were observed in SH-SY5Y cells with urate pre-treatment, although the changes were not as obvious as those at 6 h after treatment.

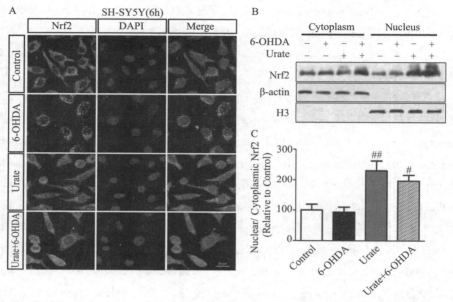

Fig.5   Effect of urate on the subcellular distribution of Nrf2 in SY-SY5Y cells. Cells were pre-incubated with urate for 30 mins prior to 6-OHDA treatment for 6 h. A, representative pictures showing the subcellular distribution of Nrf2 (FITC/green) in SH-SY5Y cells. Nuclei were stained with DAPI (blue). Scale bar = 20 μm. B and C, cytoplasmic and nuclear fractions were prepared and subjected to immunoblotting analysis. H3 and β-actin were used for nuclear and cytoplasmic protein markers respectively. Mean ± SEM, N = 4. #P < 0.05 versus 6-OHDA group; ## P < 0.01 versus control.

(6) Urate Promoted the Transcription and Protein Expression of Nrf2-target Genes

Next, we continued to study the mRNA and protein expression of Nrf2-regulated genes including γ-GCLC, γ-GCLM and ho-1. 200 μm urate treatment for 14 h was found to enhance the mRNA and protein expression of γ-gclc and ho-1 in SH-SY5Y cells (Fig.6.A, Fig.6.E). In contrast, the transcription and

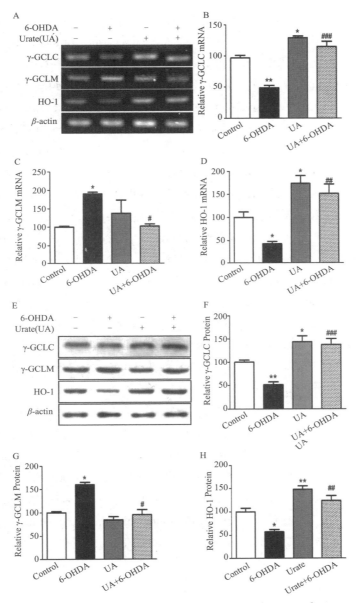

Fig. 6 Effects of urate on the mRNA and protein expression of the antioxidant genes. Cells were pretreated with 200 μmol/L urate or vehicle, followed by 6-OHDA treatment for 14 h. The mRNA (A-D) and protein (E-H) levels of γ-GCLC, γ-GCLM and HO-1 were assessed by reserve transcription PCR and immunoblotting respectively. β-actin served as loading controls. Group data were obtained by normalizing to β-actin and expressed as percentage of control values. Mean ±SEM, $N=3$. $^{*}P<0.05$, $^{**}P<0.01$ versus control; $^{\#}P<0.05$, $^{\#\#}P<0.01$, $^{\#\#\#}P<0.001$ versus 6-OHDA group.

translation of γ-gclm was not obviously altered by urate treatment. In addition, we observed the mRNA levels of γ-GCLC and HO-1 were dramatically decreased while that of γ-GCLM was increased in response to 6-OHDA treatment. However, the transcriptional changes of these genes were significantly reversed in the presence of urate pretreatment (Fig. 6. B – Fig. 6. D). Similar trends were observed at the protein levels (Fig. 6F – Fig. 6. H). Urate treatment was able to elevate the expression of γ-GCLC and HO-1 protein in both vehicle and 6-OHDA-treated cells. Meanwhile, it alleviated the increase of γ-GCLM protein expression caused by 6-OHDA in SH-SY5Y cells.

（7）Nrf2 Knockdown Abolished the Protection of Urate on SH-SY5Y Cells

To substantiate the role of Nrf2 in urate's protection, the effects of urate on cell survival and glutathione level were determined following introduction of Nrf2 siRNA into SH-SY5Y cells. Immunoblotting revealed that individual transfection with two different siRNAs against human Nrf2 (si-Nrf2-1, si-Nrf2-2) successfully reduced Nrf2 protein expression at 24 h post transfection, as compared to both untransfected (control) and mocked transfected (si-control) cells (Fig. 7. A, Fig. 7. B). The knockdown efficiency of si-Nrf2-2 appeared to be more obvious than that of si-Nrf2-1. Therefore, si-Nrf2-2 was taken in the following study.

We observed that Nrf2 siRNA-transfected cells were more susceptible to 6-OHDA-induced toxicity (12.7% reduction compared with control siRNA transfected cells, $P < 0.05$). More importantly, Nrf2 knockdown abolished the beneficial effects offered by urate pretreatment on 6-OHDA-injured cells (Fig. 7. C). The elevation of total glutathione stimulated by urate pretreatment was abolished in Nrf2 siRNA-transfected cells (Fig. 7. D).

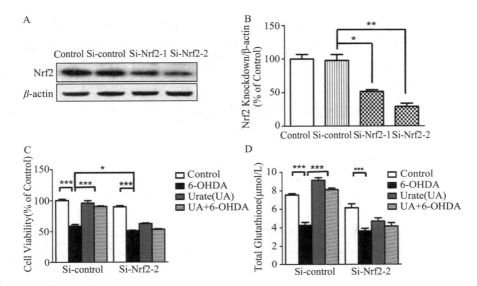

Fig.7 Nrf2-siRNA eliminated the protective effects of urate. A and B, SH-SY5Y cells were transfected with scrambled siRNA (si-control) or two different siRNAs targeting human Nrf2 (si-Nrf2-1 and si-Nrf2-2). RNA interference efficiency was determined by immunoblotting at 24 h later. Mean±SEM, $N = 3$. $^*P < 0.05$, $^{**}P < 0.01$ versus control group. C and D, cells were exposed to 6-OHDA (50 μmol/L) for 14 h, with or without urate pretreatment at 24 h after transfection. Cell viability (C) and intracellular glutathione level (D) were measured as described above. Results were presented as mean± SEM, $N=3$. $^*P<0.05$, $^{**}P<0.01$, $^{***}P<0.001$.

3. Discussion

Urate has been proposed as a neuroprotectant candidate for PD. However, the mechanisms that underlie urate's neuroprotection remains poorly understood. In this study, we showed that urate pretreatment protected dopaminergic cells against 6-OHDA-and H_2O_2-induced damage. This protection and its elevation on intracellular glutathione level was markedly abated by knockdown of Nrf2 with siRNA. We also demonstrated that urate could be accumulated into SH-SY5Y cells and exerted the protective effect intracellularly. Furthermore, we provided the evidence that urate induced Nrf2 accumulation by inhibiting its ubiquitination and degradation, and promoted Nrf2 translocation into nuclei, where it transactivated the transcription and translation of Nrf2 target genes including γ-GCLC and ho-1 (summarized in Fig.8). However, urate did not modulate Nrf2 mRNA and Keap1 protein levels, nor did it disrupt Nrf2-Keap1 association. Therefore, our findings demonstrated for the first time that Nrf2 signaling may contribute to the protection of urate on dopaminergic cells.

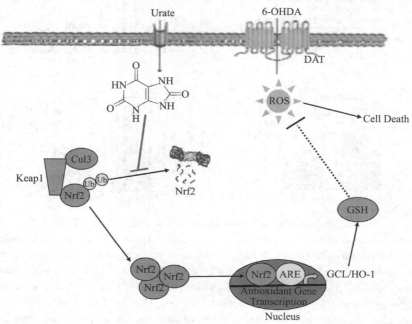

Fig. 8   Schematic representations illustrating how urate may activate Nrf2 and thus protects against oxidative stresses. Urate may be accumulated into cells via undefined transporters. It led to Nrf2 accumulation by inhibiting its ubiquitination and degradation and promoted Nrf2 translocate into nuclei, where Nrf2 may transactivate the transcription of antioxidant enzyme genes such as GCL, HO-1, and thus protected against oxidative stresses in dopaminergic cells.

Urate exists at relatively lower concentrations in the brainand are inversely related to the risk of PD. The urate levels were found to be decreased in the brains of PD patients[①]. All these indicate a beneficial effect of urate on dopaminergic neuron and PD progression. However, it remained unclear whether or not urate could be accumulated into dopaminergic neurons. Our results showed the accumulation of urate into SH-SY5Y cells. This is in line with a previous

---

①   CHURCH WH, WARD VL. Uric Acid is Reduced in the Substantia Nigrain Parkinson's Disease: Effect on Dopamine Oxidation[J]. *Brain Res Bull*, 1994, 33(04): 419-425.

report by Cipriani *et al.*①. But, Guerreiro S *et al.* claimed that urate could not be significantly accumulated into mesencephalic neuron②. This discrepancy may be explained by the difference in sensitivity of the analytic methods applied. The fluorescence-based assay with urate was used in this study. This may be more sensitive than the spectrophotometric assay. Urate may be transported into dopaminergic cells via some kind(s) of unidentified transporters. Notably, urate transporters are highly expressed in kidney and brain③.

Moreover, we demonstrated a direct protection offered by relatively high concentrations of urate ($\geqslant 200$ μmol/L) against 6-OHDA-induced toxicity on dopaminergic cells. This is consistent with some previous reports. However, there are also studies reporting that pretreatment with urate at 0-100 μmol/L tended but failed to significantly decrease H_2O_2-induced cell death in MES23.5 cells and demonstrating that urate's neuroprotection was astrocyte-dependent④⑤. To substantiate our finding, we also examined if urate protected against H_2O_2-induced damage in both SH-SY5Y and MES23.5 cells. The results consistently showed that urate tended to yield protective effects at lower concentrations (<200 μm), and significantly increased the cell viability in H_2O_2-treated dopaminergic cells at higher levels($\geqslant 200$ μmol/L) (Fig.3). Thus, both direct and indirect neuroprotection of urate may exist; however, relatively higher urate levels may be required for its direct neuroprotection. Stimulation and release of astrocyte-derived neurotrophic factor(s), although still undefined, may considerably amplify the neuroprotection of urate. Nrf2 is a critical transcription factor defending against oxidative stress. It controls and initiates the transcription

① CIPRIANI S, DESJARDINS CA, BURDETT TC, et al. Protection of Dopaminergic Cells by Urate Requires its Accumulation in Astrocytes[J]. *J Neurochem*, 2012, 123(01): 172-181.

② GUERREIRO S, PONCEAU A, TOULORGE D, et al. Protection of Midbrain Dopaminergic Neurons by the End-product of Purine Metabolism Uric Acid: Potentiation by Low-level Depolarization[J]. *J Neurochem*, 2009, 109(04): 1118-1128.

③ SPECTOR R, JOHANSON C. Micronutrient and Urate Transport in Choroid plexus and Kidney: Implications for Drug Therapy[J]. *Pharm Res*, 2006, 23(11): 2515-2524.

④ CIPRIANI S, DESJARDINS CA, BURDETT TC, et al. Protection of Dopaminergic Cells by Urate Requires its Accumulation in Astrocytes[J]. *J Neurochem*, 2012, 123(01): 172-181.

⑤ DU Y, CHEN CP, TSENG CY, et al. Astrogliamediated Effects of Uric Acid to Protect Spinal Cord Neurons from Glutamate Toxicity[J]. *Glia*, 2007, 55(05): 463-472.

of several oxidation-related genes such as γ-GCLC and HO-1[1]. Our present study showed that urate promoted Nrf2 accumulation and nuclear translocation by inhibiting its ubiquitination and degradation. It also enhanced the transcription and protein expression of Nrf2 target genes including γ-GCLC and HO-1, both of which are closely related to redox homeostasis. Furthermore, Nrf2 knockdown was observed to abolish the protection offered by urate and its stimulation on glutathione. All these evidence supports a critical role of Nrf2 signaling in urate's neuroprotection. Our previous results showed that in 6-OHDA-lesioned rat model of PD, urate's neuroprotection was linked with Akt/GSK3β signaling pathway. Many studies showed that PI3K/Akt signaling pathway was associated with Nrf2 activation and glutathione synthesis[2]. Therefore, it is likely that the Nrf2 activation was secondary to the action of urate on Akt/GSK3β signaling.

Nrf2 is primarily controlled at protein level due to the presence of two degradation domains (degrons) within its Neh2 and Neh6 regions[3]. The Neh2 domain contains a redox-sensitive degron that interacts with the redox sensor Keap1 to allow ubiquitination and subsequent degradation of Nrf2 by a Cullin3-Rbx1 complex under unstressed conditions[4][5]. Our results showed urate increased the Nrf2 protein levels; however, it did not affect Nrf2 gene transcription and Keap1 protein expression, implying urate may enhance Nrf2 stability at protein level. It has been widely accepted that chemical activation of Nrf2 results from Nrf2 dissociation from Keap1, thereby allowing Nrf2 to escape from Keap1-mediated proteasomal degradation. However, we found urate

① YU J, ZHAO Y, LI B, et al. 17β-estradiol Regulates the Expression of Antioxidant Enzymes in Myocardial Cells by Increasing Nrf2 Translocation[J]. *J Biochem Mol Toxicol*, 2012, 26(07): 264-269.

② GUNJIMA K, TOMIYAMA R, TAKAKURA K, et al. 3, 4-dihydroxybenzalacetone Protects against Parkinson's Disease-related Neurotoxin 6-OHDA through Akt/Nrf2/glutathione Pathway[J]. *J Cell Biochem*, 2014, 115(01): 151-160.

③ TOBÓN-VELASCO JC, VAZQUEZ-VICTORIO G, MACÍAS-SILVA M, et al. S-allyl Cysteine Protects against 6-hydroxydopamine-induced Neurotoxicity in the Rat Striatum: Involvement of Nrf2 Transcription Factor Activation and Modulation of Signaling Kinase Cascades[J]. *Free Radic Biol Med*, 2012, 53(05): 1024-1040.

④ FURUKAWA M, XIONG Y. BTB Protein Keap1 Targets Antioxidant Transcription Factor Nrf2 for Ubiquitination by the Cullin 3-Roc1 ligase[J]. *Mol Cell Biol*, 2005, 25(01): 162-171.

⑤ ZHANG DD, LO SC, CROSS JV, et al. Keap1 is a Redox-regulated Substrate Adaptor Protein for a Cul3-dependent Ubiquitinligase Complex[J]. *Mol Cell Biol*, 2004, 24(24): 10941-10953.

inhibited Nrf2 ubiquitination without disrupting Nrf2-Keap1 association. This is consistent with a recent study reporting the mechanisms by which 5, 6-dihydrocyclopenta-1, 2-dithiole-3-thione (CPDT) and sulforaphane activated Nrf2[①]. It is possible that urate induced conformational change of Keap1 and thus rendered Keap1-bound Nrf2 unreachable by the ubiquitin ligase. We will assess this possibility in our future study.

Glutathione is a major intracellular antioxidant. Depletion of glutathione pools is involved in PD development. Our results showed that urate enhanced the transcription and expression of the rate-limiting enzymes for glutathione biosynthesis and elevated the intracellular glutathione content in 6-OHDA-treated SH-SY5Y cells. Nrf2 knockdown attenuated urate's protection and its effect on glutathione, implying Nrf2 activation was involved in the increase of glutathione stimulated by urate. However, it should be noted that other mechanisms that contributed to the glutathione elevation may also exist. For example, urate was reported to promote cysteine uptake and enhance glutathione levels in SH-SY5Y cells and hippocampus slice cultures[②].

Interestingly, in this study 6-OHDA treatment did not elicit an obvious anti-oxidant response in cells. We examined the Nrf2 distribution at both 6 h and 14 h after 6-OHDA exposure with immunofluorescent staining and immunoblotting. We did not observed a marked nuclear translocation of Nrf2 in 6-OHDA treated cells. The intracellular glutathione level was also reduced. The occurrence of anti-oxidant response may be dependent upon the severity of cell injury. A previous study showed that 6-OHDA injection into rat striatum enhanced nuclear Nrf2 translocation, which occurred at earlier time points (0.5 h and 1 h) after lesion and gradually returning to the basal level at 4 h later[③]. This indicates a compensatory anti-oxidant response to the toxic insult may be induced but only

① LI Y, PAONESSA JD, ZHANG Y. Mechanism of Chemical Activation of Nrf2[J]. *PLoS One*, 2012, 7 (04): e35122.

② AOYAMA K, MATSUMURA N, WATABE M, et al. Caffeine and Uric Acid Mediate Glutathione Synthesis for Neuroprotection[J]. *Neuroscience*, 2011, 181: 206-215.

③ TOBÓN-VELASCO JC, LIMÓN-PACHECO JH, OROZCO-IBARRA M, et al. 6-OHDA-induced Apoptosis and Mitochondrial Dysfunction are Mediated by Early Modulation of Intracellular Signals and Interaction of Nrf2 and NF-kB Factors[J]. *Toxicology*, 2013, 304: 109-119.

detected at early time period. Long-term exposure to toxic insult may inhibit the compensatory/resistance responses. Of note, 6-OHDA increased the mRNA level of γ-GCLM, which is a modifier subunit of γ-GCL. In most cases, the catalytic subunit accounts for the activity of an enzyme. Therefore, the increase of γ-GCLM mRNA probably occurs in compensation for the γ-GCLC reduction. Despite of this, urate treatment differentially regulated the transcription of these two subunits of γ-GCL protein in 6-OHDA-treated cells. It is likely that the increase of γ-GCLC protein is sufficient for glutathione synthesis elevation since it is one of the most readily induced anti-oxidant genes and ratelimiting for its synthesis.

In fact, the antioxidant activity of urate is complex. It possesses antioxidant properties comparable to those of ascorbate and provides most of the antioxidant capacity in human fluid[1][2]. In this study, we found urate not only alleviated 6-OHDA-induced toxicity, but also protected against H_2O_2-induced toxicity. Therefore, it is more likely a general antioxidant reagent. Although it acts as a powerful scavenger of peroxynitrite, peroxide and hypochlorous acid, urate does not react with some oxidants such as superoxide. It also shows iron-chelating activity independent of its direct antioxidant actions. Notably, urate acts as a pro-oxidant in some circumstances[3][4]; however, this possibility is excluded in this study, as urate treatment did not increase protein carbonyls in SH-SY5Y cells.

In sum, this study demonstrated that urate activated Nrf2 by inhibiting its ubiquitination and degradation, and thus protected against oxidative insults to dopaminergic cells.

① YEUM KJ, RUSSELL RM, KRINSKY NI, et al. Biomarkers of Antioxidant Capacity in the Hydrophilic and Lipophilic Compartments of Human Plasma[J]. *Arch Biochem Biophys*, 2004, 430(01): 97-103.

② PROCTOR P. Similar Functions of Uric Acid and Ascorbate in Man? [J]. *Nature*, 1970, 228(5274): 868.

③ SAUTIN YY, JOHNSON RJ. Uric Acid: the Oxidant-antioxidant Paradox[J]. *Nucleosides Nucleotides Nucleic Acids*, 2008, 27: 608-619.

④ DIMITROULA HV, HATZITOLIOS AI, KARVOUNIS HI. The Role of Uric Acid in Stroke: the Issue Remains Unresolved[J]. *Neurologist*, 2008, 14(04): 238-242.

4. Supporting Information

Urate induced Nrf2 protein accumulation and its translocation from cytoplasm to nucleus in SH-SY5Y cells (14 h) and MES23.5 cells (6 h). Cells were preincubated with 200 μmol/L urate for 30 mins prior to 50 μmol/L 6-OHDA treatment for 6 h (MES23.5 cell) or 14 h (SH-SY5Y cells). (a, c) Representative images showing the subcellular distribution of Nrf2 (FITC/green) in MES23.5 cells (a) and SH-SY5Y cells (c). Nuclei were stained with DAPI (blue). Scale bar = 20 μm. (b, d) Immunoblotting analysis of Nrf2 in nuclear and cytoplasmic fractions of cells subjected to abovementioned treatments. H3 and β-actin were used for nuclear and cytoplasmic protein markers respectively.

5. Acknowledgments

We thank Dr. Rachit Bakshi (Harvard Medical School) for the improvement in English writing of our manuscript. We thank Ms Wang Fen and Wang Zheng for technical assistance in immunofluorescent study.

6. Author Contributions

Conceived and designed the experiments: CFL WFL LFH. Performed the experiments: NZ TTH QLZ XYP. Analyzed the data: NZ TTH HYS. Contributed reagents/materials/analysis tools: GQZ DL. Wrote the paper: NZ LFH.

(Ning Zhang, Hai-Yang Shu, Tingting Huang, Qi-Lin Zhang, Da Li, Guan-Qun Zhang, Xiao-Yan Peng, Chun-Feng Liu, Wei-Feng Luo, Li-Fang Hu)

(本文原载于 *Nrf2 Signaling Mediates Urate's Protection* 2014 年第 9 卷第 6 期)

Urate Promotes SNCA/α-synuclein Clearance via Regulating mTOR-dependent Macroautophagy

Abstract：Serum urate levels are reported to be significantly lowered in patients with Parkinson's disease and inversely correlated to the risk and progression of PD. However, the mechanism by which urate affects PD is poorly understood. Here we showed that treatment with uric acid resulted in an autophagy activity enhancement in PC12 cells in dose-and time-dependent manners, as indicated by LC3-Ⅱ increase and P62 decrease. Moreover, UA was still able to increase the LC3-Ⅱ level and the number of LC3 puncta in the presence of Bafilomycin A1, a lysosomal inhibitor. These changes of autophagic markers were preceded by mTOR inhibition and ULK1 activation. Co-treatment with 3-benzyl-5-(2-nitrophenoxy methyl)-dihydrofuran-2(3H)-one(3BDO), an mTOR activator, abolished the UA-induced LC3-Ⅱ increase. More importantly, UA reduced SNCA/α-synuclein accumulation in PC12 cells that overexpress wildtype or A53T mutant SNCA, and this was blocked by Bafilomycin A1 co-treatment. The *in vivo* study showed that UA administration was able to modulate the levels of autophagy markers, increase the autophagosome/autolysosome formation, and reduce SNCA accumulation in the midbrain of $SNCA^{A53T}$ transgenic mice. Taken together, our findings suggest that UA could induce autophagy activation via an mTOR-dependent signaling and ameliorate SNCA accumulation. This implicates that urate-elevating agent may become a potential strategy for PD therapy.

Keywords：urate; macroautophagy; mTOR; SNCA/α-synuclein; Parkinson's disease.

1. Introduction

Parkinson's disease is an age-related neurodegenerative disorder, probably caused by complicated interactions between genetic and environmental factors.

The exact pathogenesis of PD remains elusive. Pathologically, it is featured by the progressive loss of dopaminergic neurons in the substantia nigra (SN) pars compacta and appearance of SNCA/α-synuclein-containing Lewy bodies and neurites. SNCA is a key pathogenic protein in PD, although its physiological function is yet to be determined. The multiplication or point mutations in *SNCA* gene is linked to familial PD. Additionally, the polymorphisms in *SNCA* gene are major risk factors for sporadic PD. In recent years, SNCA aggregates are found to spread via prion-like mechanisms through neural networks, and the spreading increases with age. Therefore, promoting the clearance of misfolded or aggregated SNCA is proposed to be a potential approach that may halt or delay the progression of PD.

Autophagy-lysosome pathway is a catabolic process that recruits dysfunctional organelles and protein aggregates into autophagosomes and delivers them to lysosomes for degradation and recycling. Mutant SNCA and its aggregates are degraded via macroautophagy (referred to as autophagy thereafter). Autophagy impairment results in SNCA accumulation. Aberrant alterations in autophagy-related proteins, accompanied with SNCA aggregation, were observed in the patients with PD. Conditional knockout of autophagy-related gene leads to protein aggregates formation and progressive losses of dopaminergic neurons in the SN. Compelling evidence suggests that autophagy impairment contributes to PD pathogenesis. However, the factors that impede autophagy induction or autophagy flux are poorly understood.

Urate, the anionic form of uric acid (UA), is the end product of purine metabolism due to the *urate oxidase gene* mutation during evolution. It is a potent antioxidant and acts as the scavenger of superoxide, peroxynitrite and other free radicals. Serum urate levels were reported to be lower in patients with PD compared to healthy controls, and inversely related to the risk and progression of PD. We previously reported that intraperitoneal administration with UA exerted neuroprotection to midbrain dopaminergic neurons and alleviated the motor deficits in 6-hy-droxydopamine-lesioned rats. However, whether or not UA affects SNCA aggregation is unknown. Therefore, in this study we aimed to explore the effect of UA on SNCA aggregation and the underlying mechanism. Our findings demonstrate that treatment with UA promoted the clearance of SNCA by enhancing an mTOR-dependent autophagy activity.

2. Materials and Methods

（1）Reagents and Antibodies

Uric acid（UA，U2625），rotenone and cycloheximide（CHX）were purchased from Sigma-Aldrich（St Louis，MO，USA）.UA was dissolved in sterile water,pH-adjusted to 7.4 with sodium hydroxide.Bafilomycin A1（BafA1）was purchased from Abcam（New Territories，Hong Kong，China）.3BDO was gifted by Prof. JunYing Miao from Shandong University.

（2）Cell Lines and Cell Culture

Rat pheochromocytoma PC12 cells were purchased from Institute of Cell Biology（Chinese Academy of Sciences，Shanghai，China）.To establish SNCA over expressing cells，PC12 cells were infected with the lentivirus（titer：2×10^8 TU/mL,Genechem Shanghai，China）expressing wildtype or A53T mutant SNCA at a multiplicity of infection（MOI）of 15.Cells were cultured in RPMI1640 medium，supplemented with 10% fetal bovine serum and 1% penicillin/streptomycin in an incubator at 37 ℃.

（3）Western Blotting

Cells or tissues were lysed in chilled RIPA buffer（150 μm NaCl,25 μm Tris,5 μm EDTA,1% Nonidet P-40,pH 7.5）with protease inhibitor cocktail （Roche Diagnostics, Penzberg, Germany）. And phosphatase inhibitor cocktail tablets were additionally added into RIPA for phosphorylation analysis. The lysates were cleared by centrifugation at 13 200 rpm for 30 mins at 4 ℃.Protein samples were denatured,separated on 8% ~ 13.5% SDS-PAGE gels,and then transferred onto PVDF membranes（Millipore，Bedford，MA，USA）. Next, membranes were blocked with Tris buffered saline/Tween 20（TBST：10 μm Tris,150 μm NaCl,0.1% Tween 20,pH 7.4 ~ 7.6）containing 5% non-fat dry milk（w/v）for 1 h at room temperature,followed by incubation with the primary antibodies：LC3（1 ：4 000，Novus，NB100 − 2220），P62 （1 ：5 000，Sigma, P0067），SNCA（1 ：500，Abcam，ab1903），p-mTOR（S2448）（1 ：1 000，Cell Signaling Technology［CST］，5536S），mTOR（1 ：1 000，CST，2983S），p-

P70S6K（1∶1 000,CST,9208）,P70S6K（1∶800,CST,2708）,p-ULK1（S757; 1∶1 000,CST,6888）,p-ULK1（S555;1∶1 000,Chemicon,2,449,230）,ULK1 （1∶500,CST,4773）,Beclin 1（1∶500,Santa Cruz Biotechnology,sc11427）, ACTB/β-actin（1∶5 000, Sigma, A3854）and TUBB/β-tubulin（1∶5 000, Sigma,T0198）at 4 ℃ overnight. After that,membranes were rinsed with TBST three times and incubated with goat anti-mouse IgG（H+L）（1∶5 000,Jackson, 115-035-003）or goat anti-rabbit IgG（H+L）（1∶5 000,Jackson,111−035−003） for 1 h at 37 ℃. The protein bands were visualized by BioRad imaging system and analyzed using ImageJ software（National Institute of Health,USA）as previously reported（Wang et al.,2015）.

（4）Quantitative PCR

Total RNA was extracted using Trizol reagent（Life technologies,15596− 018）and reverse transcribed into cDNA using a cDNA synthesis kit（Thermo Scientific,K1622）. An equal volume of cDNA product was amplified using SYBR1 green PCR Master Mix（Invitrogen,Carlsbad,CA,USA）on the ABI 7500 system（Applied Biosystems, Foster City, CA, USA）. The primers used were: p62,5'-CAG GCG CAC TACCGC GAT GA-3'（forward）,5'-TCG CAC ACG CTG CAC AGG TC-3'（reverse）;SNCA,5'-CTA TGT AGG TTC CAA AAC TAA G-3'（forward）,5'-CCT CCC AAC ATT TGT CAC-3'（reverse）; and 18S, 5'- TCA ACA CGG GAA ACC TCA C-3'（forward）,5'-CGC TCC ACC AAC TAA GAA C-3'（reverse）. All primers were synthesized by Sagon（Shanghai,China）. Relative gene expressions were calculated by normalizing to those of 18S.

（5）Cell Viability Determination

Cell viability assay was performed with MTT（Sigma）. In brief,cells were treated with UA or vehicle at various concentrations for different time periods. After that,10 μL MTT（5 mg/mL）was added into each well and incubated for 4 h. Then the supernatant was discarded,followed by the addition of 100 μL Dimethyl sulfoxide to dissolve the violet crystals. Finally, the absorbance was measured at 490 nm using a microplate reader（Tecan M200,Grodig,Austria）.

（6）mRFP-GFP-LC3 Dots Quantification

The autophagic fiux was also monitored by the tandem RFP-GFP-LC3 fluorescence analysis as previously reported. In brief, cells were infected with

RFP-GFP-LC3 adenovirus (HanBio, Shanghai, China) . 24 h post-infection, cells were treated with 100 μm UA for 12 h or 25 nm BafA1 for 6 h. For co-treatment, BafA1 was added 6 h after UA treatment. After that, cells were fixed with 4% paraformaldehyde (PFA) for 10 mins, briefly washed with PBS, and then mounted with DAPI (Vector Laboratories, Burlingame, CA, USA) . Cells were observed and imaged under a confocal microscope (LSM, Zeiss, Germany) . The number of yellow and red LC3 dots (1.0 ~ 1.5 μm in diameter) per cell was counted using Image JPro software and manually corrected by independent experimenters. At least 40 cells per group were randomly selected for quantification.

（7）Animals and Treatment

Male C57BL/6J mice (8 ~ 10 weeks old) were purchased from the SLRC Laboratory (Shanghai, China) . M83 transgenic (tg) mouse lines expressing human mutant $SNCA^{A53T}$ driven by the mouse prion promoter (PrP) were purchased from Model Animal Research Center of Nanjing University (Nanjing, China) . All animals were housed in a SPF grade animal room (12 h : 12 h light/dark cycles at 70% ± 4% relative humidity) , with food and tap water ad libitum. The procedures were performed in accordance with the guidelines of the Institutional Animal Care and Use Committee of Soochow University.

The *in vivo* study consisted of two parts. In the first part, we conducted a pilot study to optimize the regimen for UA administration. A total of 18 male 8 – 10-week-old C57BL/6J mice (5 ~ 7 mice per group) were used in this part, and subjected to UA or saline treatment for one or two weeks. In the second part, we examined the effect of UA on autophagy activity and SNCA accumulation in $SNCA^{A53T}$ tg mice and the wildtype littermates (4 ~ 7 months old) . For this purpose, the mice were intraperitoneally (i. p.) injected with 250 mg/kg UA (dissolved in saline) or saline once daily for two weeks. At the end of treatment, some mice were processed as below for immunohistochemistry study, and the other were deeply anaesthetized for brain tissues harvest. Briefly, the striatum and the cortical tissue from the same coronal sections as the striatum were dissected using the mouse brain slicer matrix. The tissues were then lysed in RIPA buffer by sonication using the ultrasonic cell crusher (JY92- II DN, Ningbo, Zhejiang Province, China) and subjected to western blotting.

（8）Immunohistochemistry

Mice were anaesthetized by sodium pentobarbital and fixed with 4% paraformaldehyde（PFA）via transcardial perfusion. Brains were immediately dissected, post-fixed in 4% PFA overnight at 4 ℃, and sequentially dehydrated in a serial of 70%, 85%, 95%, and 100% alcohol solution. Next, brains were transparentized in dimethylbenzene and embedded in paraffin. Coronal sections （4 μm thick）that contain SN were cut, deparaffinized and rehydrated. For epitope retrieval, sections was boiled in citrate buffer（10 μm sodium citrate, 0.05% Tween 20, pH 6.0）in pre-warmed pressure cooker for 15 mins and cooled at room temperature for 20 mins. For immunostaining, sections were briefly washed in 0.01 M PBS and subjected to 3% H_2O_2 to block endogenous peroxidase for 15 mins. Next, non-specific bindings were blocked with 5% BSA for 15 mins, followed by incubation with the primary antibodies as follows: mouse monoclonal anti-tyrosine hydroxylase（TH, 1 : 1 000, Sigma, St.Louis, USA）, and rabbit polyclonal antiP62（1 : 200, Sigma, P0067）at 37 ℃ for 3 h.Subsequently, sections were washed in PBS and then incubated with AlexaFluor 488-and 555-conjugated secondary antibodies（Molecular Probes, 1 : 1 000）at 37 ℃ for 1 h. At last, sections were counterstained by DAPI and photographed using the microscope（Carl Zeiss, 37081, Germany）. And P62 intensity in TH positive neurons were measured by ImageJ software.

（9）Transmission Electron Microscopy

The striatum tissues were fixed in 4% glutaraldehyde phosphate buffer for 4~6 h, washed in phosphate buffer（0.1 m, pH 7.4）three times, and then post-fixed in 1% osmium tetroxide buffer for 1 h. After being washed in phosphate buffer twice, tissues were dehydrated in a gradient series of acetone（50%, 70%, 90%, and 100%）for 15 mins per step. Next, tissues were incubated in a mixture of resin and propylene oxide（1 : 1）for 2 h, and then embedded in 100% resin overnight. Next, ultrastructural sections （90 nm thick）were cut using ultramicrotomy and stained with 2% uranyl acetate and 0.3% lead citrate.Images were taken under a transmission electron microscope（JEM 1230, JOEL, Tokyo, Japan）.

（10）Statistical Analysis

All data were presented as mean ± SEM of at least three independent experiments. For western blot and quantitative PCR results, relative quantities (fold changes) were obtained after normalization to the expression of the housekeeping gene, and the values in control(untreated)group was normalized to 1. Statistical significance of differences were assessed by unpaired Student t-test for two group comparison or one-way analysis of variance(ANOVA)followed by Dunnett's or Tukey post hoc analysis when appropriate for multiple group comparisons using GraphPad Prism 5.0 software. Differences were considered significant when P value<0.05.

3. Results

（1）UA Induces Autophagy Activation in a Dose and Time-dependent Manner

Two autophagy-related markers LC3-Ⅱ and P62 protein levels were examined by western blotting in PC12 cells following UA or vehicle treatment. In response to 50 and 100 μm UA treatment for 12 h, the LC3-Ⅱ level increased (Fig.1.A), which was detected early at 3 h, and persisted till 24 h after 100 μm UA treatment(Fig.1.B). However, the autophagy substrate P62 levels remained almost unaltered within 24 h but reduced at 36 h and 48 h after UA treatment (Fig.1.B – Fig.1.C). And P62 mRNA level remained unchanged till 36 h after treatment(Fig.1.D). Of note, treatment with UA at the concentrations <200 μm for 12 h (Fig.1.E)or 100 μm UA for 48 h(Fig.1.F)did not significantly affect the cell viability of PC12 cells. This excludes the non-specific impact of UA on autophagy that may relate to cell damage or death.

To clarify if the UA-induced LC3-Ⅱ elevation was resulting from autophagosome formation increase or degradation impairment, we examined the change of LC3-Ⅱ level in the presence of bafilomycin A1(BafA1, 25 nm), a lysosomal inhibitor. Western blot analysis showed that treatment with UA was still able to enhance the LC3-Ⅱ level in BafA1 co-treated cells, implying that the UA-induced LC3-Ⅱ elevation mainly came from autophagy induction rather than lysosomal degradation impairment(Fig.2.A). This was confirmed by the tandem fluorescent RFP-GFP-LC3 assay, which is a valuable tool in studying autolysosome maturation and formation. This assay relies on the different sensitivity of RFP and GFP to the acidic environment. GFP is much more susceptible to lysosomal quenching than RFP in the acidic lysosome lumen. Thus, most of the puncta exhibit both red and green signals and appear as yellow dots if autophagosome fusion with lysosome or lysosome function is impaired. Conversely, it yields red-only puncta if autophagy flux proceeds normally. As shown in Fig.2.B and Fig.2.C, treatment with 100 μm UA for 12 h resulted in obvious increases of yellow and red dots, with more red-only dots formation in the cytoplasm compared to untreated cells. The lysosomal inhibitor BafA1 caused a dramatic increase of yellow dots in the perinuclear compartment. UA co-treatment further enhanced the number of yellow dots in BafA1-treated cells, indicating that UA can induce autophagy activation.

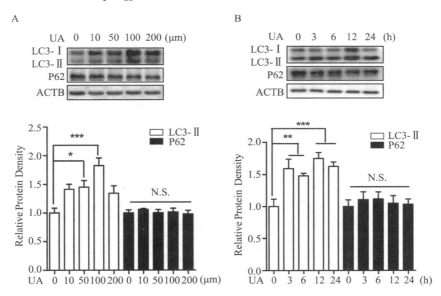

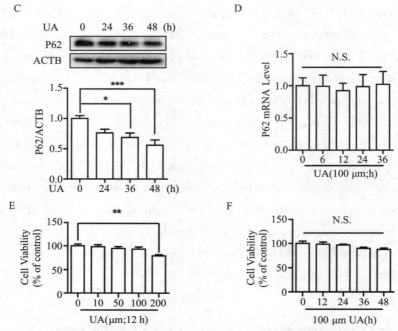

Fig.1　Dose and time-dependent effects of UA on autophagy-related proteins（LC3-Ⅱ and P62）levels in PC12 cells. A－C, dose-and time-dependent effects of UA on LC3-Ⅱ and P62 levels.Treatment with UA for a short period（＜24 h）had little effect on P62 level（$N=5\sim6$）, but did reduce P62 protein level after a prolonged（36 h and 48 h）treatment（C, $N=5$）. Actin/ACTB served as loading controls. D, UA did not affect P62 transcription.Relative values were obtained after calibration to 18S levels, and the values in control group were normalized to 1, $N=3$.E and F, at the concentrations no more than 100 μm UA had little impact on cell survival for up to 48 h treatment（$N=4$）. Cell viability was expressed as the percentage of control group. $^*P＜0.05$, $^{**}P＜0.01$, $^{***}P＜0.001$.One way ANOVA followed by Dunnett's analysis.N.S., not significant.

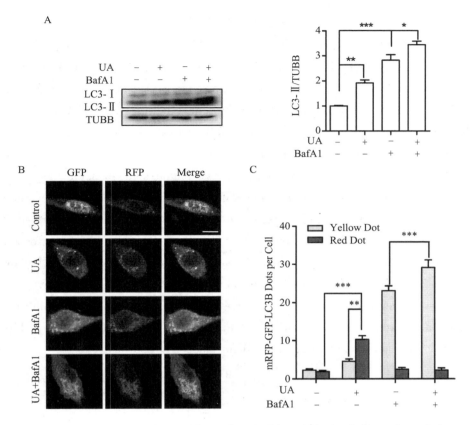

Fig.2　Effect of UA on the autophagic flux. A, UA cotreatment further enhanced the endogenous LC3-Ⅱ level compared to BafA1 alone group. PC12 cells were treated with 100 μm UA for 12 h, and 25 nm BafA1 was added 6 h before the end of UA treatment. $N = 6$. B and C, cells were infected with 3 μL RFP-GFP-LC3 adenovirus (titer: 1×10^{10} PFU/mL). 24 h after transduction, cells were treated as in A, and then fixed with 4% PFA followed by the confocal microscopy study. B, scale bar, 10 μm. The number of yellow and red LC3 dots (1.0 ~ 1.5 μm in diameter) per cell was quantified and shown in C. At least 40 cells per group were counted. One way ANOVA followed by Tukey analysis. $^*P < 0.05$, $^{**}P < 0.01$, $^{***}P < 0.001$. (For interpretation of the references to colour in this figure legend, the reader is referred to the web version of this article.)

(2) UA Activates Autophagy in an mTOR-dependent Manner

Next, we explored the molecular mechanism(s) involved. First, we studied the mTOR signaling, which is a major negative regulator of autophagy. As shown in Fig.3.A – Fig.3.C, treatment with 100 μm UA rapidly decreased the phosphorylation of mTOR, which was detected early at 0.25 h after treatment.

Accordingly, the phosphorylation of mTOR substrate P70S6K (ribosomal protein S6 kinase, 70 kDa, polypeptide 1) also declined. This process was accompanied by the dephosphorylation of ULK1 (unc-51 like autophagy activating kinase 1) S757 and increased phosphorylation of ULK1 S555 (Fig. 3. D - Fig. 3. F). These data indicate that inhibition of mTOR signaling may be involved in UA-induced autophagy activation. We then used the mTOR activator to verify this molecular event. 3BDO is a recently reported mTOR activator. It forms hydrogen bonds with TYR82A and ILE56A sites in FKBP1A, two amino acid sites for rapamycin binding, and thus serves as an antagonist of rapamycin. It has been demonstrated to inhibit autophagy in HUVECs. Here we observed that pretreatment with 3BDO abolished the LC3-II increase induced by UA (Fig. 3. G), indicating requirement of mTOR inhibition in UA-induced autophagy activation. Additionally, we examined if Beclin-1, an mTOR independent autop hagy regulator, was involved. The result showed that the Beclin-1 expression almost did not change following 100 μm UA treatment for up to 24 h (Fig. 3. H). Therefore, Beclin-1 was less likely to mediate the autophagy activation induced by UA.

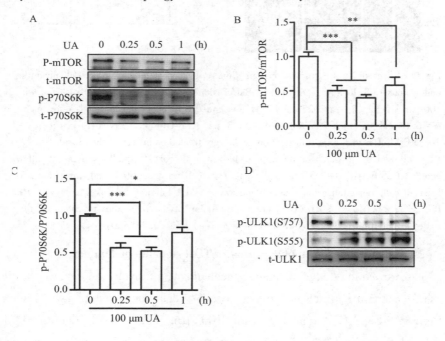

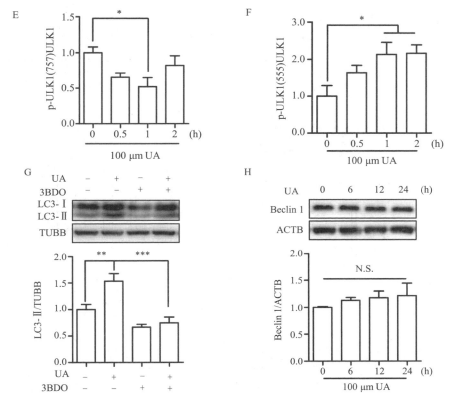

Fig.3 mTOR inhibition is required for UA-induced autophagy activation. A − F, PC12 cells were treated with 100 μm UA for different time periods. Phosphorylation of mTOR, P70S6K and ULK1 were detected with the antibodies against p-mTOR (S2488, B), p-P70S6K (C), p-ULK1 (S757, E) and p-ULK1 (S555, F) by western blotting, and normalized to the corresponding total levels of these kinase, $N = 4 \sim 6$. G, co-treatment with 60 μm 3BDO, an mTOR activator, abolished the elevation of LC3-Ⅱ level induced by UA. $N = 7$. H, UA treatment showed no significant impact on Beclin-1 protein levels ($N = 3$). One way ANOVA followed by Dunnett's (B − F, H) or Tukey (G) analysis. $^{*}P < 0.05$, $^{**}P < 0.01$, $^{***}P < 0.001$.

（3）UA Promotes SNCA Degradation in SNCA Overex-pressing Cells

Then we continued to study if UA affected SNCA degradation since it enhanced the autophagy activity. We performed an *in vitro* study in PC12 cells overexpressing wildtype SNCA (SNCA^{WT} PC12 cells). Cells were treated with 50 nm rotenone for 24 h to mimic the interaction between genetic and environmental factors. The SNCA protein level was found to be increased in rotenone-treated SNCA^{WT} PC12 cells (Fig.4.A). Treatment with UA reduced the SNCA protein but not mRNA (Fig. 4. B) level in both rotenone-treated and untreated cells, implying a post-transcriptional mechanism may be involved. We

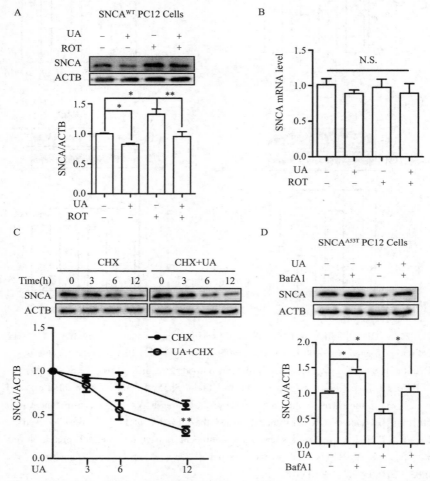

Fig.4 UA reduces SNCA accumulation *in vitro*. A, 100 μm UA treatment decreased the SNCA level in rotenone (ROT, 50 nm for 24 h)-treated and-untreated PC12 cells that overexpress wildtype SNCA. $N = 3$. But SNCA mRNA levels are not affected by the treatments (B, $N = 4$). C, CHX chase assay showed that UA accelerated the decline of SNCA protein level in the presence of CHX (1 μg/mL). Student *t*-test, $N = 5$. D, UA-induced reduction of SNCA level was blocked by BafA1 (25 nm) co-treatment. PC12 cells stably over expressing A53T mutant SNCA were treated with UA for 24 h, and 25 nm BafA1 was added 6 h before the end of UA treatment. $N = 4$. One way ANOVA followed by Tukey analysis except for panel (C). $^{*}P<0.05$, $^{**}P<0.01$.

then examined the SNCA half-life using the cycloheximide (CHX, a protein translation inhibitor) chase assay. Here, SNCA^{WT} PC12 cells were treated with or without 100 μm UA for 0, 3, 6 and 12 h in the presence of CHX (1 μg/mL), which blocked the de novo protein synthesis. Whole cell lysates were then harvested and subjected to western blotting. The results showed that the SNCA levels in UA-treated group at 6 h and 12 h were significantly lower than those in UA-untreated cells (Fig. 4. C), indicating that UA promoted the SNCA degradation and shortened its half-life.

The effect of UA on the degradation of mutant SNCA was also examined. We infected PC12 cells with A53T MUTANT SNCA using lentiviral vector (designated as SNCA^{A53T} PC12 cells) as we previously reported. It was observed that UA treatment reduced the SNCA^{A53T} levels compared to controls, and this effect was abolished by BafA1 (25 nm) co-treatment (Fig.4.D).

(4) UA Enhances Autophagy and Reduces SNCA Accumu lation in SNCA^{A53T} Transgenic Mice

Last, we tested the effect of UA on autophagy activity and SNCA degradation *in vivo*. In a pilot study, a group of male C57BL/6 mice were intraperitoneally injected with 250 mg/kg UA once daily for 7 or 14 days. Control group received saline treatment. As shown in Fig.5.A – Fig.5.B, UA administration for 14 days was sufficient to enhance the LC3-Ⅱ level (Fig.5.C); however, it had no obvious effect on P62 level (Fig.5.D) in the striatum. Similar observations were found in the cortex. This indicates that UA produces a region non-specific regulation on autophagy activity in the brains of normal mice and that LC3-Ⅱ is sensitive to UA-induced change in autophagy.

Based on these observations, we examined the effect of UA on autophagy and SNCA accumulation in a SNCA^{A53T} transgenic mouse model. SNCA^{A53T} tg mice and non-tg littermates were injected with 250 mg/kg UA or saline once daily for 14 days. The striatal tissues were then harvested for western blotting. As can be seen from Fig.6.A – Fig.6.D, there was an obvious accumulation of P62 and SNCA protein in SNCA^{A53T} tg mice compared to non-tg counterparts. Administration with UA at this regimen was able to alleviate the accumulation of P62 and SNCA proteins in the tg mice although it merely had a mild effect on LC3-Ⅱ level. The

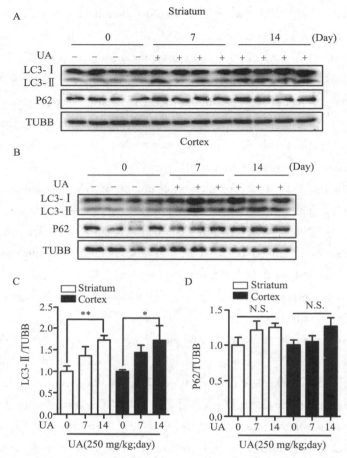

Fig.5 UA administration upregulated LC3-II levels in the brain.Adult male C57BL/6J mice were injected with 250 mg/kg(i.p.) UA or saline once daily for 7 or 14 days.The striatal and cortical lysates were subjected to western blotting.UA increased the LC3-II level in both the striatum(hollow column) and the cortex(black column) at 14 days,with a mild increase of LC3-II at 7 days after treatment.P62 protein levels in these two regions were not affected.TUBB/β-tubulin served as loading controls.$N = 5 \sim 7$ mice per group. One way ANOVA followed by Dunnett's analysis. $^{*}P<0.05$, $^{**}P<0.01$.

immunofluorescence study (Fig. 6. E) confirmed that P62 fluorescence intensity were enhanced in TH positive neurons in the SN of tg mice compare to non-tg mice. Moreover, P62 fluorescence was dispersely distributed without any aggregates formation in TH positive neurons.UA administration mitigated the P62 fluorescence intensity in the transgenic mice(Fig.6.F).Consistent with previous reports, no significant loss of TH⁺neurons was observed in the SN pars compacta of SNCA^{A53T} transgenic mice, no matter UA was given or not (Fig. 6. G). In addition, the transmission electronic micrographs showed that numerous double-membrane structured vacuoles appeared in the striatum of UA-treated transgenic

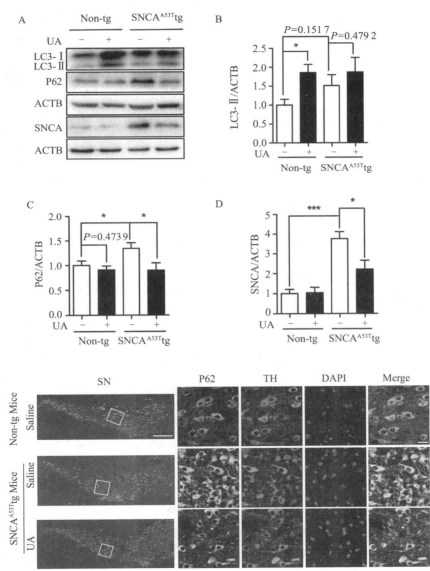

133

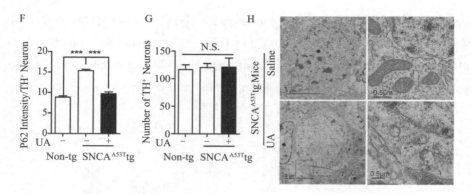

Fig.6　UA administration reduces the accumulation of P62 and SNCA in SNCA^{A53T} transgenic mice.A – D,representative gel images A and group data for striatal LC3-Ⅱ (B),P62(C) and SNCA(D) levels in male SNCA^{A53T} transgenic(tg) mice and non-tg littermates following UA(250 mg/kg,i.p.) or saline treatment once daily for 14 days.$N=$ 5.Student t-test. E,coimmunofiuorescence staining of P62 and TH in the SN of non-tg mice and SNCA^{A53T} transgenic(tg) mice(4~7-month-old) following UA or saline treatment for 14 days. F,P62 fluorescence intensity per TH^{+}neurons.The data presented the mean± SEM of P62 signals in at least 20 randomly selected TH^{+} neurons per slice from three mouse brains,with two brain slices for each mouse.Scale bar at 100 μm(overview image, left) and 10 μm(enlarged images,right). G,the number of SN TH^{+}neurons were counted by the experimenters blind to the treatments.A total of six brain slices from three mice was counted per group. One way ANOVA followed by Tukey analysis. * $P < 0.05$, ** $P <$ 0.01, *** $P < 0.001$; N. S., not significant. H, representative transmission electronic micrographs showing the autophagic vacuoles(red arrows pointed) in the striatum of saline-and UA-treated SNCA^{A53T} tg mice at 14 days. In responses to UA injection, numerous double-membrane structured vacuoles appeared in the striatum, and such vacuoles were rarely seen in saline group.(For interpretation of the references to colour in this figure legend,the reader is referred to the web version of this article.)

mice,and such vacuoles were rarely seen in saline-treated group(Fig.6.H).This also suggests the autophagy activation by UA *in vivo*,which may result in SNCA degradation.

4. Discussion

In this study we demonstrated for the first time that UA activated autophagy through inhibiting mTOR/ULK1 signaling in dopaminergic cells. More importantly,treatment with UA was able to promote SNCA^{A53T} degradation via the autophagy-lysosome pathway in both cellular and animal models with SNCA^{A53T}

overexpression. This reveals a novel mechanism for UA neuroprotection in PD and other synucleinopathies. Our study may provide the clue for explaining the association between higher serum UA levels and the slower progression of PD.

UA is the end product of purine metabolism in human. It exists in serum with a physiological range at 200 ~ 500 μm. Beyond that range, UA produces detrimental effects. For example, abnormally elevated serum urate is associated with gout, cardiovascular and renal disease. On the contrary, lower serum urate levels were reported in the patients with PD, and have been linked to a higher risk of developing PD. A recent prospective study reveals that urate could slow PD progression in men during the preclinical stage of disease. Previously, we and other groups demonstrate that UA produces neuroprotection against midbrain dopaminergic neuron losses via its antioxidant effect. In addition, Du Y et al. reported that UA protected spinal cord neurons against glutamate toxicity through an astroglia-mediated mechanism. Of note, an urate-elevating agent Inosine (a precursor of urate) is currently under investigation as a potential disease-modifying strategy in individuals with PD. Here, we identify a novel mechanism of UA neuroprotection, demonstrating that UA could promote SNCA clearance via macroautophagy. All these suggest a beneficial role of UA, if appropriately elevated, in PD.

Aberrant accumulation of SNCA as filamentous aggregates is a major pathological feature of PD. The prion-like propagation of SNCA aggregates may exacerbate the neurodegenerative process. Therefore, SNCA-targeting strategies are believed to be promising approaches for PD therapy. Autophagy is an effective way of eliminating SNCA aggregates. Chaperone-mediated autophagy is responsible for removing WT SNCA while macroautophagy degrades both WT and its mutant variants. Our *in vitro* data showed that UA reduced SNCA accumulation through enhancing autophagy flux, as the lysosomal inhibitor BafA1 was able to block UA-mediated SNCA clearance. Moreover, UA administration lowered the striatal SNCA level in SNCA^{A53T} transgenic mice. Unfortunately, we didn't observe any obvious SNCA aggregate in the SN dopaminergic neurons of this transgenic mice (<8 months old), thus limiting us to assess the effect of UA on the clearance of SNCA aggregates. In addition, we did not observe any significant loss of SN dopaminergic neurons (TH⁺) in transgenic mice. This is consistent with previous studies on the mice expressing the PrP driven human A53T mutant SNCA gene (M83). Future studies are warranted to evaluate if UA affects intraneuronal SNCA aggregates in other models, for example the platelet-derived growth factor β-driven SNCA transgenic mice.

Defective autophagy is implicated in PD pathogenesis. Several autophagy-enhancing molecules or gene-based therapies exert neuroprotection in different models of PD. Our *in vitro* and *in vivo* work consistently showed the autophagyenhancing effect of UA in both physiological (non-transgenic mice) and pathological conditions (SNCA^{A53T} transgenic). Moreover, this effect is not limited to the striatum as UA injection also enhanced the LC3-Ⅱ level in the cortex. This may have implications for other synucleinopathies such as multiple system atrophy (MSA) since serum urate levels are also reduced and correlated to its pathogenesis. Additionally, the transmission electronic micrographs identified an increase of double membraned structures, which is indicative of autophagosome and autolysosome formation increases, in UA-treated transgenic mice. This also suggests that UA enhances the autophagy activity, although only a mild increase of LC3-Ⅱ was observed in UA-treated transgenic mice. This may be due to the increased autophagy flux that leads to a partial degradation of LC3-Ⅱ associated with SNCA and P62 clearance following UA administration. Thus, the western blot data reflects a dual effect of UA on LC3-Ⅱ : the LC3-Ⅱ increase during autophagosome formation followed by a partial degradation of LC3-Ⅱ in autolysosome. Furthermore, we observed the reduction of P62 (an autophagy substrate) intensity in the SN dopaminergic neurons following UA treatment using the double immunofluorescence staining, which was confirmed by western blot analysis. However, we only detected a dispersed increase not the dots-like pattern of P62 fluorescence in the SNCA^{A53T} transgenic mice (<8 months old). This may reflect an agedependent change of this protein, just like the SNCA pathology and motor impairments which began to develop in aged (8 ~ 17 months) mice. Taken together, all the data suggest that UA could enhance the autophagy flux and thereby promote SNCA degradation.

mTOR is a highly conserved serine/threonine kinase that negatively regulates autophagy. Phosphorylation of mTOR at Thr 2446, Ser 2448 and Ser 2481 contributes to its overall higher activity. It acts in concert with AMP-activated protein kinase (AMPK) in regulating ULK1 activity and autophagy induction. When cellular energy supply is limited, AMPK is activated and mTOR is inhibited, followed by the decrease of ULK1 phosphorylation at Ser757. Meanwhile, activated AMPK interacts with and phosphorylates ULK1 Ser 555 and thus initiates autophagy. In this study we observed that UA treatment potently inhibited mTOR activity in a time-dependent manner, as indicated by the decreased phosphorylation of mTOR Ser 2488 and its substrate P70S6K. These alterations were accompanied by the decreased phosphorylation of ULK1 Ser 757 and increased phosphorylation of ULK1 Ser 555. Moreover, co-treatment with 3-BDO, an activator of mTOR, abolished the increase of LC3-II level induced by UA. These data suggest that mTOR inhibition is required for UA-induced autophagy activation. However, it remains to elucidate how UA inhibits mTOR signaling. Previous studies reported that UA resulted in mitochondrial oxidative stress and ATP depletion in endothelial cells. Given that AMPK is a central energy sensor, it is likely that the UA-mediated mTOR inhibition is secondary to AMPK activation. This deserves further investigation in future.

In sum, this study demonstrates that UA enhances autophagy activity via an mTOR-dependent signaling and promotes the clearance of SNCA *in vitro* and *in vivo*. This indicates that the urate-elevating strategy may be of value in the treatment of PD.

5. Acknowledgements

This work was supported by grants from the National Key R&D program of China (No. 2016YFC1306002) and the National Natural Science Foundation of China (81571233, 81171212). This was also partly supported by Suzhou Clinical Research Center of Neurological Disease (Szzx201503), Natural Science Foundation of Jiangsu Province of China (BK2011294), and the Priority Academic Program Development of Jiangsu Higher Education Institutions (PAPD). We thank Prof. JunYing Miao from Shandong University for kindly providing 3-BDO.

References

[1] AHMED I, LIANG Y, SCHOOLS S, et al. Development and Characterization of a New Parkinson's Disease Model Resulting from Impaired Autophagy[J].*J Neurosci*,2012,32(46): 16503−16509.

[2] ALVAREZ-ERVITI L, RODRIGUEZ-OROZ MC, COOPER JM,et al. Chaperone-mediated Autophagy Markers in Parkinson Disease Brains[J].*Arch Neurol*,2010,67(12): 1464−1472.

[3] ANGLADE P, VYAS S, JAVOY-AGID F, et al. Apoptosis and Autophagy in Nigral Neurons of Patients with Parkinson's Disease [J]. *Histol Histopathol*,1997,12(01): 25−31.

[4] BHATTACHARYYA S, BAKSHI R, LOGAN R,et al. Oral Inosine Persistently Elevates Plasma Antioxidant Capacity in Parkinson's Disease[J]. *Move Disord*,2016, 31(03): 417−421.

[5] CHURCH WH, WARD VL. Uric Acid is Reduced in the Substantia Nigra in Parkinson's Disease: Effect on Dopamine Oxidation[J].*Brain Res Bull*, 1994,33(04): 419−425.

[6] DAUER W, PRZEDBORSKI S.Parkinson's Disease: Mechanisms and Models[J].*Neuron*,2003, 39(06): 889−909.

[7] DAVIES KJ, SEVANIAN A, MUAKKASSAH-KELLY SF, et al.Uric Aecid-iron Ion Complexes. A New Aspect of the Antioxidant Functions of Uric Acid[J].*Biochem J*,1986, 235(03): 747−754.

[8] DE LAU LM, KOUDSTAAL PJ, HOFMAN A,et al.Serum Uric Acid Levels and the Risk of Parkinson Disease[J].*Ann Neurol*,2005,58(05): 797−800.

[9] DECRESSAC M, MATTSSON B, WEIKOP P,et al.TFEB-mediated Autophagy Rescues Midbrain Dopamine Neurons from Alpha-synuclein Toxicity [J].*Proc Natl Acad Sci USA*,2013,110(19): E1817−1826.

[10] DICKSON DW, BRAAK H, DUDA JE, et al. Neuropathological Assessment of Parkinson's Disease: Refining the Diagnostic Criteria[J].*Lancet Neurol*,2009,8(12): 1150−1157.

[11] DU Y, CHEN CP, TSENG CY, et al.Astroglia-mediated Effects of Uric Acid to Protect Spinal Cord Neurons from Glutamate Toxicity[J]. *Glia*,

2007, 55(05): 463-472.

[12] EGAN DF, SHACKELFORD DB, MIHAYLOVA MM, et al. Phosphorylation of ULK1(hATG1) by AMP-activated Protein Kinase Connects Energy Sensing to Mitophagy[J].*Science*,2011, 331(6016): 456-461.

[13] GAO X, O'REILLY EJ, SCHWARZSCHILD MA, et al.Prospective study of plasma urate and risk of Parkinson disease in men and women[J]. *Neurology*,2016, 86(06): 520-526.

[14] GE D, HAN L, HUANG S, et al. Identification of a novel MTOR activator and discovery of a competing endogenous RNA regulating autophagy in vascular endothelial cells[J].*Autophagy*,2014, 10(06): 957-971.

[15] GIASSON BI, DUDA JE, QUINN SM, et al. Neuronal Alpha-synucleinopathy with Severe Movement Disorder in Mice Expressing A53T Human α-synuclein[J].*Neuron*,2002, 34(04): 521-533.

[16] GONG L, ZHANG QL, ZHANG N,et al.Neuroprotection by Urate on 6-OHDA-lesioned Rat Model of Parkinson's Disease: Linking to Akt/GSK3beta Signaling Pathway[J].*J Neurochem*,2012,123(05): 876-885.

[17] HASHIMOTO M, MASLIAH E. Alpha-synuclein in Lewy Body Disease and Alzheimer's Disease[J].*Brain Pathol*,1999,9(04): 707-720.

[18] JOHNSON RJ, KANG DH, FEIG D, et al. Is there a Pathogenetic Role for Uric Acid in Hypertension and Cardiovascular and Renal Disease? [J]. *Hypertension*,2003, 41(06): 1183-1190.

[19] JOHNSON RJ, NAKAGAWA T, SANCHEZ-LOZADA LG, et al. Sugar, Uric Acid, and the Etiology of Diabetes and Obesity[J].*Diabetes*,2013, 62(10): 3307-3315.

[20] KIM J, KUNDU M, VIOLLET B,et al. AMPK and mTOR Regulate Autophagy through Direct Phosphorylation of Ulk1[J].*Nat Cell Biol*,2011,13 (02): 132-141.

[21] KOVACS GG, BREYDO L, GREEN R, et al. Intracellular Processing of Disease-associated Alpha-synuclein in the Human Brain Suggests Prion-like Cell-to-cell Spread[J].*Neurobiol Dis*,2014,69: 76-92.

[22] LIU X, HUANG S, WANG X, et al. Chaperone-mediated Autophagy and Neurodegeneration: Connections, Mechanisms, and Therapeutic Implications

［J］.*Neurosci Bull*,2015,31(04)：407-415.

［23］LUK KC, KEHM V, CARROLL J, et al. Pathological Alpha-synuclein Transmission Initiates Parkinson-like Neurodegeneration in Nontransgenic Mice［J］.*Science*,2012, 338(6109)：949-953.

［24］NI HM, BOCKUS A, WOZNIAK AL, et al. Dissecting the Dynamic Turnover of GFP-LC3 in the Autolysosome［J］.*Autophagy*,2011, 7(02)：188-204.

［25］PAUMIER KL, SUKOFF RIZZO SJ, BERGER Z,et al. Behavioral Characterization of A53T Mice Reveals Early and Late Stage Deficits Related to Parkinson's Disease［J］.*PLoS One*,2013, 8(08)：e70274.

［26］PEELAERTS W, BOUSSET L, VAN DER PERREN A, et al. Alpha-Synuclein Strains Cause Distinct Synucleinopathies after Local and Systemic Administration［J］.*Nature*,2015, 522(7556)：340-344.

［27］PERLUIGI M, DI DOMENICO F, BUTTERFIELD DA. mTOR Signaling in Aging and Neurodegeneration：at the Crossroad between Metabolism Dysfunction and Impair-ment of Autophagy［J］.*Neurobiol Dis*,2015, 84：39-49.

［28］RECASENS A, DEHAY B, BOVE J, et al. Lewy Body Extracts from Parkinson Disease Brains Trigger Alpha-synuclein Pathology and Neurodegeneration in Mice and Monkeys［J］. *Ann Neurol*,2014,75(03)：351-362.

［29］SAKUTA H, SUZUKI K, MIYAMOTO T, et al. Serum Uric Acid Levels in Parkinson's Disease and Related Disorders［J］. *Brain and Behavior*, 2017, 7(01)：e00598.

［30］SIMÓN-SÁNCHEZ J, SCHULTE C, BRAS JM. Genome-wide Association Study Reveals Genetic Risk Underlying Parkinson's Disease［J］. *Nat Genet*,2009,41(12)：1308-1312.

［31］SPENCER B, POTKAR R, TREJO M, et al.Beclin 1 Gene Transfer Activates Autophagy and Ameliorates the Neurodegenerative Pathology in Alpha-synuclein Models of Parkinson's and Lewy Body Diseases［J］. *J Neurosci*,2009, 29(43)：13578-13588.

［32］WANG JD, CAO YL, LI Q, et al.A Pivotal Role of FOS-mediated BECN1/Beclin 1 Upregulation in Dopamine D2 and D3 Receptor Agonist-induced Autophagy Activation［J］. *Autophagy*,2015, 11(11)：2057-2073.

［33］YU MA，SANCHEZ-LOZADA LG，Johnson，R.J，et al. Oxidative Stress with an Activation of the Renin-angiotensin System in Human Vascular Endothelial Cells as a Novel Mechanism of Uric Acid-induced Endothelial Dysfunction［J］. *J Hypertens*，2010，28（06）：1234-1242.

［34］ZHANG N，SHU HY，HUANG T，et al. Nrf2 Signaling Contributes to the Neuroprotective Effects of Urate against 6-OHDA Toxicity［J］. *PLoS One*，2014，9（06）：e100286.

（Yu-Lan Sheng，Xing Chen，Xiao-Ou Hou，Xin Yuan，Bao-Shi Yuan，Yu-Qing Yuan，Qi-Lin Zhang，Xian Cao，Chun-Feng Liu，Wei-Feng Luo，Li-Fang Hu）

（本文原载于 *Experimental Neurology* 2017 年第 297 卷）

Uric Acid Demonstrates Neuroprotective Effect on Parkinson's Disease Mice through Nrf2-ARE Signaling Pathway[①]

Abstract: Uric acid has neuroprotective effect on Parkinson's disease by inhibiting oxidative damage and neuronal cell death. Our previous study has shown that uric acid protected dopaminergic cell line damage through inhibiting accumulation of NF-E2-related factor 2(Nrf2). This study aimed to investigate its in vivo neuroprotective effect. PD was induced by MPTP intraperitoneally injection for 7 d in male C57BL/6 mice. Mice were treated with either uric acid (intraperitoneally injection 250 mg/kg) or saline for a total of 13 d. We showed that uric acid improved behavioral performances and cognition of PD mice, increased TH-positive dopaminergic neurons and decreased GFAP-positive astrocytes in substantia nigra. Uric acid increased mRNA and protein expressions of Nrf2 and three Nrf2-responsive genes, including γg-glutamate-cysteine ligase catalytic subunit (γ-GCLC), heme oxygenase-1 (HO-1) and NQO1. Uric acid significantly increased superoxide dismutase, CAT, glutathione(GSH) levels and decreased malondialdehyde level in SN regions of MPTP-treated mice. Uric acid inhibited the hippocampal expression of IL-1β and decreased serum and hippocampus levels of interleukin-1β(IL-1β), IL-6 and tumor necrosis factor-α (TNF-α). In conclusion, uric acid demonstrates neuroprotective properties for dopaminergic neurons in PD mice through modulation of neuroinflammation and oxidative stress.

Keywords: Parkinson's disease; uric acid; oxidative stress; neuroinflammation; NF-E2-related factor 2.

---

① This study was funded by the science and technology support program of Changzhou Wujin Social Development and Medicine(Grant No.WS201504).

1. Introduction

Parkinson's disease is one common neurodegenerative disorder, with higher incidence among people over 60 years old. The main clinical feature of PD is motor impairment, including resting tremor, muscular rigidity and bradykinesia. The pathologically features of PD are loss of dopaminergic neurons in the substantia nigra(SN) and the formation of inclusion bodies in the cytoplasm. In fact, there are about 80% of the striatal dopamine terminals are lost when patients are diagnosed with PD[1]. Though the precise mechanism of PD remains elusive, oxidative stress and neuroinflammation are two main pathogenic mechanisms which may contribute to dopaminergic neuron damage[2][3]. Therefore, injection of MPTP, a molecule targeting reactive oxygen species (ROS) and inflammation, could cause neurotoxicity and selective damage of dopaminergic neurons, and makes it a widely used method to establish PD animal model[4]. The current dopamine replacement therapy only relieves the symptoms but cannot impede neurodegenerative process. Meanwhile, its long-term use often causes side-effects motor complications and dyskinesia[5]. Therefore, identifying effective neuroprotective agents and exploring their mechanisms against dopaminergic neuron loss are still an important challenge for PD treatment.

Uric acid is the end product of diet purines. High serum uric acid levels are associated with several diseases, including hypertension, atherosclerosis, hyperlipidemia and obesity[6]. Uric acid is a strong antioxidant molecule and

① DAUER W, PRZEDBORSKI S. Parkinson's Disease: Mechanisms and Models[J]. Neuron, 2003, 39 (06):889-909.

② SURENDRAN S, RAJASANKAR S. Parkinson's Disease: Oxidative Stress and Therapeutic Approaches [J]. Neurol Sci, 2010, 31:531-540.

③ TIWARI PC, PAL R. The Potential Role of Neuroinflammation and Transcription Factors in Parkinson Disease[J]. Dialogues Clin Neurosci, 2017, 19(01):71-80.

④ YOKOYAMA H, KUROIWA H, YANO R, et al. Targeting Reactive Oxygen Species, Reactive Nitrogen Species and Inflammation in MPTP Neurotoxicity and Parkinson's Disease[J], Neurol Sci, 2008, 29(05):293-301.

⑤ BARGIOTAS P, KONITSIOTIS S. Levodopa-induced Dyskinesias in Parkinson's Disease: Emerging Treatments[J], Neuropsychiatr Dis Treat, 2013, 9:1605-1617.

⑥ SO A, THORENS B. Uric Acid Transport and Disease[J]. J Clin Invest, 2010, 120(06):1791-1799.

scavenger of ROS[1], which makes it protective in some CNS diseases. Therefore, serum uric acid levels were significantly lower in Parkinson's disease in comparison to control subjects[2]. Uric acid level was decreased in substantia nigra of PD patients, thus making dopamine susceptible to oxidative stress[3]. Therefore, the antioxidant properties of uric acid might provide neuroprotection against neuronal damage of PD and serum uric acid could serve as one biomarker to predict the risk of disease progression.

Oxidative stress closely involves the pathogenesis of PD[4] and can produce many response proteins that enhance cell survival, including the transcription factor NF-E2-related factor 2 (Nrf2). In response to oxidative stress, Nrf2 is activated and binds to antioxidant response element (ARE), thus regulating various antioxidant proteins[5]. Furthermore, Nrf2-ARE antioxidant defense pathway showed neuroprotective effects in experimental PD models through suppression of oxidative stress and neuroinflammation[6]. However, there is little literature on the interaction between uric acid and Nrf2-ARE pathway in PD.

This study investigated the neuroprotective effect of uric acid using a PD mouse model that is induced by MPTP, and the modulation of uric acid on Nrf2-ARE pathway and neuroinflammation, which may involve uric acid-mediated protection of dopaminergic neurons.

---

① SAUTIN YY, JOHNSON RJ. Uric Acid: the Oxidant-antioxidant Paradox [J]. *Nucleos Nucleot Nucl Acids*, 2008, 27(06):608-619.

② WEN M, ZHOU B, Y. H. Chen, et al. Serum Uric Acid Levels in Patients with Parkinson's Disease: a Meta-analysis [J]. *PLoS One*, 2017, 12(03):e0173731.

③ CHURCH WH, WARD VL. Uric Acid is Reduced in the Substantia Nigra in Parkinson's Disease: Effect on Dopamine Oxidation [J], *Brain Res Bull*, 1994, 33(04):419-425.

④ SURENDRAN S, RAJASANKAR S. Parkinson's Disease: Oxidative Stress and Therapeutic Approaches [J]. *Neurol Sci*, 31(05):531-540.

⑤ JAISWAL AK. Nrf2 Signaling in Coordinated Activation of Antioxidant Gene Expression [J]. *Free Radic Biol Med*, 2004, 36(10):1199-1207.

⑥ KUMAR H, KOPPULA S, KIM IS, et al. Nuclear Factor Erythroid 2-related Factor 2 Signaling in Parkinson Disease: a Promising Multi Therapeutic Target against Oxidative Stress, Neuroinflammation and Cell Death [J]. *CNS Neurol Disord Drug Targets*, 2012, 11(08):1015-1029.

2. Materials and Methods

（1）Drugs and Reagents

Uric acid and MPTP were purchased from Sigma-Aldrich（Saint Louis, MO, USA）, and dissolved in saline. Rabbit anti-mouse tyrosine hydroxylase（TH）and GFAP antibodies were purchased from DAKO（Glostrup, Denmark）. Antibody to Nrf2 was purchased from Cell Signaling Technology, Inc.（Danvers, MA, USA）.

（2）Parkinson's Disease Mice Induced by MPTP

Male C57BL/6J mice（6-8 weeks, 20 – 25 g）were purchased from the Shanghai SLAC Laboratory Animals Co Ltd（Shanghai, China）. Mice were housed in SPF conditions with an automatic 12 h/12 h light-dark cycle at a constant temperature（21 ± 1 ℃）. All animal studies were approved by the Animal Care and Use Committee of Wujin Hospital Affiliated to Jiangsu University, and these experimental protocols were performed in accordance with Guidelines for the Care and Use of Laboratory Animals（Chinese-NationalResearch-Council, 2006）. All mice were divided into three groups: control group, MPTP group, and uric acid group（uric acid+MPTP）. PD mice were induced by intraperitoneal injection of MPTP（25 mg/kg）for 7 d（once a day）. Uric acid group received intraperitoneal injection of uric acid（250 mg/kg）for a total of 13 d（3 d before the start of MPTP, 7 d during MPTP administration and 3 d after the end of MTPT）（2 h prior to intraperitoneal injection of MPTP）[①]. Control group received 0.9% saline replacing MPTP and uric acid. On day 14, behavioral and cognitive tests were measured, and then these mice were sacrificed to obtain the brain tissue for further analysis.

（3）Behavioral Testing

① Locomotor Activity

Horizontal locomotor activity was measured in an infrared photobeam activity cage system（Jiliang Ltd, Shanghai, China）. Mice were habituated in the test room for 30 mins, and then individually placed in the center of a Plexiglas/polyvinyl chloride（PVC）cage（25 cm/25 cm/30 cm）. Basal spontaneous locomotion was

---

① JIA J, XING J, DING Y, et al. Hyperuricemia Causes Pancreatic β-cell Death and Dysfunction through NF-kB Signaling Pathway[J], *PLoS One*, 2013, 8（10）: e78284.

monitored during the light phase for 50 mins. Total ambulatory counts were scored as the number of adjacent photobeam breaks and the distance travelled (m) was recorded.

② Rotarod Test

The rotarod test was applied to evaluate motor and coordination abilities. Mouse was placed in a rotarod (diameter, 7 cm) at a fixed speed of 30 rpm. The time that each mouse spent on the rod was measured. The rotarod test was performed on days 14 with repeated five experiments for each mouse. The mean duration (time on rotarod) for each mouse was recorded.

③ Pole Test

Pole test was used to evaluate bradykinesia of PD. Mice were placed head downward on the top of a vertical pole (60 cm in length and 2 cm in diameter) with a rough surface. The time for the mice to reach the floor was measured and recorded as latency (s). Latency was averaged from five repeated trials for each mouse.

(4) Cognition Measurement

The spatial learning and memory was determined by Morris water-maze test on day 14, and included place navigation test and space exploration test. In place navigation test, a transparent platform was placed within a 1/2 radius of any of the four quadrants, with the water surface 1 cm higher the top of the platform. The mice were placed at the opposite quadrant to the platform, and allowed to find and climbed onto the platform. The duration that each mouse found and climbed onto the platform was recorded as escape latency, and was averaged from the four quadrants. In space exploration test, the above platform was removed from the pool and mice were placed in water of the opposite quadrant. The swimming path of each mouse was observed for 60 s, and the number of times the mouse crossed over the original platform position was recorded as platform crossings.

(5) Immunofluorescence Staining

After the behavioral tests, mice were anesthetized with 4% chloral hydrate and then perfused with 0.9% saline for 15 mins, followed by paraformaldehyde (4%) in 0.1 mol/L PBS (pH 7.4) for 20 mins. Then the brains were collected and post-fixed in paraformaldehyde overnight at 4 ℃, followed by 30% sucrose at

4 ℃ for 72 h. The brains were serially cut into 20 μm coronal sections. Then the sections were kept in 0.1 mol/L PBS and blocked by 3% BSA. After washing in PBS, the sections were incubated with anti-TH antibody(1 ∶ 400)or anti-GFAP antibody(1 ∶ 200)at 4 ℃ for 24 h. The sections were treated with Alexa Fluor 488 conjugated goat anti-rabbit IgG(1 ∶ 400,Thermo Fisher Scientific)for 2 h at room temperature in the dark. After washing(10 mins each), the sections were mounted and imaged using a laser confocal fluorescent microscope. The numbers of TH-positive neurons and GFAP-positive astrocytes were counted respectively[①].

(6) Striatal Dopamine Levels

To determine the effect of uric acid on striatal dopamine level in Parkinsonian mice, mice were sacrificed on the last day of uric acid treatment(day 14). Both sides of striatum were isolated and homogenized by sonication in ice-cold 0.1 m $HCLO_4$ (containing 0.01% EDTA), followed with centrifuge at 10 000 g×10 mins at 4 ℃. The supernatant (10 μL) was separated and injected into the HPLC system equipped with the Electro-Chemical detector(Waters Corp., Milford, MA, USA)at a flow rate 0.8 mL/min to determine the content of dopamine[②].

(7) Quantitative Real-time Polymerase Chain Reaction(qRT-PCR)

Mice were decapitated on day 7 and day 14, and the right side of SN was isolated and put into RNase free centrifuge tubes(1.5 mL), stored at −80 ℃. Total RNA was extracted using Trizol[®] reagent(Life Technologies, Carlsbad, CA, USA). Total RNA(2μg)was reverse transcribed to cDNA using the Superscript Ⅲ enzyme (Life Technologies) to determine the mRNA expressions of target genes by qRT-PCR using SYBR Green reagent (TaKaRa, Japan). The PCR condition was as follows: 95 ℃ for 5 mins, 60 ℃ for 20 s, 40 amplification cycles. Housekeeping gene β-actin served as an internal control. The mRNA expressions of target genes were measured by 2-ΔΔCt method and normalized to

① REN ZX, ZHAO YF, CAO T, et al. Dihydromyricetin Protects Neurons in an MPTP-induced Model of Parkinson's Disease by Suppressing Glycogen Synthase Kinase-3 Beta Activity[J]. *Acta Pharmacol Sin*, 2016, 37 (10): 1315−1324.

② BORAH A, MOHANAKUMAR KP. Long-term L-DOPA Treatment Causes Indiscriminate Increase in Dopamine Levels at the Cost of Serotonin Synthesis in Discrete Brain Regions of Rats[J]. *Cell Mol Neurobiol*, 2007, 27(08): 985−996.

β-actin. All reactions were performed in triplicate. PCRs were performed using the following primers: Nrf2 primer: forward, 5'-TCTTGGAGTAAGTCGAGAAGTGT-3'; reverse, 5'-GTTGAAACTGAGCGAAAAAGGC-3'. γ-GCLC primer: forward, 5'-GGGGTGACGAG GTGGAGTA-3'; reverse: 5'-GTTGGGGTTTGTCCTCTCCC-3'. HO-1 primer: forward, 5'-AAGCCGAGAATGCTGAGTTCA-3'; reverse: 5'-GCCGTGTAGATATGGTACAAGGA-3'. NQO1 primer: forward, 5'-ATGGGAG-GTGGTCGAATCTGA-3'; reverse: 5'-GCCTTCCTTATACGCCAGAGATG-3'. β-actinprimer: forward, 5'-TGCTGTCCCTGTATGCCTCT-3'; reverse: 5'-TTGAT-GTCACGCACGATTTC-3'.

(8) Western Blot

The right side of SN was digested by RIPA lysis buffer with protease inhibitors (1 g/mL each of pepstatin, aprotinin and leupeptin) for 30 mins. Protein sample (50 μg) was separated by 8% SDS-PAGE and transferred to PVDF membranes, and blocked with 5% non-fat milk at 4 ℃ overnight. The membranes were incubated with rabbit anti-mouse Nrf2 antibody (1 ∶ 200) (1 ∶ 10 000) overnight at 4 ℃. After washing with 0.1% TBST 3 times, the membranes were incubated with HRP-labeled goat-anti rabbit secondary antibody (1 ∶ 10 000). The antigen-antibody complexes were detected by enhanced chemiluminescence (ECL Amersham Life Science, England) and visualized by Bio-Rad ChemiDoc XRS (Bio-Rad, USA).

(9) Oxidative Activity Evaluation by Biochemical Assessment

The supernatant of the midbrain tissue homogenate was prepared by centrifugation at 10 000g 10 mins at 4 ℃. A microplate reader (Ricso RK201, Shenzhen Ricso Technology Co., Ltd, Shenzhen, Guangdong, China) was used to perform spectrophotometry to determin the contents of SOD(560 nm), CAT(405 nm), GSH(420 nm), and MDA(532 nm) using assay kits (Nanjing Jiancheng Bioengineering Research Institute, Nanjing, China)[1].

---

① SHI X, CHEN YH, LIU H, et al. Therapeutic Effects of Paeonol on Methyl-4-phenyl-1, 2, 3, 6-tetrahydropyridine/probenecid-induced Parkinson's Disease in Mice [J]. *Mol Med Rep*, 2016, 14(03): 2397 – 2404.

（10）Immunohistochemical Staining

On d 14 after uric acid treatment, mice were anesthetized with 4% chloral hydrate, and the hippocampus was cut and fixed with 4% triformol overnight. After dehydration, hippocampus tissue was embedded with paraffin to make continuous sections（5 μm thickness）. Sections were treated with 3% BSA for 1 h, and then incubated with primary antibody to IL-1β（1∶100）overnight at 4 ℃, followed by PBS washing twice. The goat anti-rabbit biotinylation HRP-IgG （1∶100, second antibody）was added to sections at room temperature for 2 h. Then sections were colored with diaminobenzidine（DAB）, and counterstained with hematoxylin. The positive neurons for IL-1β were observed under an Olympus BX51 microscope（Olympus Company, Japan）, their number was counted from five randomly selected fields and converted into cell densities（cells/HP）.

（11）Serum Cytokine Analysis

The hippocampus and serum samples were obtained at 14 d after uric acid administration. The supernatant of hippocampus homogenate was prepared by centrifugation at 10000 g×10 mins at 4 ℃. The serum was immediately separated by centrifugation at 3000 g for 15 mins at 4 ℃. Their aliquots were stored at −80 ℃ for assay. Levels of IL-1β, IL-6 and TNF-α were determined by enzymelinked immunosorbent assay（ELISA）kits（R&D Systems Inc., Minneapolis, MN, USA）, by measuring optical density（OD）at 450 nm in a microplate reader.

（12）Statistical Analysis

Data were analyzed using SPSS software（version 19.0）and are expressed as the mean±standard deviation（SD）in all experiments. One-way ANOVA was used for multiple-group comparisons, followed by Q test for pairwise comparisons. $P<0.05$ was considered statistically significant.

3. Results

（1）Uric Acid Improved MPTP-induced Behavioral and Cognitive dysfunction

We first examined the effects of uric acid administration on motor function of PD mouse model. MPTP treatment induced severe motor impairments. Uric acid administration（250 mg/kg）improved locomotor activity in MPTP-treated mice, as evidenced by increased average travel speed and total distance travelled on day 14（Fig. 1. A and Fig. 1. B）. Uric acid also attenuated the MPTP-induced deficit in movement balance, with longer time on rotarod and decreased latency （Fig.1.C and Fig.1.D）.

We also performed Morris water-maze test to evaluate the cognitive function of PD mice. Place navigation test showed that the escape latency on the d 14 was

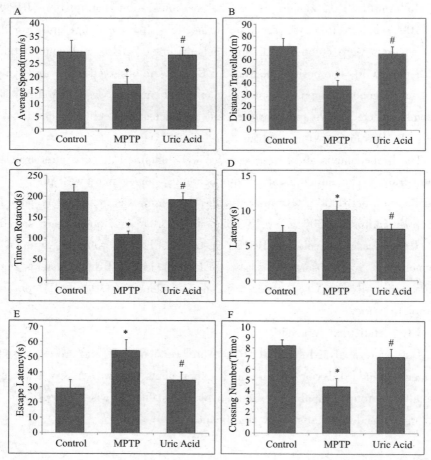

Fig. 1   Uric acid induces recovery of behavioral and cognitive function. Uric acid significantly increased average travel speed（A）, total distance travelled（B）and time on rotarod（C）, and decreased latency（D）in MPTP mice. Compared with MPTP mice, uric acid treatment significantly decreased escape latency time（E）and increased platform crossing number（F）（$N=10, x\pm s$）. $^{*}P<0.05$ versus control group; $^{\#}P<0.05$ versus MPTP group.

prolonged in MPTP mice but reduced in uric acid mice（$P<0.05$）（Fig.1.E）. Space exploration test showed that the platform crossing number was increased in MPTP mice but increased in uric acid mice（$P<0.05$）.

（2）Uric Acid Demonstrated Neuroprotective Effects on MPTP-induced PD Mice

We performed immunofluorescence staining to evaluate the dopaminergic neurons of MPTP mice.The fluorescence pictures showed TH-positive neurons and GFAP-positive astrocytes of the substantia nigra area（Fig.2.A,Fig.2.B,Fig.2.C）.

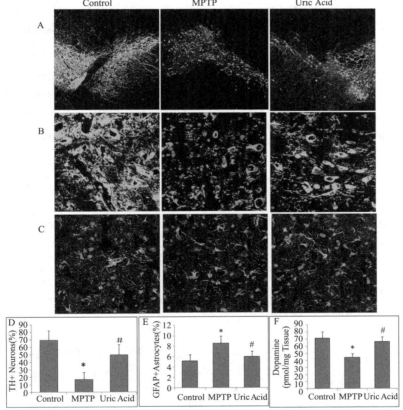

Fig.2 Uric acid shows neuroprotective properties for dopaminergic neurons. Immunofluorescence staining was performed with anti-TH antibody or anti-GFAP antibody in substantia nigra.Representative photomicrographs are shown. A,TH-positive neurons, ×10 magnification. B,TH-positive neurons,×60. C,GFAP-positive astrocytes,×10. Uric acid significantly increased TH-positive dopaminergic neurons（D）and decreased GFAP-positive astrocytes（E）.F,uric acid increased dopamine content in striatum of MPTP mice. $^*P<0.05$ versus control group;$^\#P<0.05$ versus MPTP group.

The summarized quantitative data showed that compared with the controls, the TH-positive neurons reduced in the MPTP mice, and this effect was partly restored in the uric acid mice (Fig. 2. D). Furthermore, MPTP administration increased GFAP-positive astrocytes, which could be reversed by uric acid (Fig.2.E). The content of dopamine in the striatum was significantly decreased in the MPTP mice, but was partly restored by uric acid (Fig.2.F).

（3）Uric Acid Activates Nrf2-ARE Pathway And Inhibits Oxidative Stress in MPTP Mice

Compared with controls, Nrf2 mRNA and protein levels decreased significantly in the MPTP mice. Co-treatment with uric acid significantly increased Nrf2 expression in the substantia nigra (Fig. 3. A, Fig. 3. B). Furthermore, Nrf2 mRNA and protein levels were higher in mice on d 14 compared with mice on d 7. We then analyzed the mRNA expressions of several Nrf2 target genes. The mRNA levels of γ-GCLC, HO-1 and NQO1 were significantly decreased by MPTP and uric acid administration up-regulated the mRNA expressions of these Nrf2 target genes (Fig.3.C, Fig.3.D, Fig.3.E).

We then measured oxidative activity in midbrain tissue of PD mice. The contents of SOD, CAT and GSH in the midbrain were significantly decreased by MPTP, which suggested that MPTP could disrupt antioxidant defense systems disruption in the midbrain. However, activities of SOD, CAT and GSH could be restored by uric acid administration at 250 mg/kg, respectively (Fig. 3. F, Fig.3.G, Fig.3.H). MDA level was increased in the MPTP mice but significantly decreased by uric acid (Fig.3.I).

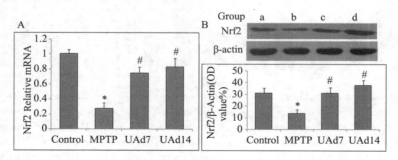

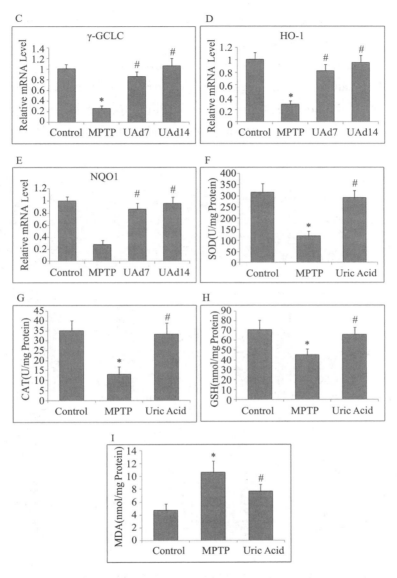

Fig.3 Uric acid activates Nrf2-ARE signaling pathway and inhibits oxidative stress in MPTP mice. Mice were sacrificed on d 7 and d 14 and substantia nigra was obtained to extract RNA and protein. Uric acid significantly increased mRNA (A) and protein (B) expressions of MPTP mice. A, control; B, MPTP; C, uric acid 7 d; D, uric acid 14 d. Uric acid also significantly increased mRNA levels of Nrf2-responsive genes γ-GCLC (C), HO-1 (D) and NQO1 (E). Uric acid significantly increased the activity of SOD (F), CAT (G) and GSH (H), and decreased MDA (I) in the midbrain of MPTP mice. * $P < 0.05$ versus control group; # $P < 0.05$ versus MPTP group.

（4）Uric Acid Suppresses Neuroinflammation and Decreases Proinflammatory Cytokines in Hippocampus and Serum

Immunohistochemistry showed IL-1β-positive neurons in hip pocampus of control MPTP and uric acid mice(Fig.4.A).Quantitative analysis showed that the number of IL-1β-positive neurons was significantly higher in MPTP mice compared to the control mice,and uric acid significantly decreased the number of IL-1β-positive neurons($P<0.05$)(Fig.4.B).

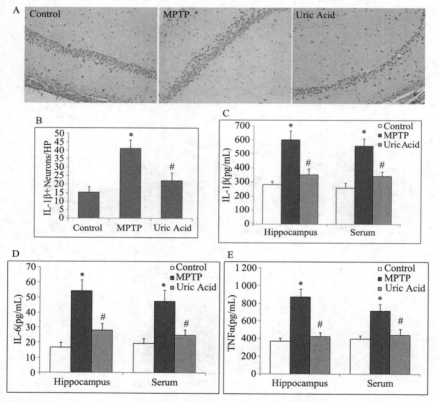

Fig.4　The effects of uric acid on neuroinflammation of MPTP mice. A, representative images of immunohistochemical staining are shown (×200).B, quantitative data showed that uric acid significantly decreased cell density of IL-1β-positive neurons in hippocampus.ELISA showed that uric acid significantly decreased hippocampus and serum IL-1β(C),IL-6(D) and TNF-α(E)levels. *$P<0.05$ versus control group;#$P<0.05$ versus MPTP group.

We measured inflammatory cytokine levels in hippocampus and serum at d 14 after uric acid administration. The hippocampus and serum levels of IL-1β, IL-6 and TNF-α were significantly increased after MPTP induction. Uric acid significantly reduced serum IL-1β, IL-6 and TNF−α levels in hippocampus and serum of PD mice(P<0.05)(Fig.4.C, Fig.4.D, Fig.4.E).

4. Discussion

The present study demonstrated that administration of uric acid significantly attenuates behavioral impairments and cognitive dysfunction in MPTP-induced PD mice, with decreased TH-positive neurons and increased GFAP-positive astrocytes in the substantia nigra area. Uric acid activates Nrf2-ARE pathway, as evidenced by increased expressions of Nrf2 mRNA and protein and transcription of Nrf2 target genes γ-GCLC, HO-1 and NQO1 in substantia nigra of PD mice. Uric acid also inhibited oxidative stress, with increased contents of SOD, CAT and GSH and decreased content of MDA in the midbrain. Uric acid administration reduced number of IL-1β-positive neurons in hippocampus and IL-1β, IL-6 and TNF-α levels in hippocampus and serum. These data provide clear evidence that uric acid elicits potent neuroprotective effects on dopaminergic neuron of PD mice. In addition, activation of Nrf2-ARE pathway, suppression of oxidative stress; neuroinflammation may contribute to this protection.

Uric acid is a degradation product from nucleic acid and its concentrations are significantly lower in serum and substantia nigra of PD patients in comparison with those of healthy controls[1][2]. In PD patients, low serum uric acid levels were associated with freezing of gait[3] and later occurrence of mild cognitive

① WEN M, ZHOU B, Y.H.Chen, et al. Serum Uric Acid Levels in Patients with Parkinson's Disease: a Meta-analysis[J]. *PLoS One*, 2017, 12(03): e0173731.

② CHURCH WH, WARD VL. Uric Acid is Reduced in the Substantia Nigra in Parkinson's Disease: Effect on Dopamine Oxidation[J]. *Brain Res Bull*, 1994, 33(04): 419−425.

③ OU R, CAO B, WEI Q, et al. Serum Uric Acid Levels and Freezing of Gait in Parkinson's Disease[J]. *Neurol Sci*, 2017, 38(06): 955−960.

impairment[1]. Therefore, raising serum uric acid level may demonstrate neuroprotection in PD animal models and patients. Our previous study showed that urate prevented oxidative injury of 6-OHDA-induced PC12 cells, which may involve mechanisms underlying the association between high serum uric acid and reduced PD risk[2]. The present study showed that uric acid pretreatment significantly attenuated behavioral and cognitive deficits induced by MPTP. We found that uric acid protected dopamine neurons, as evidenced by increased TH-positive neurons in substantia nigra and dopamine content in striatum. In the present study, we administrated uric acid through intraperitoneally injection at 250 mg/kg, and our previous study has shown that intraperitoneally injection could elevate urate(the anionic form of uric acid) in plasma and striatum by 55% and 36.8% in 6-OHDA-induced PD rats[3]. This suggests that uric acid could cross the blood-brain barrier and is a promising therapeutic strategy for Parkinson's disease.

Our present study showed that uric acid activated Nrf2-ARE signaling pathway in substantia nigra of MPTP mice. Nrf2 is a transcription factor that inhibits oxidative stress through initiating transcription of several antioxidant genes, such as γ-GCLC, HO-1 and NQO-1[4]. This is in accordance with our results that uric acid enhanced the transcription of Nrf2 target genes, including γ-GCLC, HO-1 and NQO-1, and all of which are closely associated with oxidative stress and redox homeostasis. Our previous study also showed activation of Nrf2-ARE signals by in vitro urate pretreatment in 6-OHDA-induced dopaminergic

① PELLECCHIA MT, SAVASTANO R, MOCCIA M, et al. Lower Serum Uric Acid is Associated with Mild Cognitive Impairment in Early Parkinson's Disease: a 4-year Follow-up Study [J]. *J Neural Transm* (*Vienna*), 2016, 123(12): 1399-1402.

② ZHU TG, WANG XX, LUO WF, et al. Protective Effects of Urate against 6-OHDA-induced Cell Injury in PC12 Cells through Antioxidant Action[J]. *Neurosci Lett*, 2012, 506(02): 175-179.

③ GONG L, ZHANG QL, ZHANG N, et al. Neuroprotection by Urate on 6-OHDA Lesioned Rat Model of Parkinson's Disease: Linking to Akt/GSK3β Signaling Pathway[J]. *J Neurochem*, 2012, 123(05): 876-885.

④ YANG HL, LIN SW, LEE CC, et al. Induction of Nrf2-mediated Genes by Antrodia Salmonea Inhibits ROS Generation and Inflammatory Effects in Lipopolysaccharide-stimulated RAW264.7 Macrophages[J]. *Food Funct*, 2015, 6(01): 229-240.

cell line[1].Furthermore, the anti-oxidative effect of uric acid was confirmed by significantly increased levels of SOD, CAT and GSH, and decreased levels of MDA.SOD, CAT and GSH are used to measure the oxidative stress level, as they could effectively remove oxygen free radicals and lipid peroxides[2].MDA is the most prevalent lipid peroxidation byproducts during oxidative stress lipid peroxidation and used as a biomarker of oxidative stress[3].Taken together, uric acid demonstrated a suppressive effect on MPTP-induced oxidative stress, perhaps through activating Nrf2-ARE antioxidant pathway.

Our present study showed that uric acid potently suppressed neuroinflammation of MPTP mice, as evidenced by decreased number of IL-1β-positive neurons in hippocampus.Hippocampus is a temporal lobe with functions in learning and memory, and MPTP-induced PD mice showed apoptosis in the hippocampus and deteriorated short-term memory[4], which is consistent with our results and cognitive deficits in PD patients.Furthermore, high expression of IL-1β in mouse hippocampus impairs spatial memory[5], and this is confirmed by impaired spatial reference memory and spatial working memory of MPTP mice. Astrocytes are resident innate immune cells involving the inflammatory process. Our result showed that MPTP increased GFAP-positive astrocytes in substantia nigra area, and these uncontrolled activated astrocytes indicate neuroinflammation[6].Activated astrocytes also could promote releasing various

① ZHANG N, SHU HY, HUANG T, et al. Nrf2 Signaling Contributes to the Neuroprotective Effects of Urate against 6-OHDA Toxicity[J].*PLoS One*,2014, 9(06):e100286.

② WEYDERT CJ, CULLEN JJ. Measurement of Superoxide Dismutase, Catalase and Glutathione Peroxidase in Cultured Cells and Tissue[J].*Nat Protoc*,2010,5(01):51-66.

③ ANTUS B, DROZDOVSZKY O, BARTA I, et al.Comparison of Airway and Systemic Malondialdehyde Levels for Assessment of Oxidative Stress in Cystic Fibrosis[J].*Lung*,2015, 193:597-604.

④ KIM M, CHO KH, SHIN MS, et al.Berberine Prevents Nigrostriatal Dopaminergic Neuronal Loss and Suppresses Hippocampal Apoptosis in Mice with Parkinson's Disease[J].*Int J Mol Med*,2014,33(04):870-878.

⑤ MOORE AH, WU M, SHAFTEL SS, et al. Sustained Expression of Interleukin 1β in Mouse Hippocampus Impairs Spatial Memory[J].*Neurosci*,2009, 164(04):1484-1495.

⑥ CATTS VS, WONG J, FILLMAN SG, et al. Increased Expression of Astrocyte Markers in Schizophrenia:Association with Neuroinflammation[J].*Aust N Z J Psychiatry*,2014, 48(08):722-734.

inflammatory cytokines, including IL-1β, IL-6 and TNF-α[①], which is in accordance with our results. Therefore, uric acid might directly target brain tissue, especially substantia nigra and hippocampus, thereby exerting anti-inflammatory effect on PD mice.

In conclusion, the present study confirmed that uric acid exhibited a significant neuroprotective effect for dopaminergic neurons in PD mice. The mechanism of uric acid may be associated with Nrf2-ARE-induced inhibition of oxidative damage and neuroinflammation. The study reveals that uric acid may be a promising therapeutic agent for Parkinson's disease treatment. Further investigation is needed to elucidate the mechanisms of Nrf2-ARE in neuroprotective effect by uric acid, especially in Nrf2 knock-out mice.

(Ting-Ting Huang, Dong-Lin Hao, Bo-Na Wu, Lun-Lin Mao, Jin Zhang)
(本文原载于 *Biochemical and Biophysical Research Communications* 2017 年第 1 卷第 7 期)

① MORE SV, KUMAR H, KIM IS, et al. Cellular and Molecular Mediators of Neuroinflammation in the Pathogenesis of Parkinson's Disease[J]. *Mediat Inflamm*, 2013, 2013:952375.

尿酸对 6-羟基多巴胺致大鼠黑质纹状体系统毒性的影响①

目的：评价尿酸对 6-羟基多巴胺致大鼠黑质纹状体系统多巴胺能神经元毒性的影响。

方法：30 只雄性 SD 大鼠，分为生理盐水组（10 只）、100 mg/kg 尿酸组（5 只）、200 mg/kg 尿酸组（10 只）和 250 mg/kg 尿酸组（5 只）。每天 2 次（间隔 2 h），每次腹腔注射生理盐水或尿酸 5 d，于第 6 天第 1 次腹腔注射生理盐水或尿酸后，在立体定向仪指导下，右侧纹状体内两点注射 6-羟基多巴胺。此后继续给予大鼠腹腔注射生理盐水或尿酸 5 d。于注射 6-羟基多巴胺后第 3、第 4 周分别进行自主活动计数，安非他明旋转实验，前肢功能测定。注射 6-羟基多巴胺后第 5 周进行纹状体多巴胺和高香草酸水平测定。

结果：200 mg/kg 尿酸组大鼠自主活动计数 [（14±4）次/2 mins] 明显高于生理盐水组 [（4±5）次/2 mins，$P < 0.01$]；安非他明诱导的旋转实验 100 mg/kg 尿酸组（11.2±4.2）和 200 m/kg 尿酸组每分钟旋转次数（10.8±7.5）显著低于生理盐水组（19.3±5.2，$P < 0.01$）。200 mg/kg 尿酸组前肢功能测定 5 s 内移动 90 cm 的前患肢步数（9.89±3.41）明显高于生理盐水组（4.36±3.72，$P < 0.01$）；200 mg/kg 尿酸组毁损侧纹状体多巴胺（0.29±0.19）、高香草酸水平（1.22±0.5）显著高于生理盐水组多巴胺（0.05±0.03，$P < 0.01$）、高香草酸水平（0.24±0.13，$P < 0.05$）。

结论：适当提高体内的尿酸水平能减轻 6-羟基多巴胺对 SD 大鼠黑质纹状体系统多巴胺能神经元的毒性作用。

关键词：尿酸；6-羟基多巴胺；大鼠；帕金森病；行为学；多巴胺。

———————————

① 本文系苏州市科技发展计划（社会发展及医药）项目（项目编号：200815404）；江苏省高校自然科学基础研究项目（项目编号：08KJB320012）。

Protective Effects of Uric Acid on Nigrostriatal System Injury Induced by 6-hydroxydopamine in Rats

Objective: To investigate the protective effects of uric acid on nigrostriatal system injury induced by 6-hydroxydopamine in rats.

Methods: Thirty male SD rats were divided into four groups. Uric acid of 100 mg/kg, 200 mg/kg, 250 mg/kg were injected intraperitoneally (ip) into 5, 10, 5 rats twice daily at a 2-hour interval for five days and saline was injected ip into 10 rats as controls. At day 6, 6-hydroxydopamine was injected into striatum to establish Parkinson's disease model in rats. Then uric acid was injected ip into three groups and saline into controls for five days. Locomotion test, amphetamineinduced rotation and forepaw adjusting step test were performed at weeks 3 and 4 respectively after injection of 6-hydroxydopamine. HPLC-MS/MS was performed to detect the contents of dopamine and its metabolite homovanillic acid(HVA) in striatum at week 5.

Results: The scores of locomotion in 2 minutes of 200 mg/kg uric acid group(14±4/2 min) was higher significantly than those in the saline group(4±5/2 min, $P<0.01$). The amphetamine-induced rotation number in the 200 mg/kg uric acid group(10.8±7.5) was lower significantly than those in the saline group(19.3±5.2, $P<0.01$). Forepaw adjusting step test scores of 200 mg/kg uric acid group were higher significantly than those in the saline group(9.89±3.41 vs 4.36±3.72, $P<0.01$). HPLC-MS/MS showed that the contents of DA(0.29±0.19) and HVA(1.22±0.5) in injured striatum of 200 mg/kg uric acid group were higher significantly than those in the saline group(0.05±0.03, $P<0.01$; 0.24±0.13, $P<0.05$).

Conclusion: An appropriately elevated level of uric acid may protect the dopamine neuron of nigrostriatal system from injury of 6-hydroxydopamine in rats.

Key words: uric acid; 6-hydroxydopamine; rats; behavior; Parkinson disease; dopamine.

帕金森病是一种以中脑黑质致密部多巴胺能神经元的进行性变性减少为病理特征的慢性进行性疾病。尽管多巴胺能神经元选择性死亡的确切发病机制至今不明,但流行病学、基础实验研究及临床资料均证实有多个因素与 PD 的发病密切相关,如杀虫剂、1-甲基-4-苯基-1,2,3,6-四氢吡啶;含有抗氧化剂的饮食减少及体内尤其是黑质纹状体系统清除自由基物质水平的降低所导致的氧化应激反应的增强;线粒体功能障碍;等等①②③。尿酸是一种重要的生理性的天然抗氧化剂、铁螯合剂、自由基清除剂。研究发现,PD 发病率与低血尿酸水平有关④⑤,PD 患者黑质纹状体及血尿酸水平显著降低⑥⑦⑧。为此,我们尝试适当提高大鼠尿酸水平,观察尿酸对 6-羟基多巴胺致大鼠黑质纹状体系统毒性的影响。

一、材料与方法

1. 试验分组及动物模型的制备

(1) 将 180~220 g 雄性 SD 大鼠(苏州大学实验动物中心)46 只随机分为 2 组。第一组(非造模组)16 只,随机分为生理盐水组($N=4$),100 mg/kg 尿酸组($N=4$),200 mg/kg 尿酸组($N=4$),250 mg/kg 尿酸组($N=4$)。进行干预之前尾静脉取血测定大鼠的血尿酸水平,然后按照组别进行如下操作:每天 2 次(间隔 2 h),每次腹腔注射生理盐水(0.25 mL/kg)和尿酸(100,200,250 mg/kg)10 d,于第 11 天测定活体大鼠的血尿酸水平,处死后测定纹状体尿酸水平。

(2) 第二组(造模组)30 只随机分为生理盐水组($N=10$),100 mg/kg

① LOCKWOOD AH.Pesticides and Parkinsonism: is there an Etiological Link? [J].*Curr Opin Neurol*, 2000,13(06): 687-690.

② BALLARD PA,TETRUD JW,LANGSTON JW.Permanent Human Parkinsonism Due to 1-methyl-4-phenyl-1,2,3,6-tetrahydropyridine(MPTP): Seven Cases[J].*Neurology*,1985,35(07): 949-956.

③ JANDKY R, OGITA K, PASQUALOTTO BA, et al. Glutathione and Signal Transduction in the Mammalian CNS[J].*J Neurochem*,1999,73(03):889-902.

④ DE LAU LM,KOUDSTAAL PJ,HOFMAN A,et al.Serum Uric Acid Levels and the Risk of Parkinson Disease[J].*Ann Neurol*,2005,58(05): 797-800.

⑤ WEISSKOPF MG,O'REILLY E,CHEN H,et al.Plasma Urate and Risk of Parkinson's Disease[J].*Am J Epidemiol*,2007,166(05): 561-567.

⑥ CHURCH WH,WARD VL.Uric Acid is Reduced in the Substantia Nigra in Parkinson's Disease: Effect on Dopamine Oxidation[J].*Brain Res Bull*,1994,33(04): 419-425.

⑦ ANNANMAKI T,MUURONEN A,MURROS K.Low Plasma Uric Acid Level in Parkinson's Disease [J].*Mov Disord*,2007,22(08): 1133-1137.

⑧ 王丽君,罗蔚锋,王恒会,等.帕金病患者血尿酸水平[J].中华神经科杂志,2008,41(03): 157-158.

尿酸组（$N=5$）,200 mg/kg 尿酸组（$N=10$）,250 mg/kg 尿酸组（$N=5$）。每天 2 次分别腹腔注射生理盐水或上述不同剂量的尿酸 5 d,于第 6 天第 1 次腹腔注射生理盐水或不同剂量的尿酸后,3.6% 水合氯醛 1 mL/100 g 腹腔注射麻醉 SD 大鼠。应用 KOPF 立体定向仪（KOPF 公司）,参照包新民的《大鼠脑立体定向图谱》①,确定单侧纹状体两点的坐标位置。第一点：前囟前 0.7 mm,中线右侧 3.0 mm,硬膜下 4.5 mm；第二点：前囟后 0.2 mm,中线右 2.6 mm,硬膜下 6.0 mm。分别在以上两点处各注射 3.5 μL 的 6-OHDA 盐溶液。注药速度为 0.5 μL/min,留针 5 mins 后以 1 μL/min 的速度退针。此后继续给予大鼠腹腔注射生理盐水或不同剂量的尿酸 5 d；纹状体内注射 6-OHDA 后第 3 周进行自主活动计数,第 4 周进行前肢功能测定,第 5 周检测纹状体多巴胺和高香草酸水平。

2. 大鼠（非造模组）血液、纹状体尿酸检测

大鼠断尾采血 1 mL,置于抗凝管中。以 3 000 r/min 离心 10 mins。取上清 300 μL 至于 EP 管中,置入 −70 ℃冰箱中保存。将大鼠断头处死,冰台上取出纹状体,称重。加入生理盐水（1 mg∶10 μL）,冰浴上匀浆研磨 5 mins,15 000 r/min,4 ℃离心 15 mins,取上清液 200 μL。采用全自动生化分析仪（美国 DADE Behring 公司）测定尿酸水平。

3. 大鼠（造模组）动物行为学检测

（1）自主活动计数：术后 3 周应用大鼠自主活动箱记数 2 mins 内大鼠自主活动次数,连续测 3 次,取其平均值。

（2）术后 4 周安非他明（中国药品生物制品检定所）诱发旋转试验：以 10 mg/kg 体重的剂量注射于大鼠项部皮下。相同环境下计数 60 mins 内旋转次数,从而计算平均每分钟转数。

（3）前肢功能测定：6-OHDA 注射后第 4 周采用 Chang 等②的试验方法,试验者一手固定大鼠躯体后半部和后肢,使其离地,另一手固定一侧前肢使另一前肢着地,以大鼠正手方向斜向一侧移动大鼠（5 s 内移动 90 cm）,记录移动时着地侧前肢步数,测量患侧上肢的跨步数。

---

① DE LAU LM,KOUDSTAAL PJ,HOFMAN A,et al.Serum Uric Acid Levels and the Risk of Parkinson Disease[J].*Ann Neurol*,2005,58(05)：797−800.

② CHANG JW, WACHTEL SR, YONG D, et al. Biochemical and Anatomical Character-rization of Forepaw Adjusting Steps in Rat Models of Parkinson Disease：Studies on Medial Forebrain Bundle and Striatal Lesions[J]. *Neurosci*,1999,88(02)：617−628.

4. 大鼠（造模组）纹状体多巴胺浓度的测定

6-OHDA 注射后第 5 周,每组取 5 只用高效液相色谱-质谱连用(HPLC-MS/MS)(美国 Agilent-AB 公司)检测。将大鼠迅速断头、取脑,放入预冷的生理盐水中,去除脑膜和血液,滤纸吸干水分,在冰皿上剥离纹状体,称重后置于匀浆器中,加入样本提取液(1 mg∶10 μL)在冰水浴中制成匀浆,于16 000 r/min(4 ℃)离心 15 mins,取上清液 50 μL 进样分析。

5. 统计学分析

所有数据采用"$\bar{x}\pm s$"表示,用 SPSS11.5 统计软件统计分析模块进行单因素方差分析(analysis of variance,ANOVA)。

二、结果

1. 不同组别的大鼠（非造模组）血液和纹状体尿酸的水平结果

未进行干预之前,4 组之间的大鼠血尿酸水平差异无统计学意义($P>$ 0.05)。腹腔注射尿酸 10 d 后,100 mg/kg 尿酸组、200 mg/kg 尿酸组、250 mg/kg尿酸组血尿酸水平明显高于生理盐水组($P<0.05$)。10 d 后,测定大鼠纹状体的尿酸水平,100 mg/kg 组、200 mg/kg 组、250 mg/kg 纹状体尿酸水平明显高于生理盐水组($P<0.05$,表 1)。

表 1   4 组大鼠(非造模组)尿酸水平比较(μmol/L, $\bar{x}\pm s$)

组别	动物数	干预前(血液)	第 10 天(血液)	第 10 天(纹状体)
生理盐水组	4	38.20±2.50	39.80±4.79	0.83±0.26
100 mg/kg 尿酸组	4	38.70±11.70	61.50±7.86[a]	1.60±0.41[a]
200 mg/kg 尿酸组	4	37.50±15.70	58.70±18.67[a]	2.20±0.51[a]
250 mg/kg 尿酸组	4	37.50±7.14	66.00±13.36[a]	2.90±0.30[a]

注：与生理盐水组相比,[a]$P<0.05$。

2. 大鼠自主活动计数结果

200 mg/kg 尿酸组大鼠自主活动计数[(14±4)次/2 mins]显著高于生理盐水组[(4±5)次/2 mins,$P<0.01$],100 mg/kg 尿酸组[(10±8)次/2 mins]和250 mg/kg组自主活动计数[(11±7)次/2mins]虽然高于生理盐水组,但无统计学意义($P>0.05$)。

163

3. 安非他明诱发旋转试验

安非他明诱导的旋转实验100 mg/kg尿酸组（11.2±4.2）和200 mg/kg尿酸组每分钟旋转次数（10.8±7.5）显著低于生理盐水组（19.3±5.2，$P<0.01$）。

4. 前肢功能测定结果

大鼠5 s内移动90 cm的患侧肢体平均步数200 mg/kg尿酸组（9.9±3.4）明显高于生理盐水组（4.3±3.7，$P<0.01$）。100 mg/kg尿酸组（5.4±4.4）和250 mg/kg尿酸组（2.9±2.7）分别与生理盐水组相比较差异无统计学意义。

5. 大鼠（造模组）纹状体DA水平检测结果

毁损侧纹状体较对侧纹状体多巴胺水平NS组下降约88%，100 mg/kg组下降约80%，200 mg/kg组下降约68%，250 mg/kg组下降约90%。在生理盐水组，100 mg/kg组，200 mg/kg组，250 mg/kg组，毁损侧纹状体较对侧纹状体多巴胺、高香草酸水平差异有统计学意义（$P<0.01$，$P<0.05$）。200 mg/kg组毁损侧纹状体多巴胺（0.29+0.19）、高香草酸水平（1.22±0.5）高于生理盐水组多巴胺（0.05±0.03，$P<0.01$）、高香草酸水平（0.24±0.13，$P<0.05$）。100 mg/kg，250 mg/kg组毁损侧纹状体多巴胺与生理盐水组相比差异无统计学意义（$P>0.05$）（表2）。

表2　四组大鼠纹状体多巴胺浓度和高香草酸浓度的比较（$ng/mg, \bar{x}±s$）

组别	动物数	毁损侧		对侧	
		多巴胺	高香草酸	多巴胺	高香草酸
生理盐水组	5	0.05±0.03	0.24±0.13	0.44±0.24[c]	1.88±0.24[d]
100 mg/kg 尿酸组	5	0.16±0.18	0.74±0.73	0.83±0.78[ac]	2.23±0.20[bd]
200 mg/kg 尿酸组	5	0.29±0.19[a]	1.22±0.52[b]	0.91±0.18[ac]	2.75±2.67[ad]
250 mg/kg 尿酸组	5	0.06±0.07	0.39±0.28	0.58±0.21[c]	1.93±0.28[d]

注：与生理盐水组相比，[a] $P<0.05$，[b] $P<0.05$；与毁损侧相比，[c] $P<0.01$，[d] $P<0.05$。

三、讨论

尿酸是嘌呤代谢产物，大多数哺乳动物的尿酸在肝脏经尿酸盐氧化酶分解成尿囊素,体内尿酸的浓度由嘌呤的摄入量、尿酸的生物合成及其排泄速率决定①,我们测定正常未干预大鼠(非造模组)血尿酸水平,发现各组大鼠血尿酸水平差异无统计学意义,与 Johnson 等②的研究相似。Hooper 等③研究发现通过腹腔注射尿酸来提高大鼠尿酸水平,能显著改善多发性硬化(MS)动物模型的行为表现。在对大鼠腹腔注射尿酸 10 d 后,我们发现100 mg/kg,200 mg/kg 和 250 mg/kg 尿酸组大鼠血尿酸水平、纹状体的尿酸水平均明显高于生理盐水组,说明通过腹腔注射尿酸可以提高大鼠血尿酸和基底节区的尿酸水平。

尿酸是一种天然的抗氧化剂,能清除人体内 60% 的自由基,具有抗氧化作用和神经保护作用④。200 mg/kg 组大鼠自主活动计数和患肢前肢功能测定显著高于生理盐水组,安非他明诱导的旋转实验 200 mg/kg 组每分钟旋转次数显著低于生理盐水组,提示尿酸可以改善大鼠的运动症状。200 mg/kg组毁损侧纹状体 DA、HVA 水平显著高于生理盐水组,与自主活动计数、安非他明诱导的旋转试验和前肢功测定行为学研究结果一致,提示尿酸具有对多巴胺能神经元的保护作用。Luo 等⑤研究发现适当提高脑组织中的尿酸水平,能够减轻 MPTP 对小鼠多巴胺神经元的损伤,与我们的研究结果一致。目前认为尿酸主要通过以下三种机制发挥其对多巴胺能神经元的保护作用:(1)尿酸清除超氧化物、羟基和单态氧。尿酸阻止超氧化物歧化酶的降解,有助于清除超氧化物⑥;(2)尿酸能有效清除过氧化亚硝酸盐,阻止硝基化反应及 DNA 的氧化损伤,修复 DNA 的碱基突变,对抗氧

① MOUNT DB,KWON CY,ZANDI-NEJAD K.Renal Urate Transport[J].*Rheum Dis Clin North Am*,2006,32(02):313-331.

② JOHNSON RJ,KANG DH,FEIG D,et al.Is there a Pathogenetic Role for Uric Acid In Hypertension and Cardiovascular and Renal Disease? [J]. *Hypertension*,2003,41(06): 1183-1190.

③ HOOPER DC,SCOTT GS,ZBOREK A,et al. Uric acid,a Peroxynitrite Scavenger,Inhibits CNS Inflammation,Blood CNS Barrier Permeability Changes,and Tissue Damage in a Mouse model of Multiple Sclerosis[J].*Faseb J*,2000,14(05):691-698.

④ JENNER P.Oxidative Stress in Parkinson's Disease[J].*Ann Neurol*,2003,53(Suppl 3): S26-36.

⑤ LUO WF,SCHWARZSCHILD MA,XU K.Urate attenuates MPTP Induced Dopmainergic Toxicity in Mice[C].The Society for Neuroscience 37th Annual Meeting,2007.San Diego,California,USA.

⑥ AMES BN,CATHCART R,SCHWIERS E,et al. Uric Acid Provides an Antioxidant Defense in Humans against Oxidant and Radical Caused Aging and Cancer:a hypothesis[J].*Proc Natl Acad Sci USA*,1981,78(11): 6858-6862.

化应激[1];(3) DA:Fe^{3+}复合物启动细胞膜的脂质过氧化,导致多巴胺能神经元的死亡。尿酸和铁离子形成复合物,特别是与三价铁离子,尿酸能抑制铁离子介导的氧化反应。基底节区尿酸水平的丢失,细胞内游离铁离子的增加,加速铁离子介导的氧化损伤[2]。

我们观察到 200 mg/kg 尿酸组水平行为学改善显著,多巴胺递质含量降低最少,认为 200 mg/kg 尿酸组具有最佳神经保护治疗作用。250 mg/kg 尿酸组其保护作用降低,提示尿酸发挥神经保护作用具有一定的范围,若超过此范围,其保护作用降低,甚至可能出现毒性作用,可能因为一定的条件下尿酸可通过一系列反应生成自由基,增加脂质的氧化作用,介导多种氧化前体产生毒性作用[3]。本研究提示,尿酸只有在一定的范围内才能具有多巴胺能神经元保护作用,具体机制有待于进一步研究。

本研究应用可靠的 6-OHDA 大鼠 PD 模型证实,适当提高尿酸水平能够减轻 6-OHDA 对大鼠黑质纹状体系统的毒性作用。尿酸作为抗氧化剂和自由基清除剂具有明确的生物学功能,但应如何控制尿酸水平来达到预防或延缓 PD 的发生发展,还有待于进一步的研究。

(王丽君　罗蔚锋　王恒会　倪贵华　叶　艳　李　丹　刘春风)

(本文原载于《中华医学杂志》2010 年第 90 卷第 19 期)

①　INOUE S, KAWANISHI S. Oxidative DNA Damage Induced by Simultaneous Gen-eration of Nitric Oxide and Superoxide[J]. *FEBS Lett*,1995,371(01):86-88.

②　CHURCH WH, WARD VL. Uric Acid is Reduced in the Substantia Nigra in Parkinson's Disease:Effect on Dopamine Oxidation[J].*Brain Res Bull*,1994,33(04):419-425.

③　KANNELLIS J, KANG DH. Uric Acid as a Mediator of Endothelial Dysfunction, Inflammation and Vascular Disease[J].*Semin Nephrol*,2005,25(01):39.

不同剂量尿酸保护性治疗帕金森病大鼠对炎性因子、肾、关节及血管内皮的影响①

目的：探讨不同剂量尿酸对帕金森病大鼠炎性因子、肾、关节及血管内皮的影响。

方法：将 30 只 SD 大鼠分为 5 组，分别予生理盐水、尿酸 50、100、200、400 mg/kg 连续腹腔注射 10 天，每天 2 次。于第 5 天第 1 次腹腔注射生理盐水和尿酸后，对右侧纹状体缓慢注入 6-OHDA，建立帕金森病大鼠模型。于第 5、第 10 天第 2 次注射后 1 h 采取尾静脉血；于第 10 天采血后处死大鼠，迅速取其脑、肾、踝关节、颈总动脉、腹主动脉，分别检测血、组织上清液的 CRP、IL-6、TNF-α 和肌酐。

结果：

（1）CRP、IL-6、TNF-α 和肌酐：血浆和组织上清液的 CRP、IL-6、TNF-α 水平各组之间比较无统计学差异，血浆肌酐 400 mg/kg 组较生理盐水组显著升高（$P<0.05$）。

（2）病理 HE 染色：400 mg/kg 组肾脏轻度损伤改变，其余各组病理正常；踝关节各浓度组滑膜均无明显炎症改变；颈总动脉和腹主动脉各浓度组均无明显动脉粥样硬化和炎症改变。

结论：适当尿酸水平的提高对 6-OHDA-PD 大鼠的肌酐、CRP、IL-6、TNF-α 及肾脏、关节、动脉血管无明显影响。

关键词：尿酸；帕金森病；6-OHDA；Cr；CRP；IL-6；TNF-α。

---

① 本文系江苏省自然科学基金资助项目（项目编号：BK2010229）；苏州市科技支撑计划基金资助项目（项目编号：SS201112）。

Effects of Different Doses of Uric Acid on Inflammatory Cytokines, Kidneys, Joints and Vascular Endothelium in Rats with Parkinson's Disease

Objective: To explore the effects of different doses of uric acid on inflammatory cytokines, kidneys, joints and vascular endothelium in rats with Parkinson's disease.

Methods: Thirty SD rats were divided into five groups, 6 in each group. normal saline or uric acid at 50 mg/kg, 100 mg/kg, 200 mg/kg, 400 mg/kg were intraperitoneal injected for ten days respectively in each group, 2 times a day. On the fifth day after the first intraperitoneal injection of saline or uric acid, 6-OHDA was slowly injected into the right striatum of every rat to set up Parkinson's disease models. One hour after the second injection on the fifth and tenth day, tail vein blood of every rat was drawn. All rats were killed on the tenth day after tail vein blood was drawn. Kidney, ankle, carotid artery, abdominal aorta were then quickly extracted and fixed in 10% formalin. CRP, IL-6, TNF-α, and creatinine from blood or tissue supernatant were tested.

Results:

(1) CRP, IL-6 or TNF-α, from plasma or tissue supernatant, didn't show any significant difference among different treatment groups. Plasma creatinine in the uric acid 400 mg/kg group was markedly higher than in the saline group ($P<0.05$).

(2) Kidney from the 400 mg/kg uric acid group showed mild damage while kidney from other groups were normal. Synovium of ankle from all groups showed no obvious inflammatory changes. Carotid artery and abdominal aorta from all groups showed no apparently atherosclerosis and inflammatory changes.

Conclusion: Appropriately increasing of uric acid level has no obvious influence on creatinine, CRP, IL-6, TNF-α, kidneys, joints or arterial in 6-OHDA lesioned Parkinson rats.

Key words: uric acid; Parkinson's disease; 6-OHDA; Cr; CRP; IL-6; TNF-α.

近年来流行病学及临床研究发现帕金森病发病与尿酸水平密切相关，血尿酸水平相对低的人群 PD 的发生率较高①。PD 患者血、脑脊液及黑质纹状体尿酸水平明显低于健康对照者②③④。在 PD 患者中，尿酸水平相对高的患者比尿酸水平低的患者病情进展缓慢⑤。笔者的前期体外及在体研究也进一步证明，提高尿酸水平对多巴胺能神经元具有保护作用⑥⑦。另一方面，高尿酸血症患者常伴有 IL-6、TNF-α 等炎性因子水平的升高，以及肾、关节、动脉内皮细胞的损害⑧⑨⑩。本研究观察用于保护多巴胺能神经元不同剂量的尿酸对炎性因子水平，以及肾、关节、动脉内皮的影响，报道如下。

一、材料与方法

1. 一般材料

清洁级健康雄性 SD 大鼠 30 只，体重 180~220 g，由苏州大学实验动物中心提供。

2. 主要试剂及仪器

6-OHDA（Sigma 公司），IL-6 ELISA 试剂盒（北京欣博盛生物科技有限公司），TNF-α ELISA 试剂盒（R&D Systems，USA）。酶标仪（广东丹利科技有限公司）、光学显微镜（OLYMPUS，model：BX41TF）。

---

① DE LAU LM, KOUDSTAAL PJ, HOFMAN A, et al. Serum Uric Acid Levels and the Risk of Parkinson's Diease[J]. *Ann Neurol*, 2005, 58(05)：797−800.

② 王丽君，罗蔚锋，王恒会，等. 帕金森病患者血尿酸水平[J]. 中华神经科杂志，2008, 41(03)：157−158.

③ CHURCH WH, WARD VL. Uric Acid is Reduced in the Substantia Nigra in Parkinson's Disease：Effect on Dopamine Oxidation[J]. *Brain Res Bull*, 1994, 33(04)：419−425.

④ FITZMAURICE PS, ANG L, GUTTMAN M, et al. Nigral Glutathione Deficiency is not Specific for Idiopathic Parkinson's Disease[J]. *Mov Disord*, 2003, 18(09)：969−976.

⑤ WEISSKOPF MG, O'REILLY E, CHEN H, et al. Plasma Urate and Risk of Parkinson's Disease[J]. *Am J Epidemiol*, 2007, 166(05)：561−567.

⑥ 叶艳，罗蔚锋，朱婷鸽，等. 尿酸减轻 6-羟基多巴胺对 PC12 细胞的毒性作用[J]. 中国临床神经科学，2010, 18(02)：135−139.

⑦ 王丽君，罗蔚锋，王恒会，等. 尿酸对 6-羟基多巴胺致大鼠黑质纹状体系统毒性的影响[J]. 中华医学杂志，2010, 90(19)：1362−1365.

⑧ JOHNSON RJ, KANG DH, FEIG D, et al. Is there a Pathogenetic Role for Uric Acid in Hypertension and Cardiovascular and Renal Disease? [J]. *Hypertension*, 2003, 41(06)：1183−1190.

⑨ 王庆文，刘志红. 高尿酸血症与慢性肾脏病的关系[J]. 中华医学杂志，2012, 92(08)：510−511.

⑩ ZHANG Z, BIAN L, CHOI Y. Serum Uric Acid：a Marker of Metabolic Syndrome and Subclinical Atherosclerosis in Korean Men[J]. *Angiology*, 2011, 63(06)：420−428.

3. 方法

（1）实验大鼠分组及给药方法

将 30 只 SD 大鼠分为 5 组，每组 6 只，分别予生理盐水、尿酸 50、100、200、400 mg/kg 连续腹腔注射 10 天，每天 2 次。于第 5 天第 1 次腹腔注射生理盐水后，右侧纹状体缓慢注入 6-OHDA，建立帕金森病大鼠模型。于第 5、第 10 天第 2 次注射后 1 h 采取尾静脉血；于第 10 天采血后处死大鼠，迅速取其肾、踝关节、颈总动脉、腹主动脉置于 10% 甲醛中固定以备制作石蜡切片，进行 HE 染色；取额叶、小脑皮质、纹状体、海马、中脑、中脑和肾置于 -80 ℃ 冰箱以备超声裂解提取取上清液。分别检测血及组织上清液的肌酐、CRP、IL-6、TNF-α。

（2）6-OHDA 帕金森病大鼠模型的制作

麻醉 SD 大鼠，将大鼠固定在立体定向架上，剃去大鼠头顶处毛发。用 75% 乙醇消毒头皮后，正中纵行切开头皮，分离皮下组织，暴露颅骨，找到前囟，以前囟为基准点，确定右侧纹状体坐标，选择两个位点：① 前囟后 0.7 mm，右侧 3.0 mm，进针深度 4.5 mm；② 前囟后 0.2 mm，右侧 2.6 mm，进针深度 6.0mm。每点注射 6-OHDA 5 µg（10µg 6-OHDA 加入 5 µL 含 0.02% 抗坏血酸的生理盐水中），注射速度 0.5 µL/min，注射结束留针 5 mins，撤针速度 1 mm/min，拔针后，缝合关闭伤口，消毒，放入笼中继续饲养。

（3）组织超声裂解取上清液

保存于 -80 ℃ 冰箱中的脑组织（取 20 mg 左右）和肾脏（取 100 mg 左右），溶于 RIPA 组织裂解液（1 mg : 5µL），超声裂解后静置 30 mins，再 4 ℃、2000 g、15 mins 离心后取上清液。

（4）检测肌酐（Cr）和炎症因子（CRP、IL-6、TNF-α）

Cr 采用肌氨酸氧化酶法，试剂来自日本世诺临床诊断制品株式会社，使用东芝 TBA-120FR 测定；CRP 采用免疫比浊法，试剂来自 Orion Diagnostica Oy，使用 Kone Specific 分析仪测定；IL-6 和 TNF-α 采用 ELISA 法检测（IL-6 试剂来自北京欣博盛生物科技有限公司，TNF-α 试剂来自 R&D Systems），按试剂盒说明书方法稀释、加样、洗板、孵育，测定 450 nm 波长处的吸光度（A 值），以 A 值为横坐标，标准品浓度为纵坐标，绘制标准曲线，根据标准曲线计算各样品浓度。

（5）HE 染色观察肾脏、踝关节、颈总动脉病理改变

10% 甲醛固定组织常规方法脱水、包埋、切片、HE 染色，显微镜下观察。

4. 统计学方法

采用 SPSS 17.0 软件分析实验数据,数据以均数±标准差($\bar{x}\pm s$)表示,组间比较应用单因素方差分析,以 $P<0.05$ 为差异有统计学意义。

二、结果

1. 不同剂量尿酸对血 CRP、TNF-α、Cr 水平的影响

对各组分别予生理盐水及 50、100、200、400 mg/kg 尿酸连续腹腔注射 10 天,各组第 5、第 10 天的血 CRP、TNF-α、Cr 水平见表 1。CRP 水平在各组间比较无统计学差异($P>0.05$)。随着腹腔注射尿酸剂量的增加及天数的延长,TNF-α 水平在不同的组别中有增高的趋势,但无统计学差异($P>0.05$);Cr 水平变化相对明显,第 5、第 10 天 400 mg/kg 尿酸组 Cr 水平显著高于生理盐水组($P<0.05$)。

表 1　各组第 5、第 10 天血 CRP、TNF-α、Cr 水平($\bar{x}\pm s$)

组别	CRP(mg/L)		TNF-α(pg/mL)		Cr(μmol/L)	
	5 天	10 天	5 天	10 天	5 天	10 天
生理盐水组	4.15±0.10	4.18±0.18	80.33±17.38	82.55±15.15	14.67±3.20	15.50±3.83
50 mg/kg 尿酸组	4.18±0.15	4.23±0.21	83.11±16.79	86.44±9.76	15.83±2.48	16.33±4.23
100 mg/kg 尿酸组	4.27±0.18	4.27±0.12	85.89±22.77	90.89±17.05	16.67±3.56	18.67±3.27
200 mg/kg 尿酸组	4.28±0.15	4.37±0.10	88.67±22.78	92.56±10.68	17.17±1.72	19.50±3.51
400 mg/kg 尿酸组	4.28±0.13	4.38±0.27	88.67±22.97	94.78±7.20	19.83±1.47[*]	19.67±1.86[*]

注:与生理盐水组相比,[*] $P<0.05$。

2. 不同剂量尿酸对脑组织 TNF-α 水平的影响

各组第 10 天大脑皮质、小脑皮质、左纹状体、海马、左侧中脑、右侧中脑 TNF-α 水平见表 2。不同浓度尿酸注射组大脑皮质、小脑皮质、左纹状体、海马、左侧中脑、右侧中脑组织上清 TNF-α 值分别与生理盐水对照组比较差异均无统计学意义($P>0.05$)。

表 2　各组第 10 天大脑皮质、小脑皮质、左纹状体、海马、
左右侧中脑组织上清 TNF-α 水平($\bar{x}\pm s$, pg/mg)

组别	大脑皮质	小脑皮质	左纹状体	海马	左侧中脑	右侧中脑
生理盐水组	2.04±0.81	2.25±0.89	3.22±1.07	4.31±1.60	3.22±1.60	3.57±0.94
50 mg/kg 尿酸组	2.90±1.64	2.32±0.62	3.56±1.41	3.65±1.11	3.72±1.59	3.61±0.79
100 mg/kg 尿酸组	3.15±1.72	3.10±0.75	3.72±0.82	4.58±1.87	3.92±2.18	4.09±1.77
200 mg/kg 尿酸组	3.19±1.14	3.37±1.23	4.20±0.81	5.31±2.39	4.07±1.78	4.10±2.10
400 mg/kg 尿酸组	3.24±1.18	3.48±0.16	4.31±1.60	5.38±2.30	5.40±3.41	4.78±2.77

3. 不同剂量尿酸对肾脏 CRP、IL-6、TNF-α、Cr 水平的影响

各组第 10 天肾脏组织 TNF-α、IL-6、TNF-α 和 Cr 水平见表 3。TNF-α、IL-6、TNF-α、Cr 各组之间无统计学差异($P>0.05$)。

表 3　各组第 10 天肾脏 CRP、IL-6、TNF-α、Cr 水平($\bar{x}\pm s$)

组别	CRP(mg/L)	IL-6(pg/mg)	TNF-α(pg/mg)	Cr(μmol/L)
生理盐水组	11.28±2.86	29.84±16.22	12.44±6.83	104.33±3.44
50 mg/kg 尿酸组	11.07±1.65	30.73±20.05	14.31±4.61	105.67±4.23
100 mg/kg 尿酸组	11.30±2.75	35.01±19.05	14.36±14.06	106.33±2.88
200 mg/kg 尿酸组	11.37±2.53	36.48±22.76	15.31±5.09	109.33±4.27
400 mg/kg 尿酸组	11.77±2.11	40.98±21.98	17.46±9.81	109.33±4.55

4. 不同剂量尿酸对肾脏、踝关节、颈总动脉、腹主动脉内皮 HE 染色的影响

（1）肾脏 HE 染色

各浓度肾脏组织中均无尿酸盐结晶沉积,无内皮细胞和系膜细胞增生。其中 400 mg/kg 组 HE 染色可见肾脏轻度损伤改变(肾小球毛细血管丛轻度扩张,近曲肾小管上皮细胞水变性或气球样变,管腔内可见蛋白管型或细胞管型)(图 1,图 2,图 3)。

（2）踝关节 HE 染色

踝关节各浓度组中均无尿酸盐结晶沉积,滑膜组织无充血水肿,无红细胞、中性粒细胞及纤维素渗出,滑膜上皮排列整齐,无断裂(图 4)。

（3）颈总动脉和腹主动脉 HE 染色

颈总动脉和腹主动脉各浓度组均无明显动脉粥样硬化和炎症改变。无明显内膜及肌层增厚,各层无淋巴细胞和浆细胞为主的炎性细胞浸润,无粥样硬化的脂纹和纤维斑块(图 5,图 6)。

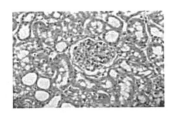

图 1 0 mg/kg 尿酸组肾脏
(HE 染色,×400)

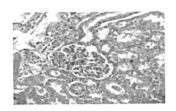

图 2 200 mg/kg 尿酸组肾脏
(HE 染色,×400)

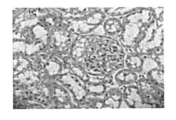

图 3 400 mg/kg 尿酸组肾脏
(HE 染色,×400)

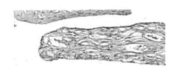

图 4 400 mg/kg 尿酸组踝关节
(HE 染色,×400)

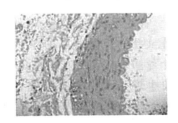

图 5 200 mg/kg 尿酸组颈总动脉
(HE 染色,×400)

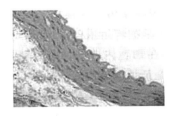

图 6 200 mg/kg 尿酸组肾脏腹主动脉
(HE 染色,×400)

三、讨论

尿酸对多巴胺能神经元具有保护作用。Chen 等①应用敲除尿酸氧化酶（urate oxidase,UOx,降解尿酸为尿囊素）基因 6-OHDA 帕金森病小鼠模型，通过测定其中脑黑质多巴胺能神经元数目、纹状体多巴胺含量和行为改变，发现尿酸水平的升高可以减轻 6-OHDA 对黑质纹状体系统多巴胺能神经元的毒性作用。相反，UOx 过表达的小鼠，尿酸水平显著降低，则加剧了 6-OHDA 对黑质纹状体多巴胺能神经元的损害，说明尿酸可以减轻 6-OHDA 对多巴胺能神经元的毒性作用；朱红灿等②研究发现，腹腔注射适当剂量的尿酸可改善 6-OHDA-PD 大鼠学习记忆能力；本研究前期的体外研究结果也表明，100~400 μmol/L 尿酸可显著减轻 6-OHDA 作用 6、12、24 h 后造成的 PC12 细胞生存率下降，减少 6-OHDA 导致 caspase-3 激活，从而降低细胞的凋亡③。Gong 等④发现腹腔注射尿酸可以提高血浆和脑组织中的尿酸水平，能够增加谷胱甘肽水平和超氧化物歧化酶活性，降低丙二醛在 6-OHDA 帕金森病 SD 大鼠纹状体内的聚积，结果提示尿酸对中脑黑质多巴胺能神经元具有保护作用，与其调节 Akt/GSK3β 信号通路功能有关。王丽君等⑤发现 100 mg/kg、200 mg/kg 尿酸处理的 6-OHDA 帕金森病 SD 大鼠组较正常生理盐水组行为学改善显著，纹状体多巴胺含量降低最少，认为 100 mg/kg、200 mg/kg 尿酸组具有最佳多巴胺能神经元保护作用，250 mg/kg 尿酸组其保护作用减弱，提示尿酸发挥神经保护作用具有一定的范围，若超过此范围，保护作用降低甚至可能出现毒性作用。

尿酸是人体主要的抗氧化剂之一，能够清除自由基及螯合金属离子，减

① Chen X, Burdett T, Desjardins C, et al. Disrupted and Transgenic Urate Oxidase Alter Urate and Dopaminergic Neurodegeneration[J].*Proc Natl Acad Sci USA*,2013,110(01)：300-305.

② 朱红灿,耿利娇,蔡春生,等.尿酸对帕金森病大鼠学习记忆能力的影响及其机制[J].中华实验外科杂志,2010,27(02)：227-229.

③ 叶艳,罗蔚锋,朱婷鸽,等.尿酸减轻 6-羟基多巴胺对 PC12 细胞的毒性作用[J].中国临床神经科学,2010,18(02)：135-139.

④ GONG L,ZHANG Q,ZHANG N,et al. Neuroprtection by Urate on 6-OHDA-lesioned Rat Model of Parkinson's Diease: Linking to Akt/GSK3β Signaling Pathway[J].*J Neurochem*,2012,123(05)：876-885.

⑤ 王丽君,罗蔚锋,王恒会,等.尿酸对 6-羟基多巴胺致大鼠黑质纹状体系统毒性的影响[J].中华医学杂志,2010,90(19)：1362-1365.

少体内氧化应激的水平①。流行病学及临床研究结果均提示尿酸对帕金森病具有保护作用,适当相对高水平的尿酸能够显著减少 PD 的发生,然而,高水平尿酸与炎症因子水平的增高、动脉粥样硬化、高血压、冠心病、脑卒中、痛风、关节和肾脏损害密切相关。在高尿酸血症(hyperuricemia,HUA)患者中,有临床症状的肾损害占 41%,但尸检几乎都有肾损害,肾小管损害较突出。本研究发现血浆肌酐 400 mg/kg 组较生理盐水组显著升高,HE 染色发现 400 mg/kg 组肾小球毛细血管丛轻度扩张,近曲肾小管上皮细胞水变性或气球样变,管腔内可见蛋白管型或细胞管型,肾脏发生轻度损伤改变,表明尿酸水平过高会对肾脏产生损坏作用。人体中 70% 的尿酸经肾脏排泄,主要通过人尿酸转运蛋白(human urate transporter protein,hUTP)在细胞内外进行跨膜转运;hUTP 基因位于第 17 号染色体的短臂上,含有 11 个外显子,分为 3 种亚型,属于贯穿细胞膜脂质的离子通道,具有高度的选择性,广泛存在于体内多种组织细胞膜中,其中在肾脏中的含量最高②。尿酸更容易在肾脏中蓄积而造成肾脏损害,可能与 hUTP 这一分布特点有关。

本研究检测的炎性因子包括 IL-6、TNF-α 和 CRP,它们分别是机体炎性反应、应激反应及非特异炎症反应的敏感标志物。高尿酸血症与炎性因子水平升高、血管内皮损害密切相关,可能与以下因素有关。

1. 尿酸在血液中物理溶解度较低,高尿酸血症时尿酸微结晶容易析出,沉积于血管壁,引起局部炎症。在炎症反应期间 IL-6 与 TNF-α 可以相互作用,TNF-α 促使 IL-6 的产生和释放,IL-6 又可以对 TNF-α 发挥调节作用;同时 IL-6、TNF-α 作为刺激物又可共同促进肝脏合成及释放急性期蛋白 CRP,从而导致 CRP 的增高③。

2. 尿酸是嘌呤、黄嘌呤氧化酶代谢途径的产物,尿酸的生成过程伴有氧自由基的产生。氧自由基增多加重氧化应激反应,而氧化应激反应是血管内皮功能损害的一个重要因素。

3. 尿酸在血管平滑肌细胞内通过激活 NF-KD 从而激活单核细胞趋化

① HINK HU,SANTANAM N,DIKALOV S,et al. Peroxidase Properties of Extracellular Superoxide Dismutase:Role of Uric Acid in Modulating in Vivo Activity[J]. *Arterioscler Thromb Vase Biol*,2002,22(09):1402-1408.

② KOEPSELL H. The SLC22 Family with Transporters of Organic Cations,Anions and Zwitterions[J]. *Mole Asp Med*,2013,34(2-3):413-435.

③ JOHNSON RI,KANG D,FEIG D,et al.Is there a Pathogenetic Role for Uric Acid in Hypertension and Cardiovascular and Renal Disease? [J].*Hypertension*,2003,41(06):1183-1190.

因子,尿酸也可直接刺激单核细胞释放 IL-1、IL-6 和 TNF-α。本研究发现,不同浓度尿酸处理后 SD 大鼠血浆和组织上清液的 CRP、IL-6、TNF-α 水平各组之间无统计学差异,血浆肌酐 200 mg/kg 及以下尿酸组与生理盐水组比较无统计学差异,病理提示肾脏 200 mg/kg 及以下尿酸组、踝关节各浓度组、颈总动脉和腹主动脉各浓度组均无明显炎症改变,提示尿酸水平的适当提高对 6-OHDA-PD 大鼠肌酐、CRP、IL-6、TNF-α 及肾脏、关节、动脉血管无明显影响。

总之,本研究结果提示尿酸对 6-OHDA 帕金森病大鼠黑质纹状体系统多巴能神经元具有显著保护作用,100 mg/kg、200 mg/kg 尿酸组,以及更小剂量尿酸组对炎性因子 IL-6、TNF-α、CRP,以及血管内膜、肾脏和关节滑膜无明显影响。这些研究结果为今后从实验室到临床的转化,适当提高尿酸水平,预防帕金森病及优化帕金森病的治疗提供了一定的依据。

(缪桂华　张　宁　舒海洋　张琪林　刘　晶　罗蔚锋)

(本文原载于《医学研究杂志》2014 年第 43 卷第 4 期)

帕金森病与尿酸的临床研究

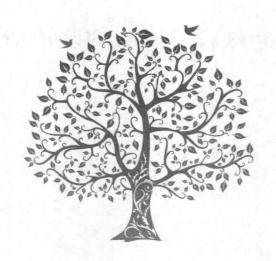

帕金森病患者血尿酸水平

帕金森病患者多巴胺能神经元选择性死亡的原因目前仍不完全清楚,氧化应激和线粒体功能障碍与 PD 发病密切相关①。尿酸是人体中主要的抗氧化剂之一,能清除自由基及螯合金属离子,减少体内氧化应激的水平②。PD 动物模型研究显示,尿酸具有对抗氧化应激及保护多巴胺能神经元的作用③。尸检研究显示,PD 患者大脑基底节区尿酸水平是降低的④。在本研究中,我们通过观察 PD 患者血尿酸的水平,探讨其与血红蛋白之间的关系。

一、资料与方法

1. 研究对象

121 例 PD 患者均系苏州大学附属第二医院 1999—2007 年的住院及门诊患者,所有患者的诊断均符合英国帕金森病协会的诊断标准⑤,其中男 62 例,女 59 例,年龄在 50~87 岁,平均年龄(68.8±7.9)岁。按病情 H-Y 分为五级:Ⅰ级 6 例、Ⅱ级 29 例、Ⅲ级 57 例、Ⅳ级 24 例、Ⅴ级 5 例。病程为 1~10 年。临床上排除脑血管疾病、脑炎等原因所导致的帕金森综合征,排除心、肺、肝和肾等疾病。同时收集同期 121 名健康者作为对照组,其性别、年龄构成与 PD 组相匹配。两组年龄及性别差异无统计学意义。所有研究对象均为本地区居民,饮食结构及生活习惯相似。所有受试者被告知并取得

---

① JENNER P. Oxidative Stress in Parkinson's Disease[J]. *Ann Neurol*, 2003, 53(Suppl 3): S26-36.

② HINK HU, SANTANAM N, DIKALOV S, et al. Peroxidase Properties of Extracellular Superoxide Dismutase: Role of Uric Acid in Modulating in Vivo Activity[J]. *Arterioscler Thromb Vasc Biol*, 2002, 22(09): 1402-1408.

③ DUAN W, LADENHEIM B, CUTLER RG, et al. Dietary Folate Deficiency and Elevated Homocysteine Levels Endanger Dopaminergic Neurons in Models of Parkinson's Disease[J]. *J Neurochem*, 2002, 80(01): 101-110.

④ FITZMAURICE PS, ANG L, GUTTMAN M, et al. Nigral Glutathione Deficiency is Not Specific for Idiopathic Parkinson's Disease[J]. *Mov Disord*, 2003, 18(09): 969-976.

⑤ MEARA J, BHOWMICK BK, HOBSON P. Accuracy of Diagnosis in Patients with Presumed Parkinson's Disease[J]. *Age Ageing*, 1999, 28(02): 99-102.

知情同意。

2. **方法**

所有受试对象均采用早晨空腹抽取肘正中静脉血 4 mL,应用美国 DADE Behring 公司全自动生化分析仪测定血尿酸,应用美国 SYSEMX 公司 XE2100 全自动血球分析仪测定血红蛋白。

3. **统计学分析**

应用 SPSS 11.0 统计学分析软件,统计结果用"$\bar{x}\pm s$"表示,两组比较用 t 检验,多组比较用方差分析 SNK 检验,相关关系用直线相关分析。

二、结果

1. **PD 患者血尿酸和血红蛋白的变化**

PD 组的血尿酸水平[(261±90)μmol/L]低于健康对照组的血尿酸水平[(337±60)μmol/L],差异有统计学意义($t=7.738,P<0.01$)。PD 组血红蛋白水平[(132±91)g/L]与健康对照组血红蛋白水平[(135±13)g/L]相比较差异无统计学意义($t=0.369,P>0.05$)。

2. **PD 患者不同性别之间血尿酸水平的变化**

健康对照组男性血尿酸水平[(350±54)μmol/L]与女性血尿酸水平[(322±63)μmol/L]的差异有统计学意义($t=2.576,P<0.05$)。PD 组男性血尿酸水平[(274±102)μmol/L]与女性血尿酸水平[(247±75)(μmol/L]的差异无统计学意义($t=0.499,P>0.05$)。

3. **PD 组不同 H-Y 分级组各项指标的变化**

PD 组 H-Y 分级的升高,与血尿酸水平无直线相关关系。健康对照组与Ⅰ-Ⅱ组、Ⅲ组、Ⅳ-Ⅴ组之间的差异均有统计学意义($P<0.01$)(表1)。

表1　PD 组不同 H-Y 分级组与健康对照组各项指标的变化($\bar{x}\pm s$)

分组	例数	血尿酸(μmol/L)	血红蛋白(g/L)
健康对照组	121	337±60	135±13
Ⅰ-Ⅱ级组	35	258±80[a]	128±16
Ⅲ级组	57	252±104[a]	142±132
Ⅳ-Ⅴ级组	29	282±71[a]	118±14

注:与健康对照组比较,[a]$F=21.068,P<0.01$。

4. PD 组与健康对照组血尿酸和血红蛋白相关性的比较

PD 组血尿酸与血红蛋白无相关性（$r=0.065$，$P>0.05$）。健康对照组血尿酸与血红蛋白无相关性（$r=0.177$，$P>0.05$）。

三、讨论

尿酸是嘌呤代谢产物，大多数哺乳动物的尿酸在肝脏经尿酸盐氧化酶分解成尿囊素，从尿中排出。近年来一些研究从多个方面证实了尿酸具有抗氧化作用，表现为：（1）尿酸盐能清除过氧化物、羟基与氧自由基，螯合转移金属离子。（2）硝基过氧化物是一氧化氮与过氧化氢离子结合的产物，能使蛋白的酪氨酸硝基化而损害细胞，尿酸能阻断硝基化反应。（3）尿酸能防止细胞外超氧歧化酶降解，超氧歧化酶是使超氧负离子变成无害的 H_2O_2 的重要催化剂。超氧负离子能使一氧化氮失活，超氧歧化酶能消除超氧负离子，保持一氧化氮水平，保护细胞。（4）健康人做有氧运动，体内超氧化合物的 8-异前列腺素浓度增高。如同时滴注尿酸可消除强度有氧运动引起的 8-异前列腺素升高，使机体抗氧化能力增强。（5）已有实验证明，适当提高脑组织中的尿酸水平，能够减轻 1-甲基-4 苯基-1，2，3，6-四氢吡啶对小鼠多巴胺能神经元的损害。

低血尿酸水平与 PD、阿尔兹海默病（AD）、多发性硬化（MS）等神经变性疾病有关[1][2][3]。在神经变性疾病中，尿酸不能阻止氧自由基和氮基的毒性损害，从而造成神经元功能和结构的改变，最终引起神经元凋亡，其中毒性作用最大的是过氧化硝酸盐[4]。Church 和 Ward[5] 发现 PD 患者黑质中的尿酸水平显著低于健康对照组。Kim 等[6]发现 AD 患者的血尿酸水平显著

① CHURCH WH，WARD VL. Uric Acid is Reduced in the Substantia Nigra in Parkinson's Disease：Effect on Dopamine Oxidation［J］.*Brain Res Bull*，1994，33（04）：419−425.

② KIM TS，PAE CU，YOON SJ，et al. Decreased Plasma Antioxidants in Patients with Alzheimer's Disease［J］.*Int J Geriatr Psychiatry*，2006，21（04）：344−348.

③ RENTZOS M，NIKOLAOU C，ANAGNOSTOULI M，et al.Serum Uric Acid and Multiple Sclerosis［J］.*Clin Neurol Neurosurg*，2006，108（06）：527−531.

④ PACHER P，BECKMAN JS，LIAUDET L.Nitric Oxide and Peroxynitrite in Health and Disease［J］.*Physiol Rev*，2007，87（01）：315−424.

⑤ CHURCH WH，WARD VL. Uric Acid is Reduced in the Substantia Nigra in Parkinson's Disease：Effect on Dopamine Oxidation［J］.*Brain Res Bull*，1994，33（04）：419−425.

⑥ KIM TS，PAE CU，YOON SJ，et al. Decreased Plasma Antioxidants in Patients with Alzheimer's disease［J］.*Int J Geriatr Psychiatry*，2006，21（04）：344−348.

低于健康对照组。*Rentzos* 等①研究发现 MS 患者的血尿酸水平显著低于健康对照组。

流行病学提示低血尿酸水平是 PD 的一个危险因素②。有尸检研究表明,PD 组和对照组大脑基底节区的尿酸水平差异有统计学意义③。在 PD 模型鼠中,尿酸治疗组可以减少氧化应激的水平,保护多巴胺能神经元④。我们的研究表明,PD 组的血尿酸水平较健康对照组低可能与下列因素有关:(1) 尿酸是一种主要的抗氧化物质和自由基清除剂,能对抗自由基引起的脂质过氧化和 DNA 损伤。尿酸在自由基损伤 DNA 之前与自由基相结合,减少甚至阻止自由基对 DNA 的损伤。PD 患者细胞内抗氧化系统受损后,细胞很容易受到自由基和金属离子的损伤。随着氧化损伤水平的升高,对抗氧化应激消耗的尿酸量增加,从而降低血尿酸水平⑤。(2) PD 患者体内氧化应激水平增加,导致红细胞内氧化氨基硫增加,氧化自由基广泛产生,生物转化功能加速,体内含氮产物大量排出体外,引起血尿酸水平下降⑥。

我们的研究表明,健康对照组男性与女性的血尿酸水平差异有统计学意义,PD 组男女患者之间的血尿酸水平差异无统计学意义。健康群体中,女性体内的雌激素可使磷脂膜抵抗尿酸盐结晶沉淀,促进肾脏排泄尿酸。随着女性年龄的增加,其体内雌激素水平下降,血尿酸水平也相应升高。而在 PD 患者中,可通过氧化应激及自由基减少女性体内的雌激素,导致 PD 患者男女之间的血尿酸水平可能无差别⑦。我们的研究表明,PD 患者血尿

① RENTZOS M,NIKOLAOU C,ANAGNOSTOULI M,et al.Serum Uric Acid and Multiple Sclerosis[J].*Clin Neurol Neurosurg*,2006,108(06):527−531.

② ANNANMAKI T,MUURONEN A,MUNOS K.Low Plasma Uric Acid Level in Parkinson's Disease[J].*Mov Disord*,2007,22(08):1133−1137.

③ FITZMAURICE PS,ANG L,GUTTMAN M,et al. Nigral Glutathione Deficiency is Not Specific for Idiopathic Parkinson's Disease[J].*Mov Disord*,2003,18(09):969−976.

④ DUAN W,LADENHEIM B,CUTLER RG,et al.Dietary Folate Deficiency and Elevated Homocysteine Levels Endanger Dopaminergic Neurons in Models of Parkinson's Disease[J].*J Neurochem*,2002,80(01):101−110.

⑤ ANDERSON RF,HARRIS TA.Dopamine and Uric Acid Act as Antioxidants in the Repair of DNA Radicals:Implications in Parkinson' Disease[J].*Free Radlc Res*,2003,37(10):1131−1136.

⑥ SIEMS WG,VAN KUIJK FJ,MAASS R,et al. Uric Acid and Glutathione Levels during Short-term Whole Body Cold Exposure[J].*Free Radic Biol Med*,1994,16(03):299−305.

⑦ SUMINO H,ICHIKAWA S,KANDA T,et al.Reduction of Serum Uric Acid by Honnone Replacement Therapy in Postmenopausal Women with Hyperuricaemia[J].*Lancet*,1999,354(9179):650.

酸的水平与 PD 的严重程度无相关性。研究结果提示,尿酸是 PD 发病的危险因素,但血尿酸水平不能作为判断 PD 患者疾病严重程度的一个指标。

　　动物实验表明,铁的增加会导致血尿酸水平的降低;临床研究显示,尿酸和血清铁蛋白有着显著的相关性[1]。低尿酸水平会削弱螯合铁离子的能力,血尿酸水平能够反映大脑包括基底节区的尿酸水平,大脑中低尿酸水平使多巴胺能神经元暴露在含铁较多的细胞中,导致神经元死亡[2]。我们进行了 PD 组血尿酸与血红蛋白的相关性研究,结果表明尿酸与血红蛋白无相关性,分析可能原因为血清铁蛋白与血红蛋白有一定的差异性。因此,血红蛋白还不能作为 PD 分析的相关指标。

（王丽君　罗蔚锋　王恒会　刘春风）

（本文原载于《中华神经科杂志》2008 年第 41 卷第 3 期）

　　[1]　MEARA J, BHOWMICK BK, HOBSON P. Accuracy of Diagnosis in Patients with Presumed Parkinson's Disease[J]. *Age Ageing*, 1999, 28(02): 99-102.

　　[2]　GHIO AJ, FORD ES, KENNEDY TP, et al. The Association between Serum Ferritin and Uric Acid in Humans[J]. *Free Radic Res*, 2005, 39(03): 337-342.

老年男性帕金森病患者血尿酸水平的研究

基础实验研究及临床资料提示,黑质纹状体系统清除自由基物质水平的降低,引起的氧化应激反应增强,线粒体功能障碍与帕金森病(PD)的发病密切相联系①②,PD与尿酸的关系日益受到人们的重视③。在本研究中,我们通过观察老年男性PD患者的血尿酸水平,探讨PD患者血尿酸水平改变的特点及意义。

一、对象和方法

1. 对象

65例男性PD患者均系苏州大学附属第二医院1999年1月至2008年1月的住院及门诊患者,如果是多次在苏州大学附属第二医院住院和门诊就诊的患者均采用第一次就诊资料。所有患者的诊断均符合英国帕金森病协会的诊断标准④,年龄在62~87岁,平均年龄(71.9±6.3)岁。其中早期(H-Y分级Ⅰ~Ⅱ级)17例、中期(H-Y分级Ⅲ级)34例、晚期(H-Y分级Ⅳ~Ⅴ级)14例。病程为6个月~10年。临床上排除脑血管疾病、脑炎等原因所导致的帕金森综合征,排除心、肺、肝和肾等重大疾病患者。以同期64例性别、年龄匹配在该院进行常规体检的健康者作为对照组,年龄60~84岁,平均年龄(70.2±6.1)岁。

2. 方法

收集PD组和对照组的血尿酸。所有受试对象均为苏州地区居民,采用早晨空腹抽取上肢肘静脉血4 mL,应用美国DADE Behring公司全自动生化分析仪测定血尿酸。

① SARAVANAN KS, SINDHU KM, SENTHILKUMAR KS, et al. Mohanakumar P. L-deprenyl Protects against Rotenone-induced, Oxidative Stress-mediated Dopaminergic Neurodegeneration in Rats[J]. *Neurochem Int*, 2006, 49(01): 28-40.

② JENNER P. Oxidative Stress in Parkinson's Disease[J]. *Ann Neurol*, 2003, 53(Suppl 3): S26-36.

③ 罗蔚锋, 刘春风. 尿酸水平与帕金森病[J]. 中华神经科杂志, 2008, 41(08): 552-533.

④ MEARA J, BHOWMICK BK, HOBSON P. Accuracy of Diagnosis in Patients with Presumed Parkinson's Disease[J]. *Age Ageing*, 1999, 28(02): 99-102.

3. 统计学方法

应用 SPSS 统计分析软件 11.0，统计结果用"$\bar{x}\pm s$"表示，两组比较采用 t 检验，多组比较采用方差分析。

二、结果

1. 老年男性 PD 患者组与对照组的年龄差异无统计学意义，两组受试者均来自同一地区，饮食习惯相似。老年男性 PD 患者组的血尿酸水平 [64.1±97.0）μmol/L]明显低于对照组的血尿酸水平[（344.6±54.2）μmol/L]（$t = 5.802, P < 0.01$）。

2. 老年男性 PD 患者早期组血尿酸（259.2±71.0）μmol/L，中期组（268.0±115.2）μmol/L，晚期组（260.2±77.7）μmol/L，分别与正常对照组比较，均显著降低，差异有统计学意义（均为 $P < 0.01$）。老年男性 PD 患者早、中、晚各期之间的血尿酸水平差异无统计学意义。

三、讨论

腺苷在腺苷脱氨酶、嘌呤核苷磷酸化酶的作用下依次转化为肌苷、次黄嘌呤。次黄嘌呤进一步在黄嘌呤氧化酶的作用下生成黄嘌呤和尿酸。70% 的尿酸经肾脏排泄，30% 的尿酸经胆道和肠道排泄。

尿酸是人体内特有的天然水溶性抗氧化剂。对 18 000 例男性在 1993—1995 年检测血尿酸，对其进行随访，2000 年有 84 例被诊断为 PD，按 1 : 2 的比例与年龄、种族、检测时间相配对的对照组比较，PD 组的血尿酸水平 [339.2μmol/L（5.7 mg/dL）]显著低于对照组的血尿酸水平[363.0 μmol/L（6.1 mg/dL）]。血尿酸水平处于高四分之一位值范围的人群 PD 发病率与血尿酸水平处于低四分之一位值范围的人群 PD 发病率之比为 0.43（$P = 0.017$），提示在一定的范围内，血尿酸水平越高，PD 的发病率越低[1]。Church 等[2]对死亡后 PD 患者的黑质和尾状核组织中的尿酸、多巴胺、抗坏血酸进行测定，发现其尿酸、多巴胺的水平显著低于年龄相匹配的对照组。对患有 PD、进行性核上性麻痹及多系统萎缩的患者在其死亡后进行黑质尿

① WEISSKOPF MG, O'REILLY E, CHEN H, et al. Plasma Urate and Risk of Parkinson's Disease[J]. *Am J Epidemiol*, 2007, 166(05): 561-567.

② CHURCH WH, WARD VL. Uric Acid is Reduced in the Substantia Nigra in Parkinson Disease: Effect on Dopamine Oxidation[J]. *Brain Res Bull*, 1994, 33(04): 419-425.

酸水平测定,发现各病例组的黑质尿酸水平较对照组降低 19%~30%,另一种抗氧化剂谷胱音肽降低 20%~30%[①]。

本研究结果提示,老年男性 PD 患者的血尿酸水平较正常组低。低尿酸水平是老年男性患 PD 的一个原因,或仅是 PD 的一个生物标志,尚不能完全确定。我们以 C57BL/6 雄性小鼠为研究对象,利用微透析技术,给予小鼠左侧脑室持续灌注尿酸 24 h,腹腔注射 1-甲基-4-苯基-1,3,3,6 四氢吡啶(MPTP)40 mg/kg,再维持相同的治疗 24 h。1 周后取纹状体,应用高效液相电化学方法测定纹状体组织中的多巴胺水平,发现尿酸组纹状体组织中的多巴胺水平显著高于人工脑脊液对照组,表明适当提高脑组织中的尿酸水平,能够减轻 MPTP 对小鼠多巴胺能神经元的损害。支持低尿酸水平很可能是 PD 的一个原因,Duan 等[②]的实验结果亦证实,适当提高尿酸水平能够减轻鱼藤酮所致的多巴胺能神经元凋亡,对其有明显的保护作用。

(罗蔚锋　王丽君　王晓君　王恒会　毛成洁　刘春风)
(本文原载于《中华老年医学杂志》2009 年第 28 卷第 1 期)

① FITZMAURICE PS, ANG L, GUTTMAN M, et al. Nigral Glutathione Deficiency is Not Specific for Idiopathic Parkinson's Disease[J]. *Mov Disord*, 2003, 18(09): 969-976.

② DUAN W, LADENHEIM B, CUTLER RG, et al. Dietary Folate Deficiency and Elevated Homocysteine Levels Endanger Dopaminergic Neurons in Models of Parkinson Disease[J]. *J Neurochem*, 2002, 80(01): 101-110.

女性帕金森病患者血尿酸水平的研究

目的：分析女性帕金森病患者的血尿酸水平，探讨血尿酸水平在女性帕金森病患者的改变特征。

方法：选取苏州大学附属第二医院诊断为帕金森病的门诊女性患者81例，以该院同期保健科随机选取年龄、性别和体重匹配的81名健康体检人群为对照组，检测其血尿酸和肌酐水平，并对两组的血尿酸和内生肌酐清除率进行对比分析。

结果：女性帕金森病患者组的血尿酸水平显著低于健康对照组（$P<0.01$）。帕金森病患者 H-Y 分级 I - II 组、IV 组、III - V 3 组之间的血尿酸水平均无统计学差异（$P>0.05$）。

结论：女性帕金森病患者的血尿酸水平降低，低血尿酸水平很可能与女性帕金森病患者的发病有关。

关键词：帕金森病；尿酸。

帕金森病是最常见的神经变性病之一，目前我国的帕金森病患者已经超过200万人。其病理改变主要是黑质内多巴胺能神经元渐进性受损。患者黑质内存在明显的氧化应激，总铁增多而铁蛋白水平下降及线粒体复合体 I [1] 缺乏，这些均提示氧化损伤在 PD 患者的多巴胺能神经元死亡过程中发挥着一定的作用。尿酸是一种重要的生理性的天然抗氧化剂、铁螯合剂、自由基清除剂，PD 与 UA 的关系日益受到人们的重视 [2]。流行病学研究发现，低尿酸水平是 PD 的危险因素 [3][4]，而这些研究的对象主要是男性，目前还没有对女性 PD 患者尿酸水平的研究。在本研究中，我们通过观察女性

① LIANG LP, PATEL M. Iron-sulfur Enzyme Mediated Mitochondrial Superoxide Toxicity in Experimental Parkinson's Disease[J].*J Neurochem*,2004,90(05)：1076-1084.

② 罗蔚锋,刘春风.尿酸水平与帕金森病[J].中华神经科杂志,2008,41(08)：552-553.

③ DAVIS JW,GRANDINETTI A,WASLIEN CI,et al.Observations on Serum Uric Acid levels and the Risk of Idiopathic Parkinson Disease[J].*Am J Epidemiol*,1996,144(05)：480-484.

④ ASCHERIO A,WEISSKOPF MG,CHEN H,et al.Plasma Urate and Risk of Parkinson's Disease[J].*Am J Epidemiol*,2007,166(05)：561-567.

PD 患者的血尿酸水平,探讨女性 PD 患者血尿酸水平改变的特点及意义。

一、对象与方法

1. 研究对象

81 例 PD 患者均是苏州大学附属第二医院 2007 年 9 月至 2008 年 10 月的门诊病人,如果是多次在该院门诊就诊的患者均采用第一次就诊的资料。所有患者的诊断均符合英国帕金森病协会的诊断标准[①],年龄在 39~89 岁,平均年龄(64.83±10.2)岁。其中早期(H-Y 分级 Ⅰ~Ⅱ级)28 例、中期(H-Y 分级Ⅲ级)31 例、晚期(H-Y 分级Ⅳ~Ⅴ级)22 例。病程为 1~22 年。临床上排除脑血管疾病、脑炎等原因所导致的帕金森综合征,排除心,肺,肝和肾等重大疾病患者,并排除高血压、糖尿病、心脏病、脑卒中和痛风等影响血尿酸水平的患者。以同期 81 名性别、年龄(±3 岁)、体重(±2 kg)匹配在该院进行常规体检的健康者作为对照组,年龄在 41~89 岁,平均年龄(66.1±10.0)岁。所有研究对象均为本地区常住居民,饮食结构及生活习惯相似。

2. 方法

（1）临床特征调查

通过问卷调查的形式收集患者的一般资料,内容包括个人信息、病程、现病史和既往史等;用修订 Hoehn 和 Yahr(H-Y)分期对疾病的严重程度进行评分。

（2）血液标本收集及测定

所有受试对象均采用早晨空腹抽取肘正中静脉血 4 mL,应用美国 DADE Behring 公司全自动生化分析仪测定血尿酸和肌酐。内生肌酐清除率(Ccr)用以下公式计算:[(140-年龄)×体重(kg)]/[85×血肌酐浓度(mg/mL)]。本研究的仪器正常值参考范围:血尿酸 89~420 μmol/L;肌酐 43~135 μmol/L。

3. 统计学方法

采用 SPSS 11.5 进行统计学分析,统计结果用"$\bar{x}±s$"表示,两组比较采用 t 检验,多组比较采用方差分析。以 $P<0.05$ 为有统计学意义。

---

① KLEMP P,STANSFIELD SA,CASTLE B,et al. Gout is on the Increase in New Zealand[J]. *Ann Rheum Dh*,1997,56(01):22-26.

二、结果

1. 女性 PD 患者血尿酸水平和内生肌酐清除率与正常对照组比较

女性 PD 患者组与健康对照组的年龄、体重相比无显著性差异,女性 PD 患者组的血尿酸水平明显低于健康对照组($t = -6.20, P < 0.01$),而两组之间的内生肌酐清除率无差异($t = -0.79, P > 0.05$)(表 1)。

表 1   女性 PD 患者组与健康对照组的血尿酸水平和内生肌酐清除率($\bar{x} \pm s$)

组别	N	UA(μmol/L)	Ccr(mL/min)
PD 组	81	244.63±67.47	75.29±19.60
健康对照组	81	302.17±49.18[1)	78.95±21.63

注:与健康对照组相比 $P < 0.01$。

2. 女性 PD 患者早、中、晚各期组与健康对照组的血尿酸水平比较

女性 PD 患者早期组、中期组、晚期组的血尿酸水平分别与健康对照组相比较,均显著性降低($F = 3.21, P < 0.05; F = 5.54, P < 0.01; F = 4.76, P < 0.01$)。女性 PD 患者早、中、晚各期之间的血尿酸水平无显著性差异($F = 2.44, P > 0.05$)(表 2)。

表 2   女性 PD 患者早、中、晚各期组与健康对照组的血尿酸水平比较

组别	N	尿酸(μmol/L)
健康对照组	81	302.17±49.18
女性 PD 患者 I - II组	28	266.57±72.30
女性 PD 患者III组	31	229.71±63.91
女性 PD 患者IV - V组	22	237.73±61.36

三、讨论

尿酸是一种弱酸,以尿酸盐的形式分布于细胞外液中。血液中尿酸盐的量取决于嘌呤的摄入、尿酸的合成及排泄速率。血尿酸水平由肾脏系统的滤过、重吸收及分泌等三大作用决定[①]。70% 的 UA 经肾脏排泄,30% 的 UA 经胆道和肠道排泄。

---

① MOUNT DB, KWON CY, ZANDI-NEJAD K. Renal Urate Transport [J]. *Rheum Dis Clin North Am*, 2006, 32(02): 313-331.

尿酸是一种天然的抗氧化剂和自由基清除剂,能够清除人体中达60%的自由基。尿酸能清除O_2^-,OH^-和单态氧[①]。尿酸阻止SOD的降解,清除O_2^-。SOD阻止NO与O_2^-反应生成过氧化亚硝酸盐。尿酸能有效阻止蛋白的硝基化[②],能螯合转移铁离子并且抑制铁依赖的抗坏血酸氧化所导致的氧化损伤[③]。实验研究表明,鱼藤酮和铁能引起培养的人类多巴胺能神经元凋亡,而尿酸能完全阻止高同型半胱氨酸、鱼藤酮和铁共同引起的细胞凋亡,最大限度地阻止与鱼藤酮和铁共同引起的线粒体膜的去极化;适当提高脑组织中的尿酸水平,能够减轻MPTP对小鼠多巴胺能神经元的损伤[④]。

低尿酸水平与帕金森病的发生和发展有关。国外流行病学研究发现,低尿酸水平是PD的危险因素之一。[⑤] 对8 000名男性在进行常规的血清UA水平测定后,进行长达30年的跟踪随访,有92例被相继诊断为PD,经年龄、吸烟危险因素纠正后发现,入组时血清水平高于平均值的人群其PD发病率降低40%[⑥]。对18 000名的男性人群进行前瞻性的流行病学研究[⑦],8年后发现血浆UA水平处于高四分位值范围的人群相对于血浆UA水平处于低四分位值范围的人群,其PD发病率降低55%,PD发病率的降低与诊断为PD者至少前4年的血浆UA水平的关系更为密切,提示低水平的血浆UA会增高PD的发病率。经年龄、吸烟、饮咖啡及其他与PD和血浆UA水平有关的因素纠正后,血浆UA水平与PD的发病率仍呈显著的负相关性,提示在一定的范围内,血浆UA水平越高,帕金森病的发病率越低。

① AMES BN, CATHCART R, SCHWIERS E, et al. Uric Acid Provides an Antioxidant Defense in Humans aginst Oxidant and Radical-caused Aging and Cancer: a Hypothesis[J]. *Proc Natl Acad Sci USA*, 1981, 78(11): 6858–6862.

② PACHER P, BECKMAN JS, LIAUDET L. Nitric Oxide and Peroxynitrite in Health and Disease[J]. *Physiol Rev*, 2007, 87(01): 315–424.

③ DAVIES KJ, SEVANIAN A, MUAKKASSAH-KELLY, et al. Uric Acid-iron Ion Complexes. A New Aspect of the Antioxidant Functions of Uric Acid[J]. *Biochem J*, 1986, 235(03): 747–754.

④ LUO WF, SCHWARZSCHILD MA, XU K. Urate Attenuates MPTP-induced Dopaminergic Toxicity in Mice[C]. The Society for Neuroscience 37th Annual Meeting, 2007. San Diego, California, USA.

⑤ DE LAU LM, KOUDSTAAL PJ, HOFMAN A, et al. Serum Uric Acid Levels and the Risk of Parkinson Disease[J]. *Ann Neurol*, 2005, 58(05): 797–800.

⑥ DAVIS JW, GRANDINETTI A, WASLIEN CI, et al. Observations on Serum Uric Acid Levels and the Risk of Idiopathic Parkinson Disease[J]. *Am J Epidemiol*, 1996, 144(05): 480–484.

⑦ ASCHERIO A, WEISSKOPF MG, CHEN H, et al. Plasma Urate and Risk of Parkinson's Disease[J]. *Am J Epidemiol*, 2007, 166(05): 561–567.

临床资料证实,PD 患者的黑质纹状体系统,脑脊液,血尿酸水平显著性降低[①②]。Annanmaki 等[③]以 40 例 PD 患者和 29 名健康者为研究对象,对其血尿酸、血清铁蛋白、体重指数及乳制品饮食等进行检测评价,结果提示 PD 患者的血尿酸水平显著性降低,尿酸水平的改变与血清铁蛋白的变化密切相联系。

本研究结果提示女性 PD 患者的血尿酸水平较正常组低。为了排除肾功能水平对尿酸结果的影响,我们同时对两组受试者的内生肌酐清除率进行了比较,结果显示无统计学差异。我们还对女性 PD 患者不同 H-Y 分级之间的血尿酸水平进行了比校,结果表明,女性 PD 患者的血尿酸水平与疾病的严重程度无相关性。这些研究结果提示,在一定范围内适当提高血尿酸水平对降低 PD 的发病率可能有一定的作用,虽然 PD 患者中的血尿酸水平低,但不能作为判断 PD 患者疾病严重程度的一个指标。

（王晓君　罗蔚锋　王丽君　刘春风）

（本文原载于《中国神经精神疾病杂志》2009 年第 35 卷第 5 期）

① CHURCH WH,WARD VL.Uric Acid is Reduced in the Substantia Nigra in Parkinson's Disease：Effect on Dopamine Oxidation[J].*Brain Res Bull*,1994,33(04)：419-425.

② 王丽君,罗蔚锋,王恒会,等.帕金森病患者血尿酸水平[J].中华神经科杂志,2008,41(03)：157-158.

③ ANNANMAKI T,MUURONEN A,MURROS K.Low Plasma Uric Acid Level in Parkinson's Disease[J].*Mov Disord*,2007,22(08)：1133-1137.

尿酸水平和高血压病与帕金森病
关系的病例对照研究

目的：探讨尿酸水平和高血压病与帕金森病的关系。

方法：采用病例对照研究，收集门诊或住院的 PD 患者 372 例（PD 组），另选择性别、年龄与 PD 组匹配的对照者 372 名（对照组）为研究对象。采用 Mantel-Haenszel（M-H）x^2 检验等统计学方法分析两组的一般情况、尿酸水平、高血压病病史、高血压病病程（分为<10 年和≥10 年）和高血压病级别（按收缩压：Ⅰ级=140~159 mmHg、Ⅱ级=160~179 mmHg，Ⅲ级≥180 mmHg）与 PD 症状（UPDRS Ⅱ／Ⅲ）和严重程度（H-Y 分级）的关系。

结果：PD 组中，与非高尿酸血症者比较，高尿酸血症患者患 PD 的危险性降低（$OR=0.24$，95%CI：$0.15~0.37$）；与非高血压病患者比较，高血压病患者患 PD 的危险性降低（$OR=0.50$，95%CI：$0.37~0.70$）。对高血压病患者分别按高血压病级别（Ⅰ~Ⅲ级）及高血压病病程（分为<10 年和≥10 年）分层后进行单因素分析，依然存在负相关（$P<0.05$）。此外，PD 组随着 H-Y 分级的增加，高血压病患病率和尿酸水平均呈下降趋势，且 PD 合并高血压病患者的 UPDRS Ⅱ／Ⅲ 评分明显低于 PD 非合并高血压病患者，均值差异有统计学意义（$P<0.01$）。

结论：高尿酸血症和高血压病与 PD 存在负相关性。

关键词：尿酸；高尿酸血症；高血压病；帕金森病；负相关联。

高血压病（hypertension）和帕金森病均是老年人的常见疾病，其患病率和发病率随年龄增加而升高。据世界卫生组织报道，中国老年人（≥60 岁）高血压病的患病率达 39.7%。Zhang 等[1]的流行病学调查结果提示，中国 65 岁以上人群的 PD 患病率约为 1.7%。高血压病患者中约有 30%并发高尿

① ZHANG ZX，ROMAN GC，HONG Z，et al.Parkinson's Disease in China：Prevalence in Beijing，Xian，and Shanghai［J］.*Lancet*，2005，365（9459）：595-597.

酸血症(high uric acid hematic,HUA)①。流行病学研究②③提示,相对低尿酸水平人群的 PD 发生率增高,尿酸水平与 PD 关系的基础④⑤和临床⑥⑦研究结果亦支持适当高水平的尿酸对 PD 患者具有一定的保护作用。但有关高血压病与 PD 的研究不多,为此本研究对 HUA、高血压病和 PD 的患病率进行调查,通过病例对照研究探讨尿酸水平、高血压病与 PD 的关系。

一、资料与方法

1. 研究对象来源

收集 2011 年 1 月至 2013 年 1 月在苏州大学附属第二医院和江苏大学附属昆山医院门诊或住院的 372 例老年 PD 患者为 PD 组,平均年龄(70.89±6.62)岁,平均发病年龄(65.45±7.71)岁,其中男性 204 例,女性 168 例。另选择同期居住在苏州市社区老年人健康调查或在苏州大学附属第二医院体检中心体检的人群,性别、年龄[(±3)岁]与 PD 组匹配的 372 名对照者为对照组,无锥体外系疾病史。对照组与 PD 组的民族构成、居住地比较差异无显著性。

2. PD 诊断标准

均符合英国帕金森病协会的诊断标准⑧:行动迟缓;至少有下列症状之一——肌强直、静止性震颤(4~6 Hz)、姿势步态异常。同时排除继发性帕金森综合征和帕金森叠加症。

---

① 党爱民,刘国仗.尿酸与心血管事件[J].中华心血管病杂志.2003,31(06):478-480.

② 王丽君,罗蔚锋,王恒会,等.帕金森病患者血尿酸水平[J].中华神经科杂志,2008,41(03):157-158.

③ ZHANG HN,GUO JF,HE D,et al.Lower Serum UA Levels in Parkinson's Disease Patients in the Chinese Population[J].*Neurosci Lett*,2012,514(02):152-155.

④ 朱婷鸽,张琪林,黄婷婷,等.尿酸减轻 6-OHDA 介导 PC12 细胞 SOD 活性下降和损伤的实验研究[J].分子诊断与治疗杂志,2011,3(02):96-99.

⑤ 朱红灿,蔡春生,耿利娇,等.尿酸对帕金森病模型大鼠多巴胺能神经元氧化应激的影响[J].中华老年医学杂志,2010,29(04):319-323.

⑥ DE LAU LM,KOUDSTAAL PJ,HOFMAN A,et al.Serum Uric Acid Levels and the Risk of Parkinson Disease[J].*Ann Neurol*,2005,58(05):797-800.

⑦ WEISSKOPF MG,O'REILLY E,CHEN H,et al.Plasma Urate and Risk of Parkinson's Disease[J].*Am J Epidemiol*,2007,166(05):561-567.

⑧ MEARA J,BHOWMICK BK,HOBSON P. Accuracy of Diagnosis in Patients with Presumed Parkinson's Disease[J].*Age Ageing*,1999,28(02):99-102.

3. 高血压病判定标准

收缩压(SBP)≥140 mmHg(1 mmHg = 0.133 kPa)或舒张压(DBP)≥90 mmHg判定为高血压病。高血压病级别：Ⅰ级为 SBP 140～159 mmHg，DBP 90～99 mmHg；Ⅱ级为 SBP 160～179 mmHg，DBP 1 100～109 mmHg；Ⅲ级为 SBP≥180 mmHg，DBP≥110 mmHg。

4. HUA 标准

男性≥420 μmol/L^{-1}，女性≥360 μmol/L^{-1}。

5. 资料收集

由经过培训的神经内科专科医生和研究生对 PD 组及对照组人群进行采访记录。记录内容包括社会人口学资料：姓名、年龄、性别；是否有 HUA；是否有高血压病病史、高血压病级别(以受访者的即时血压值评定)和高血压病病程(分为<10 年和≥10 年，PD 患者的高血压发病时间均早于 PD 发生)。另外，对 PD 患者还记录 PD 日常活动能力及运动功能评估[分别采用统一 PD 评定量表Ⅱ，Ⅲ部分(UPDRSⅡ，UPDRSⅢ)]；PD 病情严重度评估[采用 Hoehn-Yahr(H-Y)分期评估]，H-Y 分为 5 期：轻度=1～2 期，中度=2.5～3 期，重度=4～5 期。

6. 血压、血尿酸测定方法

(1) 血压

受试者在安静环境下休息5～10 mins，采用坐位，上臂伸直轻度外展，肘部与心脏同一水平测量。

(2) 尿酸

早晨空腹上肢肘静脉抽血4 mL，应用美国 DADE Behring 公司全自动生化分析仪酶偶联法测定血尿酸水平。

7. 统计学方法

对所有的资料进行整理、编码，并用 Foxpro 6.0 软件建立数据库，应用 SPSS17.0 统计软件完成资料分析，计量数据用"$\bar{x}\pm s$"表示，应用 Mantel-Haenszel(M-H)x^2 检验对计量资料计算比值比(OR)值、OR(95%CI)及 P 值，P<0.05 为差异有统计学意义。

二、结果

1. 两组一般情况分析

见表 1。PD 组与对照组的性别（$P=1$）和年龄（$P=0.094$）比较，差异无统计学意义。PD 组 UPDRS Ⅱ／Ⅲ 评分平均为（36.34 ± 11.85）分，H-Y 分期平均为（2.84 ± 1.22），病程 1～30 年［平均（5.26±2.16）年］。PD 组尿酸水平平均为（286.16±87.74），与对照组（337.57±89.01）比较，以及 PD 组 HUA 比率与对照组比较，均值差异有显著统计学意义（$P<0.01$）。

表 1　PD 组和对照组的一般情况（$\bar{x}\pm s$）

项目	PD 组			对照组		
	平均/总	男	女	平均/总	男	女
年龄	70.89±6.62	70.70±6.54	71.13±6.72	70.05±7.16	70.12±7.32	69.96±6.97
性别［例（%）］	372	204/372（54.84）	168/372（45.16）	372	204/372（54.84）	168/372（45.16）
尿酸（μmol/L）	286.16±87.74[1]	298.45±86.72[1]	271.23±86.90[1]	337.57±89.01	355.15±90.76	316.22±82.17
HUA 例［（%）］	30/372（8.06）[2]	10/30（33.33）	20/30（66.67）	101/372（27.15）	52/101（51.48）	49/101（48.51）
高血压病［例（%）］	130/372（34.95）	77/130（59.23）	53/130（40.77）	193/372（51.88）	106/193（54.92）	87/193（40.08）
UPDRS Ⅱ/Ⅲ评分	36.34±11.85	34.20±10.95	38.47±12.74			
H-Y 评级	2.84±1.22	2.65±1.24	3.03±1.19			

注：PD 组尿酸均值及 HUA 比率与相应对照组比较，[1]$P<0.01$，[2]$P<0.01$，PD 组其余各项目与相应对照比较，均 $P>0.05$。

2. HUA 和高血压病与 PD 关系的单因素分析

见表 2。PD 组中，与非 HUA 患者比较，HUA 患者患 PD 的危险性降低（$OR=0.24$，95%CI：0.15～0.37）；与非高血压病患者比较，高血压病患者 PD 的危险性降低（$OR=0.50$，95%CI：037～0.70）；按照高血压病级别顺序 Ⅰ～Ⅲ级，OR 值依顺序降低，分别为 0.85、0.40、0.20（均 $P<0.01$），按照高血压病病程划分，<10 年和 ≥10 年后，OR 值也降低，分别为 0.56 和 0.35（均 $P<0.01$）。

表2 两组HUA和高血压病与PD相关性的单因素分析(M-H/x^2检验)

影响因素		PD组(例)	对照组(例)	OR(95%CI)	P值
是否HUA	否	342	271	1.00	
	是	30	101	0.24(0.15~0.37)	0.000
是否高血压病	否	242	179	1.00	
	是	130	193	0.50(0.37~0.70)	0.000
高血压病级别	Ⅰ	78	68	0.85(0.58~1.24)	0.000
	Ⅱ	37	69	0.40(0.26~0.62)	0.000
	Ⅲ	15	56	0.20(0.11~0.36)	0.000
高血压病病程	<10年	105	140	0.56(0.40~0.76)	0.000
	≥10年	25	53	0.35(0.21~0.58)	0.000

注:拟非HUA患者患PD的风险为1,拟非高血压病患者患PD的风险为1。

3. PD组尿酸水平、高血压病与H-Y分级和UPDRS评分的关系分析

见表3。随着PD患者H-Y分级的增加,PD患者高血压病患病率呈下降趋势,差异有显著统计学意义($x^2=428.03$,$P<0.01$);尿酸水平呈下降趋势,差异有显著统计学意义($P<0.01$)。此外,PD合并高血压病患者的UPDRS Ⅱ/Ⅲ评分平均为(26.30 ± 6.48),明显低于PD无合并高血压病患者的评分(41.41 ± 10.85),差异有显著统计学意义($F=84.03$,$P<0.01$)。

表3 PD组尿酸水平、高血压病与H-Y分级和
UPDRS评分的关系分析(M-Hx^2检验)

因素		合并高血压病	无合并高血压病	高血压病患病率(%)	尿酸水平
H-Y分级(例)	轻度	105	49	68.18	299.87±93.34
	中度	15	86	14.85	290.35±86.58
	重度	10	108	8.47[1]	264.70±77.13[2]
UPDRS评分($\bar{x}\pm s$)	UPDRSⅡ	10.85±2.65	14.02±3.24		
	UPDRSⅢ	15.45±4.31	27.39±8.14		
	UPDRSⅡ/Ⅲ	26.30±6.48[3]	41.41±10.85		

注:H-Y分级重度与轻度比较,高血压病患病率和尿酸水平分别为[1]$P<0.01$,[2]$P<0.01$;UPDRS Ⅱ/Ⅲ评分合并高血压病与无合并高血压病比较,[3]$P<0.01$。

三、讨论

PD是老年人中枢神经系统常见神经退行性疾病之一,其病理学改变特征是黑质纹状体系统多巴胺能神经元的变性、减少,多巴胺水平显著下降,残留的神经细胞中有路易体形成等[1]。导致黑质多巴胺能神经元变性死亡的确切机制目前尚不完全清楚,但已知氧化应激、线粒体功能损害等与之密切相关。尽管应用多巴胺替代疗法、多巴胺受体激动剂等药物治疗,以及脑深部电刺激术(deep brain stimulation,DBS)等外科治疗对于改善PD患者症状取得了显著疗效,但尚无确切的可以阻止甚至减缓PD进行性进展和减少、预防PD发生的方法。因此PD发病的影响因素成为这一领域的研究热点之一。

本研究结果显示,尿酸水平和高血压病及PD呈负相关,且与高血压病级别和病程具有负性关联。对PD组高血压病和尿酸水平进行单因素分析的结果显示,高血压病患者患PD的危险性几乎占无高血压病患者的1/2($OR=0.50,P<0.01$),HUA患者占非HUA患者的1/4($OR=0.24,P<0.01$),提示HUA和高血压病对PD可能有保护作用($P<0.05$),Miyake等[2]、Gao等[3]和Noyce等[4]的研究结果亦支持本研究结果。

相对的高尿酸水平对PD具有保护作用。基础实验表明:尿酸对多巴胺能神经元具有保护作用。本研究组先前的研究[5]结果显示,尿酸水平在$10\sim400\ \mu mol/L^{-1}$可显著减轻6-OHDA作用6、12、24 h后造成的PC12细胞生存率下降,并减少6-OHDA导致的caspase-3激活,从而减少细胞凋亡。Chen等[6]应用敲除尿酸氧化酶(urate oxidase,UOx;降解尿酸为尿囊素)基因的6-OHDA小鼠PD模型,通过测定小鼠中脑黑质多巴胺能神经元数目、

① AGID Y.Parkinson's Disease:Pathophysiology[J].*Lancet*,1991,337(8753):1321-1324.

② MIYAKE Y,TANAKA K,FUKUSHIMA W,et al.Case-control Study of Risk of Parkinson's Disease in Relation to Hypertension,Hypercholesterolemia,and Diabetes in Japan[J].*J Neurol Sci*,2010,293(1-2):82-86.

③ GAO X,CHEN H,CHOI HK,et al.Diet,Urate,and Parkinson's Disease Risk in Men[J].*Am J Epidemiol*,2008,167(07):831-838.

④ NOYCE AJ,BESTWICK JP,SILVEIRA-MORIYAMA L,et al.Meta-analysis of Early Nonmotor Features and Risk Factors for Parkinson's Disease[J].*Ann Neurol*,2012,72(06):893-901.

⑤ 叶艳,罗蔚锋,朱婷鸽,等.尿酸减轻6-羟基多巴胺对PC12细胞的毒性作用[J].中国临床神经科学.2010,18(02):135-139.

⑥ CHEN X,BURDETT TC,DESJARDINS CA,et al.Disrupted and Transgenic Urate Oxidase Alter Urate and Dopaminergic Neurodegeneration[J].*Proc Natl Acad Sci USA*,2012,110(01):300-305.

纹状体多巴胺含量及行为改变,发现升高的尿酸水平可以减轻 6-OHDA 对黑质纹状体系统多巴胺能神经元的毒性作用;相反,在 UOx 过表达小鼠,尿酸水平显著降低,加剧了 6-OHDA 对黑质纹状体多巴胺能神经的损害,说明尿酸在减轻 6-OHDA 对多巴胺能神经元的毒性方面具有重要作用。Gong 等①研究发现,腹腔注射尿酸可以提高大鼠血浆和脑组织中的尿酸水平,增加谷胱甘肽水平和超氧化物歧化酶活性,降低丙二醛在 6-OHDA PD 大鼠纹状体内的聚积,结果提示尿酸对大鼠中脑黑质多巴胺能神经元具有保护作用,与其对 Akt/GSK3β 信号通路的调节有关。流行病学和临床研究也证明相对高尿酸水平对 PD 具有保护作用。对 4 695 例 55 岁以上(包括 55 岁)人群进行前瞻性研究,平均随访 9.4 年,有 68 例被诊断为 PD。发现血清尿酸水平升高可以明显降低 PD 发病率②。对 18 000 例的男性人群进行前瞻性的流行病学研究,8 年后发现血浆尿酸水平处于高五分位值范围的人群相对于尿酸水平处于低五分位值范围人群,PD 发病率降低 55%③。Winquist 等④进行横向社区流行病学研究调查发现,无论是男性还是女性,尿酸水平处于平均值或高于平均值人群的 PD 患病率显著低于尿酸水平处于平均值以下的人群。Schwarzschild 等⑤通过对 797 例早期确诊但尚未接受治疗的 PD 患者进行多巴胺转运体显像发现,尿酸水平越高的 PD 患者,其多巴胺缺失的程度就越低;研究进一步证实,血尿酸水平对 PD 患者的病情进展有明确的影响,血尿酸水平越高,PD 患者的病情进展越慢。

高血压病患者患 PD 的风险明显降低,可能与高血压病患者的血尿酸水平相对较高有关。高血压病通过肾素-血管紧张素-醛固酮系统(renin-angiotensin-aldosteronesystem,RAAS)对肾血流动力学产生影响,从而使肾血流量减少,由此导致肾小球滤过率降低,对尿酸盐的排泄减少;另外,肾血流量减少导致肾缺氧,从而使乳酸生成增多,堆积的乳酸与尿酸竞争排泄,也

① GONG L,ZHANG QL,ZHANG N,et al.Neuroprotection by Urate on 6-OHDA-lesioned Rat Model of Parkinson's Disease: Linking to Akt/GSK3β Signaling Pathway[J].J Neurochem,2012,123(05):876-885.

② DE LAU LM,KOUDSTAAL PJ,HOFMAN A,et al.Serum Uric Acid Levels and the Risk of Parkinson Disease[J].Ann Neurol,2005,58(05):797-800.

③ WEISSKOPF MG,O'REILLY E,CHEN H,et al.Plasma Urate and Risk of Parkinson's Disease[J].Am J Epidemiol,2007,16(05)6:561-567.

④ WINQUIST A,STEENLAND K,SHANKAR A.Higher Serum Uric Acid Associated with Decreased Parkinson's Disease Prevalence in a Large Community-based Survey [J].Mov Disord,2010,25(07):932-936.

⑤ SCHWARZSCHILD MA,MAREK K,Eberly S,et al.Serum Urate and Probability of Dopaminergic Deficit in Early "Parkinson's Disease" [J].Mov Disord,2011,26(10):1864-1868.

使血液尿酸水平升高①。腾飞等②检测 8415 名健康体检人群的血压、尿酸等指标,探讨血尿酸水平与高血压病的关系,结果显示高血压病风险随血尿酸水平的升高而增加,血尿酸水平与高血压病风险有关。樊晓寒等③通过阶段性随机整群抽样入选 5 235 例 40~75 岁高血压病患者,进行问卷调查、体检、生化指标测定等,对结果进行分析发现,降压药物、吸烟、饮酒等均显著增加 HUA 患病率及血尿酸水平。本研究结果也显示两组高血压病患者的平均尿酸水平[(338.56±98.69)μmol/L/(323 例)]明显高于无高血压病患者[(291.38±80.83)μmol/L(421 例)],$P<0.01$。高血压病人群患 PD 风险低还可能与其他因素有关,包括:① 高血压病尤其是高(systolic blood pressure,SBP)使脑的有效灌注压升高、交感肾上腺素能活性上调,不易出现自主神经功能衰竭等,而自主神经功能衰竭被认为是神经退行性疾病(如 PD)的早期表现④;② 高血压病患者脑内 RAAS 活性升高,其中血管紧张素 Ⅱ 受体和血管紧张素 Ⅳ 受体的激活可抑制炎症反应、抗氧化应激、增加脑血流,从而减少 PD 的发生和延缓 PD 的进展⑤。

本研究结果还显示,随着 PD 患者 H-Y 分级的增加,其尿酸水平有下降趋势,差异有统计学意义,但无直线相关关系,尿酸水平不能反映 PD 患者病情的严重程度,符合既往的研究⑥。此外,随着 PD 患者 H-Y 分级的增加,高血压病患病率有下降趋势,且 PD 合并高血压病患者的 UPDRS Ⅱ/Ⅲ 评分(26.30±6.48)明显低于 PD 无合并高血压病患者(41.41±10.85),表明随着 PD 症状及病情的加重,高血压病的患病率有下降趋势,可能与 PD 患者随着病情的进展,自主神经功能衰竭越来越重,更易出现血压调节障碍有关,尤其是直立性低血压和餐后低血压。PD 患者出现血压调节障碍与年

① 党爱民,刘国仗.尿酸与心血管事件[J].中华心血管病杂志.2003,31(06):478-480.

② 腾飞,邹彩艳,薛莹,等.血尿酸与代谢危险因素交互作用对高血压的影响[J].中华内分泌代谢杂志,2011,27(07):573-574.

③ 樊晓寒,孙凯,汪一波,等.中国农村高血压患者高尿酸血症患病率及相关因素分析[J].中华医学杂志,2009,89(38):2667-2670.

④ MIYAKE Y,TANAKA K,FUKUSHIMA W,et al.Case-control Study of Risk of Parkinson's Disease in Relation to Hypertension,Hypercholesterolemia,and Diabetes in Japan[J].*J Neurol Sci*,2010,293(1-2):82-86.

⑤ WRIGHT JW,KAWAS LH,HARDING JW.A Role for the Brain RAS in Alzheimer's and Parkinson's Diseases[J].*Front Endocrinol(Lausanne)*,2013,4:158-164.

⑥ 王丽君,罗蔚锋,王恒会,等.帕金森病患者血尿酸水平[J].中华神经科杂志,2008,41(03):157-158.

龄、病程、疾病严重度、抗 PD 药物及抗高血压药物的使用等有关。Velseboer 等①进行 Meta 分析发现,PD 患者直立性低血压的发生率约为 30%,餐后低血压的发生率高达 80%。PD 的病理特征是脑内多巴胺能神经元的丢失和路易体的形成,此外,岛叶皮质、下丘脑、小脑、迷走神经背侧核、交感神经节以及肠肌层和黏膜下层亦出现相似的病理变化。这些控制自主神经功能区域的病理变化与单纯自主神经功能障碍的病理变化非常相似,可以使血压下降。餐后低血压的发病机制不清,一般认为与压力感受器反射灵敏度下降、餐后交感神经反应不足及餐后胰岛素、生长抑素或血管活性肠肽等体液因素改变等有关。直立性低血压和餐后低血压作为潜在的危险因素,可引起 PD 患者因血压短时间迅速降低而心脑供血不足,引起头晕、心悸、跌倒等缺血性心脑血管不良事件的发生②。

综上所述,尿酸水平和高血压病与 PD 存在负相关联。有关尿酸水平和高血压病与 PD 的相互关系及可能机制,仍有待更大样本量及更深入的研究证实。

(张　炎　缪桂华　罗蔚锋)
(本文原载于《中国临床神经科学》2016 年第 24 卷第 5 期)

---

① VELSEBOER DC, DE HAAN RJ, WIELING W, et al. Prevalence of Orthostatic Hypotension in Parkinson's Disease: a Systematic Review and Meta-analysis [J]. *Parkinsonism Relat Disord*, 2011, 17 (10): 724-729.

② UMEHARA T, TOYODA C, OKA H. Postprandial Hypotension in De Novo Parkinson's Disease: a Comparison with Orthostatic Hypotension [J]. *Parkinsonism Relat Disord*, 2014, 20 (06): 573-577.

帕金森病患者认知功能与尿酸及相关因素分析

目的：探讨帕金森患者认知功能和血尿酸水平的关系并对认知功能相关因素进行分析。

方法：对 104 例 PD 患者进行认知功能评分和抑郁评分，收集其空腹血尿酸标本，对有认知功能障碍组和无认知功能障碍组的血尿酸水平进行比较，并用多重线性回归对认知功能相关因素进行分析。

结果：

（1）有认知功能障碍组的血尿酸水平（249 μmol/L±59 μmol/L）低于无认知功能障碍组（323 μmol/L±52 μmol/L），差异有统计学意义。（$t=-6.78, P<0.001$）。

（2）PD 患者的认知功能水平与教育水平、血尿酸水平、年龄、H-Y 分期和抑郁程度有相关性，与性别、吸烟、身高体重指数（BMI）和病程无相关性。

结论：

（1）PD 患者认知功能障碍与血尿酸水平降低有关，血尿酸水平越低，认知功能水平越低。

（2）PD 患者的教育水平、年龄、H-Y 分期和抑郁严重程度影响认知功能的改变。

关键词：帕金森病；认知功能障碍；尿酸；相关因素。

Study on Uric Acid and the Related Factors Associated with Cognition in the Patients with Parkinson's Disease

Objective：To explore the relation of cognition and uric acid in Parkinson's disease and analyze the related factors of cognition.

Methods：A total of 104 patients with Parkinson's disease were divided into two groups：those with cognitive impairment and those without.Every patient was subject to the cognitive and depression function assessment, and the fasting blood uric acid samples.Then compare the serum uric acid levels of two groups and analyze the related factors of the cognitive with multiple linear.

Results：

（1）The serum uric acid level in the group with cognitive impairment（249 μmol/L±59 μmol/L）is lower than that without cognitive impairment（323 μmol/L±52 μmol/L），and there was marked statistical significance（$t = -6.78, P<0.001$）.

（2）In PD patients，the cognitive scores correlated with serum uric acid levels，education，age，H-Y stages and the depression levels，but didn't with gender，disease duration，smoking and BML.

Conclusion：

（1）There was correlation between the serum uric acid and the cognitive impairment.Low serum uric acid level predicted worse cognitive scores.

（2）In PD，the change of the cognitive function was impacted by their education，age，H-Y stages and depression levels.

Key words：Parkinson's disease；cognition；uric acid；related factors.

目前我国的帕金森病患者已超过 200 万人。国外流行病学调查显示，PD 患者中有 40% 的患者会伴发认知功能障碍①。有研究表明，低尿酸水平是 PD 的一种危险因素②③④，但对 PD 患者血尿酸水平和认知功能关系的研究还非常少。因此，我们有必要对 PD 患者进行认知功能评分，观察他们的血尿酸水平，探讨 PD 患者的认知功能与血尿酸水平的关系。

一、对象与方法

1. 对象

104 例 PD 患者均是苏州大学附属第二医院神经内科 2007 年 9 月至

① LIEBERMAN A. Are Dementia and Depression in Parkinson's Disease Related？［J］.*J Neurol Sci*，2006，248(1-2)：138-142.

② DE LAU LM，KOUDSTAAL PJ，HOFINAN A，et al. Serum Uric Acid Levels and the Risk of Parkinson Disease［J］. *Ann Neurol*，2005，58(05)：797-800.

③ WEISSKOPF MG，O'REILLY E，CHEN H，et al. Plasma Urate and Risk of Parkinson's Disease［J］. *Am J Epidemiol*，2007，166(05)：561-567.

④ 罗蔚锋，刘春风.尿酸水平与帕金森病［J］.中华神经科杂志，2008，41(08)：552-553.

2008 年 9 月的门诊患者,均符合英国 帕金森病协会的诊断标准①:缓慢起病;具有静止性震颤、强直和运动迟缓等 3 项症状中的至少 2 项;左旋多巴治疗试验有反应,临床上排除脑血管疾病、脑炎等原因所致的帕金森综合征和帕金森叠加综合征,排除高血压病、糖尿病及心、肺、肝和肾等疾病患者。所有研究对象均为本地区居民,饮食结构及生活习惯相似,均签署知情同意书,研究经医院伦理委员会批准。

2. 临床特征调查

(1)通过问卷调查形式收集患者的一般资料,内容包括个人信息、病程、现病史、用药史、既往史和家族史等。

(2)用修订 Hoehn-Yahr(H-Y)分期对疾病的严重程度进行评分。

3. 神经精神症状调查

(1)用《汉密尔顿抑郁量表(HAMD)》对抑郁程度进行评分。

(2)用《蒙特利尔认知评估量表(MoCA)(北京版)》对患者的认知功能水平进行评分,如果受教育年限≤12 年则加 1 分,最高分为 30 分;总分≥26 分为无认知障碍,<26 分为有认知障碍。

4. 血液标本收集及测定

所有受试对象均采用早晨空腹抽取肘正中静脉血 4 mL,应用美国 DADE Behring 公司全自动生化分析仪测定血尿酸、肌酐和尿素氮。内生肌酐清除率(Ccr)用以下公式计算:男性[(140−年龄)×体重(kg)]/[72×血肌酐浓度(mg/mL)];女性[(140−年龄)×体重(kg)]/[85×血肌酐浓度(mg/mL)]。

5. 统计学处理

采用 SPSS 11.5 统计分析软件,采用两个独立样本的 t 检验对两组受试者的血尿酸和内生肌酐清除率进行比较,采用逐步法多重线性回归对认知功能障碍的相关因素进行分析。

二、结果

1. 对象一般情况

有认知功能障碍组 54 例(51.92%),无认知功能障碍组 50 例(48.08%),其中男 57 例,女 47 例,平均年龄(65±9)岁。H-Y 分期:1 期 28

---

① MEARA J, BHOWNICK BK, HOBSON P. Accuracy of Diagnosis in Patients with Presumed Parkinson's Disease[J]. *Age Ageing*, 1999, 28(02): 99−102.

例,2 期 43 例,3 期 24 例,4 期 9 例,病程为 1～22 年。两组的性别、病程差异无统计学意义。

2. 两组 PD 患者血尿酸水平和内生肌酐清除率

有认知功能障碍组的血尿酸水平(249 μmol/L±59 μmol/L)明显低于无认知功能障碍组(323 μmol/L±52 μmol/L)($t=-6.78$,$P<0.001$),有认知功能障碍组的内生肌酐清除率(81 mL/min±27 mL/min)与无认知功能障碍组(88 mL/min±20 mL/min)相比差异无统计学意义($t=-1.39$,$P>0.05$)。

3. PD 患者认知功能与相关因素的回归分析

PD 患者的认知功能评分与其受教育水平、血尿酸、年龄、H-Y 分期和抑郁程度有显著的相关性,与性别、是否吸烟、身高体重指数和病程长短无相关性,其中认知功能评分与教育水平、血尿酸水平呈正相关,与年龄、H-Y 分期和抑郁程度呈负相关(表 1)。

表 1　PD 患者认知功能与相关因素的回归分析

相关因素	R^2	t 值	P 值
受教育水平	0.604	8.216	0.000
血尿酸水平	0.713	2.773	0.007
年龄	0.694	−3.826	0.000
H-Y 分期	0.376	−4.843	0.000
抑郁程度	0.654	−3.667	0.000

三、讨论

研究发现,PD 患者的认知功能与其血尿酸水平有关,这个发现考虑与尿酸神经保护作用的性质有关。目前已知,氧化损伤在帕金森病和认知功能障碍的形成机制中都起着重要的作用。动物实验和临床研究提示氧化损伤与认知功能障碍密切相关[1][2]。尿酸是一种重要的抗氧化剂和自由基清

① FARR SA, POON HF, DOGRUKOL-AK D, et al. The Antioxidants Alphalipoic Acid and N-acetylcysteine Reverse Memory Impairment and Antioxidative Stress in Aged SAMP8 Mice[J]. *J Neurochem*, 2003, 84(05): 1173-1183.

② FUKUI K, ONODERA K, SHINKAI T. Impairment of Learning and Memory in Rats Caused by Oxidative Stress and Aging, and Changes in Antioxidative Defense Systems[J]. *Ann NY Acad Sci*, 2001, 928(01): 168-175.

除剂,能够清除过氧化物、羟基、氧自由基,阻断硝基化反应,并螯合铁离子,减少体内的氧化应激水平。实验研究表明,适当提高脑组织中的尿酸水平,能够减轻1-甲基-4-苯基-1,2,3,6-四氢吡啶(MPTP)对小鼠多巴胺能神经元的损伤①。当PD患者细胞内抗氧化系统受损后,细胞很容易受到自由基和铁离子的损伤,随着氧化损伤水平的升高,对抗氧化应激消耗的尿酸量增加,导致血中尿酸水平的降低②,可能会引起认知功能的损伤。

PD伴发认知功能障碍的发生率各家报道不一,国外报道为17%～57%③④⑤,国内报道为31.9%～59.5%⑥⑦。发生率差异较大,分析主要有以下几方面原因:(1)使用认知功能评定的量表不同。(2)调查人群的来源不同——我们的研究人群是门诊帕金森病患者。(3)样本量不同。我们的研究发现PD患者的认知功能障碍发生率为51.92%,与国内外相似。

对相关因素的回归分析结果显示,PD患者的认知功能障碍与其受教育水平、血尿酸水平呈正相关,而与年龄、H-Y分期及抑郁程度呈负相关。PD患者的受教育水平越高,本身的逻辑思维越丰富,越善于从周围事物中寻找联系和规律,来弥补疾病本身带来的影响。而年龄越大,增龄性的因素也就越多,如动脉硬化和脑萎缩等,这些都会加重PD患者的认知功能障碍。PD患者的认知功能水平与H-Y分期呈负相关而与病程无相关性,这可能是因为在这104例PD患者中,其病程长短差异较大,有的患者病程虽长,但病情较轻,病情发展慢,损害小,而有的患者虽然病程很短,但已经处于疾病的中晚期,病情发展较快,损害大。这说明并不是病程长的患者就一定比病程短的患者损害严重。有关PD的抑郁和认知功能的关系,经双变量分析发

① LUO WF, SCHWARZSCHILD MA, XU K.Urate Attenuates MPTP-induced Dopmainergic Toxicity in Mice[J].The Society for Neuroscience 37th Annual Meeting, 2007.San Diego, California, USA.

② ANDERSON RF, HAMS TA.Dopamine and Uric Acid Act as Antioxidants in the Repair of DNA Radicals: Implications in Parkinson' Disease[J].*Free Radic Res*, 2003, 37(10): 1131−1136.

③ AARSLAND D, ZACCAI J, BRAYNE C.A Systematic Review of Prevalence Studies of Dementia in Parkinson's Disease[J].*Mov Disord*, 2005, 20(10): 1255−1263.

④ LIEBERMAN A.Are Dementia and Depression in Parkinson's Disease Related? [J].*J Neurol Sci*, 2006, 248(1−2): 138−142.

⑤ WILLIAMS-GRAY CH, FOLTYNIE T, BRAYNE CE, et al.Evolution of Cognitive Dysfunction in an Incident Parkinson's Disease Cohort[J].*Brain*, 2007, 130(Pt 7): 1787−1798.

⑥ 唐峥华, 梁华忠.帕金森氏病患者认知功能的研究[J].中国临床心理学杂志, 1998, 6(02): 91−93.

⑦ 蔡晓杰、陈海波、王新德、等.帕金森病的智能障碍——瑞文测验的应用及意义[J].脑与神经疾病杂志, 1997, 5(02): 94−96.

现,抑郁程度与发生痴呆症有关,抑郁愈严重,发生痴呆症的危险性愈高①。Lieberman②曾对美国106例PD患者的神经精神症状进行调查,结果显示抑郁与痴呆有显著的相关性。这与我们的研究结果相一致。有关PD抑郁情绪影响记忆成绩的机制较为复杂,有待于进一步研究探讨。

PD患者的认知功能水平与血尿酸水平呈正相关,即认知功能水平越低,其血尿酸水平也越低,这与国外的研究结果一致③。同时,为了排除肾功能水平对血尿酸结果的影响,我们同时对两组患者的内生肌酐清除率进行了比较,结果显示无统计学差异,这就排除了因肾功能而导致的血尿酸异常。

Schretlen等④在对健康人群的调查研究中发现,血尿酸水平高对认知功能有害。这种认知缺损的机理被认为是脑血管方面的问题,高尿酸水平是引起脑血管疾病的危险因素,尿酸水平显著增高容易引起脑血管病变,从而导致认知功能的减退。表面上看我们的研究与上述结果相反,但是实际并非如此。这种相反的结果与以下原因有关:(1)两项研究的研究对象不同。Schretlen等⑤的研究是将PD患者排除在外。(2)PD患者的血尿酸水平低于正常健康人群⑥,所以PD患者与正常健康人群的尿酸水平是完全不同的。研究提示,我们可以通过测定PD患者的血尿酸水平对其发生认知功能障碍的风险性进行预测评估,从而进行膳食指导,使其在一定范围内适当提高血尿酸水平,以达到预防或延缓发生痴呆的目的。

（王晓君　罗蔚锋　王丽君　毛成洁　王　兰　刘春风）

（本文原载于《中华医学杂志》2009年第89卷第23期）

① HUGHES TA, ROSS HF, MUSA S, et al. A 10-year Study of the Incidence and Factors Predicting Dementia in Parkinson's Disease[J]. *Neurology*, 2000, 54(08): 1596-1602.

② LIEBERMAN A. Are Dementia and Depression in Parkinson's Disease Related? [J]. *J Neurol Sci*, 2006, 248(1-2): 138-142.

③ ANNANMAKI T, PESSALE DA, HOKKANEN L, et al. Uric Acid Associates with Cognition in Parkinson's Disease[J]. *Parkinsonism Relat Disord*, 2008, 14(07): 576-578.

④ SCHRETLEN DJ, INSCORE AB, JINNAH HA, et al. Serum Uric Acid and Cognitive Function in Community-dwelling Older Adults[J]. *Neuropsychology*, 2007, 21(01): 136-140.

⑤ SCHRETLEN DJ, INSCORE AB, JINNAH HA, et al. Serum Uric Acid and Cognitive Function in Community-dwelling Older Adults[J]. *Neuropsychology*, 2007, 21(01): 136-140.

⑥ 王丽君,罗蔚锋,王恒会,等,帕金森病患者血尿酸水平[J].中华神经科杂志,2008,41(03): 157-158.

尿酸对帕金森病患者不同认知功能域影响分析①

帕金森病认知功能损害近年来受到人们的关注,大约40%的PD患者会发展为痴呆,发生率高于健康人群6倍②③,但目前其确切发病机制还不清楚。有研究显示,氧化应激损伤在PD认知功能损害中起到重要作用。低血尿酸水平人群的PD发病率显著升高,高血尿酸水平人群的PD发病率显著降低,PD患者组的血尿酸水平低于健康对照组④⑤。我们以往的研究结果显示,PD患者的血尿酸水平与其认知功能呈正相关,即相对高水平血尿酸的PD患者有较好的认知功能⑥。我们此次的研究旨在进一步探讨血尿酸水平与哪些认知功能域有相关性及其可能的机制。

资料和方法

一、研究对象

1. 诊断标准

所有患者的诊断均符合英国帕金森病协会的诊断标准⑦:缓慢起病;具有静止性震颤、强直和运动迟缓等3项症状中的至少2项;左旋多巴治疗有效。

———————————

① 本文系江苏省高校自然科学基础研究资助项目(项目编号:08KJB320012);苏州市科技发展计划(社会发展及医药)资助项目(项目编号:200815404)。

② HUGHES TA,ROSS HF,MUSA S,et al.A 10-year Study of the Incidence of and Factors Predicting Dementia in Parkinson's Disease[J].*Neurology*,2000,54(08): 1596-1602.

③ EMRE M.Dementia Associated with Parkinson's Disease[J].*Lancet Neurol*,2003,2(04): 229-237.

④ DE LAU LM,KOUDSTAAL PJ,HOFMAN A,et al.Serum Uric Acid Levels and the Risk of Parkinson Disease[J].*Ann Neurol*,2005,58(05): 797-800.

⑤ ANNANMAKI T,MUURONEN A,MURROS K.Low Plasma Uric Acid Level in Parkinson' Disease [J].*Mov Disord*,2007,22(08): 1133-1137.

⑥ 王晓君,罗蔚锋,王丽君,等.帕金森病患者认知功能与尿酸及相关因素分析[J].中华医学杂志,2009,89(23): 1633-1635.

⑦ MEARA J,BHOWMICK BK,HOBSON P. Accuracy of Diagnosis in Patients with Presumed Parkinson's Disease[J].*Age Ageing*,1999,28(02): 99-102.

2. 纳入标准

（1）临床神经专科医师明确诊断原发性 PD 患者,无家族史。

（2）140 例 PD 患者均是苏州大学附属第二医院神经内科 2007 年 9 月至 2009 年 10 月的门诊患者,为本地区居民,饮食结构及生活习惯相似,均签署了知情同意书,本研究经医院伦理委员会批准。

（3）患者年龄大于 30 岁,病程在半年以上。

（4）所有患者均早晨预约至门诊,就诊前一天晚上停服左旋多巴和苄丝肼、左旋多巴和卡比多巴等治疗 PD 的药物,PD 严重程度评分在“关”期进行。

3. 排除标准

排除脑血管疾病、脑炎、中毒、脑外伤和药物引起的具有帕金森样症状的帕金森综合征和帕金森叠加综合征;排除小脑疾病、记忆混乱、语言行为异常等早期严重痴呆的 PD 患者;排除有高血压、糖尿病、心脏病、脑卒中、痛风、肾炎等影响尿酸代谢的患者;排除服用利尿剂和其他影响尿酸代谢药物的患者。所有患者均行头颅 CT 和(或)核磁共振成像(nuclear magnetic resonance image,MRI)检查,排除明显的双侧基底节钙化、明显的纹状体腔隙性梗死、脑积水和脑白质异常者。

二、研究方法

1. 资料收集

记录患者的一般资料,包括性别、年龄、身高、体重、受教育程度、病程、现病史、用药史、既往史和家族史等。

2. 调查工具

（1）运动功能评价:采用 PD 统一评分量表第三部分(UPDRS Ⅲ)和 Hoehn-Yahr(H-Y)分级对患者运动症状严重程度进行评价。

（2）认知量表:采用《蒙特利尔认知评估量表(MoCA)(北京版)》对患者的认知功能进行评分,并记录其视空间和执行能力、命名能力、记忆能力、注意能力、语言流畅能力、抽象能力和定向能力等 7 个认知域的总分及各认知域的分值。受教育年限 ≤12 年则加 1 分,最高分为 30 分;≥26 分为正常。

（3）精神症状评价:采用《汉密尔顿抑郁量表(HAMD)》对抑郁程度进行评分,HAMD≤8 分无抑郁,HAMD>8 分有抑郁。所有量表评分一次完成,调查过程患者及家属共同参与,对回忆不清的地方参照既往病史。

3. 血液样本收集和测定

所有受试者均于晨起空腹抽取肘正中静脉血 4 mL,应用 DADE Behring 公司全自动生化分析仪测定血尿酸。

4. 统计学分析

采用 SPSS 17.0 统计分析软件,首先采用逐步多重线性回归法对认知功能的相关因素进行分析,然后将年龄、教育年限、UPDRS III、抑郁(HAMD 评分)等进入回归方程的影响因素作为控制变量,采用 Partial 相关性分析血尿酸水平与 MoCA 各认知域间的关系。

三、结果

1. 研究对象一般情况

140 例 PD 患者中男 74 例,女 66 例,58 例受教育年限≥12 年,82 例受教育年限<12 年。男性患者中 54%(40/74)接受过 12 年以上教育,女性患者中仅 27%(18/66)接受过 12 年以上教育。平均发病年龄(59±10)岁。H-Y 分期:1～3 期 133 例,4～5 期 7 例。认知功能障碍组 77 例(77/140,55%),无认知功能障碍组 63 例(63/140,45%)。

2. PD 患者的认知功能与其相关因素的分析

用逐步多元回归分析法在回归方程中引入年龄、性别、病程、受教育年限、UPDRS III 评分、HAMD 评分、血尿酸值和体重指数等可能影响 PD 认知功能的因素,其中受教育年限、血尿酸水平、HAMD 评分、年龄、性别和 UPDRS III 评分与认知功能评分存在显著相关性被选入方程,而与病程及体重指数无明显相关性。PD 患者的认知功能水平与受教育年限、血尿酸水平呈正相关,而与 HAMD 评分、年龄和 UPDRS III 评分呈负相关,而女性患者较男性患者认知功能下降(表 1)。

表 1　140 例 PD 患者认知功能与相关因素的回归分析

项目	x^2值	t 值	P 值
受教育年限	0.243	5.118	0.000
尿酸水平	0.377	3.360	0.001
年龄	0.431	−3.841	0.000
UPDRS III 评分	0.325	−3.381	0.001
性别	0.456	−2.477	0.014
HAMD 评分	0,148	−2.219	0.028

3. PD 患者的血尿酸水平与各个认知域的相关性

进行 Partial 相关性分析发现,在控制变量年龄、UPDRS Ⅲ 评分、受教育年限、HAMD 评分和性别后,PD 患者的血尿酸水平与记忆能力及抽象概括能力均有相关性 $P<0.01$(表 2)。

表 2　140 例 PD 患者的血尿酸水平与各认知域的相关性分析

检测项目	分值	平均分值	r 值	P 值
记忆能力	0~5	2.65±1.43	0.260	0.002
抽象概括能力	0~2	1.17±0.77	0.236	0.006
注意能力	0~6	5.02±1.29	0.169	0.051
语言流畅能力	0~3	2.00±0.91	0.168	0.052
命名能力	0~3	2.60±0.58	0.153	0.076
视空间和执行能力	0~5	3.12±1.53	0.141	0.102
定向能力	0~6	5.67±0.83	0.116	0.180

四、讨论

PD 是一种隐性起病、缓慢进展的神经系统变性疾病,主要病理特征为黑质致密部多巴胺能神经元进行性减少,除常见的运动症状外,还伴随非运动症状,如认知功能障碍①、抑郁和感觉异常等,其中认知功能损害是 PD 非运动症状的主要表现之一。我们之前对 104 例 PD 患者的研究结果显示,PD 患者的认知功能与其受教育水平、血尿酸水平呈正相关,与其年龄、H-Y 分级、HAMD 评分呈负相关②,我们的研究是在以往的基础上对 PD 患者的血尿酸水平与各认知功能区域的相关性进行更深入的探讨。

认知功能是指个体熟练运用知识的能力,包括语言和非语言技能,记忆新知识的能力和从丰富的知识库中追忆知识的能力,计算能力,抽象概括能力,判断事物间相似性与差别的能力③。我们使用 MoCA 评定 PD 患者的

① 姚明,陈先文,孙中武.帕金森病患者轻度认知功能损害[J].中华神经科杂志,2009,42(05):296-300.

② 王晓君,罗蔚锋,王丽君,等.帕金森病患者认知功能与尿酸及相关因素分析[J].中华医学杂志,2009,89(23):1633-1635.

③ 贾建平.临床痴呆病学[M].北京:北京大学医学出版社,2008:33-35.

认知功能,其敏感性为 90%,特异性为 100%①②,能够全面评价多个认知域,可发现存在认知功能损害的早期 PD 患者。MoCA 包括 7 个方面的认知域:视空间执行能力、命名能力、注意力、语言流畅能力、抽象概括能力、记忆力和定向力。

多元回归分析结果与我们之前的研究结果相似,140 例 PD 患者的认知功能与其受教育水平和血尿酸水平呈正相关,与其年龄、UPDRS Ⅲ 评分和 HAMD 评分呈负相关,表明血尿酸水平相对高的 PD 患者有较好的认知功能,这可能与尿酸本身是自由基清除剂,可以清除过氧化物、羟基、氧自由基,阻断硝基化反应,减少体内的氧化应激水平有关。UPDRSⅢ评分越高表明疾病越严重,对患者认知功能的损害越明显,其原因为病情严重的患者运动功能明显受损、语言表达能力下降、对周围事物观察能力下降影响了其执行能力和注意力。抑郁和焦虑症状是原发性 PD 患者最为常见的伴随症状,伴痴呆患者的抑郁症状更为常见。有关 PD 的抑郁与认知功能的关系,经双变量分析显示,抑郁愈严重,发展为痴呆的危险性愈高③。

目前 PD 患者认知功能损害的确切机制还不清楚,伴认知功能损害的 PD 患者基底核神经元丢失较无认知功能损害者严重,在多巴胺能神经元丢失达到一定程度时,乙酰胆碱代谢受影响,上行性胆碱能通路变性造成的胆碱能通路缺陷可能是导致认知功能损害的原因之一。PD 患者的记忆力、抽象概括能力和视空间执行能力下降可能与基底节和额叶之间的皮质-皮质-多巴胺环路受到损害,纹状体内及前额叶内多巴胺耗竭有关④⑤。5-羟色胺、谷氨酸等神经递质水平的改变亦参与了 PD 患者认知功能的损害。

氧化应激损伤是 PD 患者认知功能损害的主要机制之一,正常情况下氧自由基的产生和清除处于动态平衡之中,病理状态时氧自由基产生过多,

① NAZEM S,SIDEROWF AD,DUDA JE,et al.Montreal Cognitive Assessment Performance in Patients with Parkinson's Disease with"normal"Global Cognition According to Mini-mental State Examination Score[J].*J Am Geriatr Soc*,2009,57(02):304-308.

② ISMAIL Z,RAJJI TK,SHULMAN KI.Brief Cognitive Screening Instruments:an Update[J].*Int J Geriatr Psychiatry*,2010,25(02):111-120.

③ HUGHES TA,ROSS HF,MUSA S,et al.A 10-year Study of the Incidence of and Factors Predicting Dementia in Parkinson's Disease[J].*Neurology*,2000,54(08):1596-1602.

④ 陈海波.帕金森病认知和行为障碍[J].中华神经科杂志,2009,42(05):289-292.

⑤ ZGALJARDIC DJ,BOROD JC,FOLDI NS,et al.A Review of the Cognitive and Behavioral Sequelae of Parkinson's Disease:Relationship to Frontostriatal Circuitry[J].*Cogn Behav Neurol*,2003,16(04):193-210.

抗氧化系统物质大量消耗,自由基损伤生物膜,破坏细胞完整性,损伤线粒体造成细胞能量不足最终引起神经元代谢紊乱、变性、坏死,导致患者认知功能损害①②。铁离子是自由基生成的主要催化剂,PD 和阿尔兹海默患者脑部均存在铁代调异常。已有研究显示,PD 和阿尔兹海默病患者外周血氧化指标增加,而抗氧化指标维生素 E、谷胱甘肽过氧化物酶等减少③。我们以往的研究也显示,与健康对照组比较,老年男性 PD 患者的血尿酸水平明显降低,伴有认知功能障碍的 PD 患者尿酸水平更低④,表明 PD 患者及伴认知功能下降的 PD 患者外周抗氧化剂水平明显降低,从而氧化应激损伤增强。而外源性补充抗氧化剂或相关促氧化物代谢的酶可部分逆转氧化应激损伤,改善认知功能⑤。

最近 Ascherio 等⑥和 Irizarry 等⑦的研究显示,基础血尿酸水平相对高的 PD 患者病情进展相对要慢,还发现相对高尿酸水平的轻度认知功能损害(MCI)患者进展为痴呆的速度减缓,这些均显示尿酸作为抗氧化剂具有潜在的神经保护作用。此次在控制其他影响认知功能的因素后,进行血尿酸水平与 PD 患者各认知域 Partial 相关分析,发现血尿酸水平与 PD 认知域中记忆力和抽象概括能力呈显著正相关,推测其机制与黑质,基底节区尿酸减少致过多 Fe^{2+} 积聚,过(氧化)亚硝酸盐介导的硝化反应增强及抗氧化酶如 SOD 活性降低,氧自由基生成增多及其活性增强,最终导致基底节区神经元细胞过氧化变性死亡,从而破坏基底节和额叶之间的皮质-皮质-多巴

① DE LA MONTE SM, GANJU N, FEROZ N, et al. Oxygen Free Radical Injury is Sufficient to Cause Some Alzheimer-type Molecular Abnormalities in Human CNS Neuronal Cells[J]. *J Alzheimers Dis*, 2000, 2(3-4): 261-281.

② MAIESE K, CHONG ZZ. Insights into Oxidative and Potential Novel Therapeutic Targets for Alzhermer Disease[J]. *Restor Neurol Neurosci*, 2004, 22(02): 87-104.

③ CHEN CM, LIU JL, WU YR, et al. Increased Oxidative Damage in Peripheral Blood Correlates with Severity of Parkinson's Disease[J]. *Neurobiol Dis*, 2009, 33(03): 429-435.

④ 罗蔚锋,王丽君,王晓君,等,老年男性帕金森患者血尿酸水平的研究[J].中华老年医学杂志,2009,28(01): 60-61.

⑤ LIU R, LIU IY, BI X, et al. Reversal of Age-related Learning Deficits and Brain Oxidative Stress in Mice with Superoxide Dismutase/Catalase Mimetics[J]. *Proc Natl Acad Sci USA*, 2003, 100(14): 8526-8531.

⑥ ASCHERIO A, LEWITT PA, XU K, et al. Urate as a Predictor of the Rate of Clinical Decline in Parkinson Disease[J]. *Arch Neurol*, 2009, 66(12): 1460-1468.

⑦ IRIZARRY MC, RAMAN R, SCHWARZSCHILD MA, et al. Plasma Urate and Progression of Mild Cognitive Impainment[J]. *Neurodegenerative Dis*, 2009, 6(1-2): 23-28.

胺环路有关①。

我们的研究显示,PD 患者的血尿酸水平与认知域中的记忆力、抽象概括力相关,高尿酸水平患者的记忆力、抽象概括力相对较好,其确切机制还有待于进一步探讨。结合 MoCA 量表,血尿酸水平有可能成为 PD 患者早期认知功能障碍的预测因素之一,从而有助于早期发现 PD 患者的轻度认知功能障碍(mild cognitive impairment, MCI)症状,并通过饮食调整或药物治疗等途径,在一定范围内提高其尿酸水平,从而延缓 PD 患者由 MCI 向 PD 痴呆的发展。

(李　丹　王晓君　罗蔚锋　朱婷鸽　胡伟东　毛成洁　刘春风)
　　(本文原载于《中华神经科杂志》2010 年第 43 卷第 6 期)

---

① 　罗蔚锋,刘春风.尿酸水平与帕金森病[J].中华神经科杂志,2008,41(08):552-553.

附　录

腺苷 A_{2A} 受体拮抗剂治疗帕金森病的研究进展

　　摘　要：　腺苷 A_{2A} 受体拮抗剂具有治疗帕金森病的作用。本文就腺苷 A_{2A} 受体及腺苷 A_{2A} 受体拮抗剂的特性,腺苷 A_{2A} 受体拮抗剂类药物治疗帕金森病的研究进展做一综述。

　　关键词：　帕金森病;腺苷 A_{2A} 受体;腺苷 A_{2A} 受体拮抗剂。

　　左旋多巴制剂是治疗帕金森病的基本药物,但长期使用左旋多巴制剂疗效会明显减退,并出现运动障碍(dyskinesia)、开—关现象(on-off phenomenon)等一系列难以忍受的不良反应。这促进了其他类型药物的研制开发。

　　流行病学调查提示茶碱和咖啡能降低帕金森病的发病概率。研究①发现咖啡是非选择性腺苷受体拮抗剂(adenosine receptor antagonist),作用在于阻断了腺苷 A_{2A} 受体(adenosine A_{2A} receptor)。这一发现促使人们进一步研制选择性 A_{2A} 受体拮抗剂。

一、腺苷 A_{2A} 受体的分布

　　腺苷受体主要有4个亚型:A_1、A_{2A}、A_{2B}、A_3。A_{2A} 是治疗帕金森病的靶受体。A_{2A} 受体主要和多巴胺 D_2 受体共表达于纹状体—苍白球的中间棘状神经元(medium spiny neurons,MSNs),但是不和多巴胺 D_1 受体共表达②,后来

　　① 　FREDHOLM BB.Connection between Caffeine,Adenosine Receptors and Dopamine:Coffee Reduces the Risk of Parkinson Disease[J].*Lakartidningen*,2004,101(34):2552-2555.

　　② 　FINK JS,WEAVER DR,RIVKEES SA, et al.Molecular Cloning of the Rat A_2 Adenosine Receptor:Selective Co-expression with D_2 Dopamine Receptors in Rat Striatum[J].*Brain Res Mol BRAIN rES*,1992,14(03):186-195.

又发现 A_{2A} 受体主要和多巴胺 D_2 受体共表达于伏隔核的核心区和壳区及嗅结节①,也分布于免疫细胞等外周部分②。

二、腺苷 A_{2A} 受体的信号转导

腺苷 A_{2A} 受体是一种 G 蛋白偶联受体,有 7 个跨膜区域,主要与 Gs 蛋白偶联,激活 A_{2A} 受体能够激活腺苷酸环化酶和蛋白激酶 A(PKA),使 c-Fos、前脑啡肽、神经加压素、调节多巴胺和 1c AMP 的磷酸化蛋白(dopamine and cAMP-regulated phosphoprotein,DARPP-32)表达增加,而 DARPP-32③ 和 c-Fos④ 的表达增加是细胞激活的重要标志。

三、腺苷 A_{2A} 受体和多巴胺 D_2 受体形成异聚体

研究⑤表明,腺苷 A_{2A} 受体和多巴胺 D_2 受体能够形成异源二聚体(heterodimer)和/或异源低聚体(hetero-oligomer),此异源二聚体能够降低多巴胺 D_2 受体的活性,腺苷 A_{2A} 受体激动剂能够促进异源二聚体形成,而腺苷 A_{2A} 受体拮抗剂能够抑制异源二聚体形成。

四、腺苷 A_{2A} 受体和多巴胺 D_2 受体相互作用的机制

1. 受体水平的相互作用

腺苷 A_{2A} 受体和多巴胺 D_2 受体形成异源二聚体和/或异源低聚体,通过腺苷 A_{2A} 受体的段基端(the carboxyl terminus of the A_{2A} receptor)和多巴胺 D_2

---

① SVENNINGSSON P,LE MOINE C,KULL B, et al. Cellular Expression of Adenosine A_{2A} Receptor Messenger RNA in the Rat Central Nervous System With Special Reference to Dopamine Inervted Areas[J]. *Neurosci*,1997,80(04):1171-1185.

② SITKOVSKY MV,LUKASHEV D,APASOV S, et al.Physiological Control of Immune Response and Inflammatory Tissue Damage by Hypoxia-inducible Factors and Adenosine A_{2A} Receptors[J].*Ann Rev Immun*, 2004,22:657-682.

③ SVENNINGSSON P, LINDSKOG M, LEDENT C, et al. Regulation of the Phosphorylation of the Dopamine and cAMP-regulated Phosphoprotein of 32 kDa in Vivo by Dopamine D_1, Dopamine D_2, and Adenosine A_{2A} Receptors[J].*Proc Natl Acad Sci USA*,2000,97(04):1856-1860.

④ CHINENOV Y,KERPPOLA TK.Close Encounters of Many Kinds:Fos-Jun Interactions that Mediate Transcription Regulatory Specificity[J].*Oncogene*,2001,20(19):2438-2452.

⑤ FUXE K,FERRE S,CANALS M, et al. Adenosine A_{2A} and Dopamine D_2 Heteromeric Receptor Complexes and their Function[J].*J Mol Neurosci*,2005,26(2-3):209-220.

受体的 5,6 跨膜区相互作用,改变多巴胺 D_2 受体的表位,降低多巴胺 D_2 受体与其配体的亲和力,通过腺苷 A_{2A} 受体的羧基端(the carboxyl terminus of the A_{2A} receptor)和细胞内的 I3 氮末端部分(N-terminal part of I3 of the D_2 receptor)(精氨酸富集表位)(arginine-rich epitope)相互作用,降低多巴胺 D_2 受体与 G 蛋白的偶联,降低多巴胺 D_2 受体激活后促进 K^+ 外流和抑制钙内流的作用,从而降低多巴胺 D_2 受体的活性。

2. 腺苷环化酶水平的相互作用

腺苷 A_{2A} 受体是一种 G 蛋白偶联受体,有 7 个跨膜区域,主要与 Gs 蛋白偶联,激活 A_{2A} 受体能够激活腺苷酸环化酶,对细胞产生兴奋性作用[1]。而多巴胺受体主要与 Gi/o 蛋白偶联,激活 D_2 受体能够抑制腺苷酸环化酶的激活,从而促进 K^+ 外流,抑制钙内流,引起细胞的超级化,对细胞产生抑制性作用[2]。

3. 基因水平的相互作用

研究发现:长期使用左旋多巴治疗的帕金森病患者,其壳核和外侧苍白球的腺苷 A_{2A} 受体 mRNA 和腺苷 A_{2A} 受体明显高于未经左旋多巴治疗的帕金森病患者;异动症的帕金森病患者,其外侧壳核的腺苷 A_{2A} 受体 mRNA 和腺苷 A_{2A} 受体高于经左旋多巴治疗但未发生异动症的患者。因此考虑左旋多巴可能通过对多巴胺受体的长期作用影响 A_{2A} 受体的表达[3]。

五、腺苷 A_{2A} 受体和谷氨酸 mGluRs 受体

腺苷 A_{2A} 受体和谷氨酸 $mGluR_5$ 受体能够形成异源二聚体,主要分布在苍白球的中间棘状神经元[4]。腺苷 A_{2A} 受体激动剂和 $mGluR_5$ 受体激动剂能够促进此异源二聚体形成。实验表明,此异源二聚体有利于腺苷 A_{2A} 受体和谷氨酸 $mGluR_5$ 受体发挥协同作用,从而降低多巴胺 D_2 受体与其激动剂

① FREDHOLM BB.Connection between Caffeine, Adenosine Receptors and Dopamine: Coffee Reduces the Risk of Parkinson Disease[J].*Lakartidningen*,2004,101(34): 2552-2555.

② MISSALE C,NASH SR,ROBINSON SW,et al.Dopamine Receptors: from Structure to Function[J]. *Physiol Rev*,1998,78(01): 189-225.

③ CALON F,DRIDI M.HOMYKIEWICZ O,et al.Increased Adenosine A2A Receptors in the Brain of Parkinson's Disease Patients with Dyskinesias[J].*Brain*,2004,127(Pt5): 1075-1084.

④ FERRÉ S,KARCZ-KUBICHA M,HOPE BT, et al.Synergistic Interaction between Adenosine A_{2a} and Glutamate mGlu5 Receptors: Implications for Striatal Neuronal Function[J].*Pro National Acad Sci USA*,2002, 99(18): 11940-11945.

的亲和力,对多巴胺 D_2 受体起拮抗作用。而在腺苷 A_{2A} 受体基因敲除后使用 $mGluR_5$ 受体激动剂不能对多巴胺 D_2 受体发挥拮抗作用①。

六、腺苷 A_{2A} 受体对基底节通路的作用发挥

　　基底节是调节运动的重要的皮质下中枢,主要包括两条通路:直接通路(纹状体—黑质网状部/苍白球内侧—丘脑—皮质环路),间接通路(纹状体—苍白球外侧—底丘脑核—黑质网状部/苍白球内侧—丘脑—皮质环路)。纹状体作用于直接通路的传出神经元主要含 D_1 受体,作用于间接通路的传出神经元主要含 D_2 受体。激活直接通路易化丘脑皮质神经元的活动,而激活间接通路抑制丘脑皮质神经元的活动。多巴胺对 D_1 受体有兴奋作用从而激活直接通路,对 D_2 受体有抑制作用从而抑制间接通路,保持直接通路和间接通路平衡。帕金森病患者黑质致密部的 DA 神经元损伤后,对直接通路的激活作用及间接通路的抑制作用减弱,直接通路和间接通路失衡,对丘脑皮质神经元的抑制作用加强,出现运动减少、运动迟缓、僵硬、震颤等现象②。

　　1. 腺苷 A_{2A} 受体对基底通路的作用

　　腺苷 A_{2A} 受体主要通过对间接通路的调节发挥作用。

　　(1)在纹状体内 CABA 能神经元的腺苷 A_{2A} 受体被激活能够提高纹状体 GABA 能神经元兴奋性,从而抑制苍白球外侧 GABA 能神经元的兴奋性。

　　(2)激活纹状体 GABA 能神经元轴突端的腺苷 A_{2A} 受体能够促进 GABA 的释放,抑制苍白球外侧 GABA 能神经元的兴奋性③

　　2. 其作用机制

　　(1)激活腺苷 A_{2A} 受体能够激活 Gs 型腺苷酸环化酶(cAMP)和蛋白激酶 A(PKA),提高纹状体 GABA 能神经元的兴奋性。

　　(2)激活腺苷 A_{2A} 受体能够增强对多巴胺 D_2 受体的拮抗作用,降低 D_2 受体激活后对纹状体 GABA 能神经元的抑制作用。

　　① KACHROO A,ORLANDO LR,GRANDY DK, et al.Interactions between Metabotropic Glutamate 5 and Adenosine A_{2A} Receptors in Normal and Parkinsonian Mice[J].*J Neurosci*,2005,25(45):10414-10419.

　　② LANG AE,LOZANO AM.Parkinson's Disease:Second of Two Parts[J].*N Engl J Med*,1998,339(16):1130-1143.

　　③ SHINDOU T,RICHARDSON PJ,Mori A,et al.Adenosine Modulates the Striatal GABA Ergic Inputs to the Globus Palli-dus via Adenosine A_{2A} Receptors in Rats[J].*Neurosci Lett*,2003,352(03):167-170.

（3）激活腺苷 A_{2A} 受体能够协同谷氨酸 $mGluR_5$ 受体的作用，增强对多巴胺 D_2 受体的抑制作用。

（4）激活纹状体 GABA 能神经元末端的腺苷 A_{2A} 受体能够激活 Gs 型腺苷酸环化酶（cAMP）和蛋白激酶 A（PKA），提高纹状体 GABA 能神经元纹状体 GABA 能神经元轴突端的兴奋性。

其中（1）和（4）由 A_{2A} 受体本身所介导，（2）和（3）通过和其他受体相互作用介导。

七、腺苷 A_{2A} 受体拮抗剂

研究发现，茶碱和咖啡能降低帕金森病的发病概率，并且主要因为其阻断了腺苷 A_{2A} 受体，从而促进了对选择性腺苷 A_{2A} 受体拮抗剂的研究。迄今已研制出多种选择性腺苷 A_{2A} 受体拮抗剂，其中对 KW6002 的报道较多，KW6002 通过调节基底节的 GABA 的释放，平衡间接通路和直接通路。研究[1]发现 KW6002 还具有神经保护作用，阻止多巴胺能细胞及其轴树突终末的丢失，抑制黑质致密部小胶质细胞的激活。其机制主要有以下 5 个方面。

1. 抑制基底节的非多巴胺能神经元的过度兴奋。腺苷 A_{2A} 受体拮抗剂降低纹状体 GABA 能神经元兴奋性，降低对苍白球外侧 GABA 能神经元的抑制，从而增强对底丘脑核的抑制作用，使底丘脑核释放到黑质致密部的谷氨酸减少。

2. 缓解多巴胺由于自身的氧化作用而对纹状体多巴胺能神经元终末环境的影响。腺苷 A_{2A} 受体拮抗剂能够抑制多巴胺细胞外释放，同时还有可能促进多巴胺进入囊泡。

3. 调节炎症反应。腺苷 A_{2A} 受体在小胶质细胞和星形胶质细胞上也有表达，腺苷 A_{2A} 受体拮抗剂抑制环氧化酶 2（COX-2）的表达，而环氧化酶 2（COX-2）能够合成前列腺素（PGs）在炎症反应中发挥重要作用，腺苷 A_{2A} 受体拮抗剂还能够抑制纹状体星形胶质细胞的增生[2]。腺苷 A_{2A} 受体拮抗剂

---

① IKEDA K，KUROKAWA M，AOYAMA S，et al.Neuroprotection by Adenosine A_{2A} Receptor Blockade in Experimental Models of Parkinson's Disease［J］.*J Neurochem*，2002，80（02）：262-270.

② PIERRI M，VAUDANO E，SAGER T，et al. KW-6002 Protects from MPTP Induced Dopaminergic Toxicity in the Mouse［J］.*Neuropharmacology*，2005，48（04）：517-524.

KW6002 在体外有阻断单胺氧化酶 B(MAO-B)的作用①,但体内试验没能证明其对 MAO-B 的阻断作用②。

4. 腺苷 A_{2A} 受体拮抗剂减少小胶质细胞 NO 的产生③。

KW6002 的治疗效果:Hauser 等④进行了为期 12 周的、随机的、安慰剂对照的探究性临床试验,共 83 例伴有异动症和剂末效应的 PD 患者,其中 29 例为安慰剂治疗组,26 例为 KW60025/10/20mg 剂量组,28 例为 10/20/40 mg 剂量组。试验发现:KW6002 能降低关期在觉醒期所占百分比(缩短 7.1%±2.0%)(缩短关期 1.2±0.3 h),而安慰剂组关期延长 2.2%±2.7%(延长关期 0.5±0.5 h),并且不增加异动症的严重程度。患者对 KW6002 有较好的耐受性,恶心是最常见的不良反应,但随着时间的推移反应减轻。

Pinna 等⑤在用 SD 大鼠进行的实验中发现腺苷 A_{2A} 受体拮抗剂。ANR82 特别是其衍生物 ANR94 和 ANR152 能明显逆转氟哌啶醇所引起的强直性木僵,且 ANR94 和 ANR152 能诱导 6 羟多巴单侧毁损的左旋多巴敏感的大鼠产生对侧旋转行为,从而使其有可能成为新的治疗帕金森病的药物。

八、腺苷 A_{2A} 受体拮抗剂的不良反应

虽然腺苷 A_{2A} 受体主要与多巴胺 D_2 受体分布于纹状体中,但是在中枢神经系统的其他部分和机体的其他部分,如心血管系统、免疫系统、呼吸系统、肾脏、肝脏、皮肤等也有少量分布。阻断腺苷 A_{2A} 受体拮抗剂对这些部分会造成不良反应。

1. 腺苷 A_{2A} 受体是有利于睡眠的重要内源性因子。据报道,使用腺苷 A_{2A} 受体拮抗剂可以加重 PD 鼠的睡眠障碍,而帕金森病患者本身就常伴有睡眠障碍。

---

①　PETZER JP,STEYN S,CASTAGNOLI KP, et al.Inhibition of Monoamine Oxidase B by Selective Adenosine A_{2A} Receptor Antagonists[J].*Bioorg & Med Chem*,2003,11(07)1299−1310.

②　IKEDA K,KUROKAWA M,AOYAMA S, et al.Neuroprotection by Adenosine A_{2A} Receptor Blockade in Experimental Models of Parkinson's Disease[J].*J Neurochem*,2002,80(02):262−270.

③　SAURA J,ANGULO E,EJARQUE A, et al.Adenosine A_{2A} Receptor Stimulation Potentiates Nitric Oxide Release by Activated Microglia[J].*J Neurochem*,2005,95(04):919−929.

④　HAUSER RA,HUBBLE JP,TRUONG DD.Istradefylline US-001 Study Group:Randomized Trial of the Adenosine A(2A)Receptor Antagonist Istradefylline in Advanced PD[J].*Neurology*,2003,61(03):297−303.

⑤　PINNA A,VOLPINI R,CRISTALLI G, et al.New Adenosine A_{2A} Receptor Antagonists:Actions on Parkinson's Disease Models[J].*Euro J Pharmacol*,2005,512(2−3):157−164.

2. 多巴胺 D_2 受体的长期过度刺激会引起精神症状,腺苷 A_{2A} 受体拮抗剂的使用导致腺苷 A_{2A} 受体对多巴胺 D_2 受体的拮抗作用减弱,从而有可能加重精神症状。

3. 腺苷 A_{2A} 受体拮抗剂可能加重抑郁和引起疼痛。

4. 阻断腺苷 A_{2A} 受体可以抑制腺苷的抗炎作用,从而有可能加重中枢和外周器官的损害①②。同时腺苷 A_{2A} 受体拮抗剂对 A_1、A_{2B}、A_3 也有一定的亲和力,也会产生一些不良反应。

九、结语

基础和临床研究表明,腺苷 A_{2A} 受体拮抗剂有可能成为治疗帕金森病的一类新药。如何寻找一些对 A_{2A} 受体亲和力强,在体内也能很好发挥疗效,不良反应少的药物,成为腺苷 A_{2A} 受体拮抗剂研究的一个重要课题。

主要参考文献

［1］AGNATI LF，FERRE S，LLUIS C，et al. Molecular Mechanisms and Therapeutical Implications of Intramembrane Receptor/Receptor Interactions among Heptahelical Receptors with Examples from the Striatopallidal GABA Neurons［J］. *Pharmacological Reviews*，2003，55（03）：509-550.

［2］XU K，BASTIA E，SCHWARZSCHILD M. Therapeutic Potertial of Adenosine A2A Receptor Antagonists in Parkinson's Disease［J］. *Pharmacology & Therapeutics*，2005，105（03）：267-310.

［3］WEISS SM，WHAWEEL E，Upton R，et al. Potential for Antipsychotic and Psychotomimetic Effects of A2A Receptor modulation［J］. *Neurology*，2003，61（11 Suppl 6）：S88~93.

（王恒会综述　罗蔚锋审校）

（本文原载于《国外医学·老年医学分册》2006 年第 27 卷第 6 期）

---

① SITKOVSKY MV，LUKASHEV D，APASOV S，et al. Physiological Control of Immune Response and Inflammatory Tissue Damage By Hypoxia-inducible Factors and Adenosine A_{2A} Receptors［J］. *Ann Rev Immunology*，2004，22（01）：657-682.

② CHINENOV Y，KERPPOLA TK. Close Encounters of Many Kinds：Fos-Jun Interactions that Mediate Transcription Regulatory Specificity［J］. *Oncogene*，2001，20（19）：2438-2452.

尿酸水平与帕金森病

帕金森病是老年人神经系统常见的运动障碍性疾病之一,严重地影响着老年人的生活质量。PD 的主要病理特征为中脑黑质致密部多巴胺能神经元的进行性变性减少,引起黑质纹状体系统多巴胺水平降低。尽管多巴胺能神经元选择性死亡的确切发病机制至今不明,流行病学、基础实验研究及临床资料证实,由于接触一些毒素(如杀虫剂、MPTP),含有抗氧化剂的饮食减少及体内尤其是黑质纹状体系统清除自由基物质水平的降低,而引起的氧化应激反应增强,线粒体功能障碍与 PD 的发病密切相联系[1][2][3][4]。尿酸是一种重要的生理性的天然抗氧化剂、铁螯合剂、自由基清除剂。PD 与尿酸的关系日益受到人们的重视。

一、尿酸的生理代谢及作用

尿酸是体内腺苷、鸟苷和饮食中细胞内核糖核酸嘌呤代谢的终末产物,两者分别占体内尿酸总量的 80% 和 20%。腺苷在腺苷脱氨酶、嘌呤核苷磷酸化酶、黄嘌呤氧化酶的作用下生成黄嘌呤和尿酸。食用蔬菜、水果、巧克力及饮茶、饮葡萄酒会不同程度地提高人体血浆中的尿酸水平[5]。大多数哺乳动物和禽类动物体内含有尿酸酶,可将尿酸分解成尿囊素。人和猿类动物体内缺乏尿酸酶,人类血尿酸水平远远高于其他哺乳动物和禽类动物(健康人血尿酸浓度为 300 pmol/L 左右,而牛血尿酸仅为 20 pmol/L)[6]。尿酸及其盐类在水中溶解度很低,70% 的尿酸经肾脏排泄,30% 的尿酸经胆道

① LIOU HH,TSAI MC,CHEN CJ,et al.Environmental Risk Factors and Parkinson's Disease:a Case-control Study in Taiwan[J].*Neurology*,1997,48(06):1583−1588.

② LOCKWOOD AH.Pesticides and Parkinsonism:is there an Etiological Link? [J].*Curr Opin Neurol*,2000,13(06):687−690.

③ BALLARD PA,TETRUD JW,LANGSTON JW.Permanent Human Parkinsonism due to 1-methyl-4-phenyl-1,2,3,6-tetrahydropyridine(MPTP):Seven Cases[J].*Neurology*,1985,35(07):949−956.

④ JANHKY R,OGITA K,PASQUAIOTTO BA,et al.Glutathione and Signal Transduction in the Mammalian CNS[J].*J Neurochem*,1999,73(03):889−902.

⑤ LOTITO SB,FREI B.Consumption of Flavonoid-rich Foods and Increased Plasma Antioxidant Capacity in Humans:Cause,Consequence,or Epiphenomenon? [J].*Free Radic Biol Med*,2006,41(12):1727−1746.

⑥ WU XW,MUZNY DM,LEE CC,et al.Two Independent Mutational Events in the Loss of Urate Oxidase During Hominoid Evolution[J].*J Mol Evol*,1992,34(01):78−84.

和肠道排泄。尿酸主要通过 hUTP 在人体细胞内外进行跨膜运动。hUTP 基因位于第 17 号染色体的短臂上,含有 11 个外显子。hUTP 可分为 3 种亚型,属于贯穿细胞膜脂质的离子通道,具有高度的选择性,广泛存在于人体内多种组织细胞膜中①。

尿酸是人体内特有的天然水溶性抗氧化剂,抑制过(氧化)亚硝酸盐介导的硝化反应②,具有清除氧自由基和其他活性百由基的作用,比抗坏血酸有更显著的增强红细胞膜脂质抗氧化、防止细胞溶解凋亡的作用,可增强 SOD 活性,延长其生存时间,防止细胞过氧化。Fe^{2+} 能够促使更多的活性氧自由基的产生,加重氧化损伤,尿酸与 Fe^{2+} 具有很强的结合能力。

二、流行病学

对 8 000 名男性血清尿酸水平检测后,进行长达 30 年的随访,有 92 例相继被诊断为 PD,经年龄、吸烟危险因素纠正后发现,入组时血清尿酸水平高于平均值的人群,PD 发病率降低 40%③。对 4 695 例≥55 岁的人群进行前瞻性研究,平均随访 9.4 年,有 68 例被诊断为 PD。血清尿酸水平升高可以明显降低 PD 的发病率(校正后每标准差风险率升高 0.71,95% 可信区间为 0.51~0.98),且有明显的剂量相关性($P<0.05$)④。对 18 000 例的男性人群在 1993—1995 年检测其血尿酸水平,并进行随访,2000 年有 84 例被诊断为 PD,按 1∶2 的比例与年龄、种族、检测时间相配对的对照组比较,PD 组血尿酸水平(5.7 μmol/L)显著低于对照组(6.1 μmol/L)。血尿酸水平处于高四分之一位值范围的人群,PD 的发病率与尿酸水平处于低四分之一位值范围人群,PD 发病率之比为 0.43($P=0.017$)。提示低水平的血尿酸会增高 PD 的发病率,经年龄、吸烟、饮咖啡及其他与 PD 和血尿酸水平有关的因素

① LIPKOWITZ MS, LEAL-PINTO E, RAPPOPORT JZ, et al. Functional Reconstitution, Membrane Targeting, Genomic Structure, and Chromosomal Localization of a Human Urate Transporter[J]. *J Clin Invest*, 2001,107(09): 1103-1105.

② HOOPER DC, SCOTT GS, ZBOREK A, et al. Uric acid, a Peroxynitrite Scavenger, Inhibits CNS Inflammation, Blood-CNS Barrier Permeability Changes, and Tissue Damage in a Mouse Model of Multiple Sclerosis[J]. *FASEB J*, 2000,14(05): 691-698.

③ DAVIS JW, GRANDINETTI A, WASLIEN CI, et al. Observations on Serum Uric Acid Levels and the Risk of Idiopathic Parkinson's Disease[J]. *Am J Epidemiol*, 1996,144(05): 480-484.

④ DE LAU LM, KOUDSTAAL PJ, HOFMAN A, et al. Serum Uric Acid Levels and the Risk of Parkinson Disease[J]. *Ann Neurol*, 2005,58(05): 797-800.

纠正后,尿酸与 PD 的发病率仍呈显著的负相关。即在一定的范围内,血清尿酸水平越高,PD 的发病率越低[1]。

三、PD 患者黑质纹状体系统及血清尿酸水平的改变

临床资料证实,PD 患者黑质纹状体系统、血清尿酸水平发生了有意义的变化。Church 与 Ward[2] 对死亡后 PD 患者的黑质和尾状核组织中的尿酸、多巴胺、抗坏血酸进行测定,发现其尿酸、多巴胺的水平显著低于年龄相匹配的健康对照组。在黑质中两者分别降低 54%、85%。PD 患者组尾状核组织匀浆液中多巴胺氧化速度常数(表示各种组织氧化应激程度的指标)是 $4.20 \times 10^{-2}/min$,健康对照组仅为 $0.34 \times 10^{-2}/min$。黑质匀浆液中多巴胺氧化速度常数在 PD 患者组和对照组中分别是 4.57×10^{-2}、$2.82 \times 10^{-2}/min$。在 PD 患者组尾状核、黑质组织匀浆液中加入尿酸或过氧化氢酶,会使多巴胺氧化速度常数降低,将尿酸氧化酶加入健康对照组的匀浆液中能提高其氧化速度常数。对 PD、进行性核上性麻痹及多系统萎缩的患者,在其死亡后进行黑质尿酸水平的测定,发现各病例组较健康对照组降低 19%~30%,谷胱甘肽降低 20%~30%[3]。PD 患者组的铁代谢发生异常,尽管血浆中的铁浓度与健康对照组相比无区别,但其铁蛋白和转铁蛋白显著性升高($P <$ 0.05),转铁蛋白的饱和度显著性降低($P < 0.05$)[4]。Annanmaki 等[5]以 40 例 PD 患者和 29 名健康者为研究对象,对其血尿酸、血清铁蛋白、体重指数及乳制品饮食等进行检测评价,结果提示 PD 患者的血尿酸水平显著性降低,尿酸水平的改变与血清铁蛋白变化密切相联系。我们发现,121 例 PD 患者的血尿酸水平[(260.76±90.42)μmol/L]显著低于年龄、性别配对的健康人

① WEISSKOPF MG,O'REILLY E,CHEN H,et al. Plasma Urate and Risk of Parkinson's Disease[J]. *Am J Epidemiol*,2007,166(05):561-567.

② CHURCH WH,WARD VL. Uric Acid is Reduced in the Substantia Nigra in Parkinson's Disease:Effect on Dopamine Oxidation[J].*Brain Res Bull*,1994,33(04):419-425.

③ FITZMAURICE PS,ANG L,GUTTMAN M,et al. Nigral Glutathione Deficiency is not Specific for Idiopathic Parkinson's Disease[J].*Mov Disord*,2003,18(09):969-976.

④ LARUMBE ILUNDDIN R,FERRER VALLS JV,VIFIES RUEDA JJ,et al. Case-control Study of Markers of Oxidative Stress and Metabolism of Blood Iron in Parkinson's Disease[J].*Rev Esp Salud Publica*,2001,75(01):43-53.

⑤ ANNANMAKI T,MUURONEN A,MURROS K. Low Plasma Uric Acid Level in Parkinson's Disease [J].*Mov Disord*,2007,22(08):1133-1137.

$[(336.95\pm59.64)\,\mu mol/L,P<0.01]$①。

四、尿酸对多巴胺能神经元的保护作用

尿酸能够降低高浓度的多巴胺引起的 PC12 细胞的氧化产物,防止凋亡的发生②。鱼藤酮是一种对多巴胺能神经元具有毒性作用的杀虫药剂,通过抑制线粒体复合酶Ⅰ,导致能量衰竭,氧自由基增多,诱导细胞发生凋亡,与其接触会增加 PD 的发病风险。PD 患者的多巴胺能神经元的铁离子水平显著增高,铁离子通过促进羟自由基的产生及细胞膜发生脂质过氧化作用而诱导凋亡。同型半胱氨酸能增强鱼藤酮和 Fe^{2+} 对人体多巴胺能神经元线粒体膜去极化的发生和氧自由基的产生,加重凋亡,而尿酸对其有明显的保护作用③。

尿酸是人体嘌呤代谢的终产物,嘌呤代谢途径中不同产物的不同浓度对多巴胺的代谢作用是不同的。分别以不同浓度的腺苷、腺嘌呤、鸟苷、鸟嘌呤、次黄嘌呤、黄嘌呤、尿酸作用于 PC12 细胞 24 h,腺苷能够升高多巴胺的前体 3,4-二羟苯丙氨酸多巴(3,4-dihydroxyphenylalanine,DOPA)和多巴胺的分解产物二羟苯乙酸(3,4-dihydroxyphenylacetic acid,DOPAC)及高香草酸(homovanillic acid,HVA)。腺嘌呤使 DOPA 降低。高浓度的鸟苷使 DOPA、多巴胺、DOPAC 水平降低,而低浓度的鸟苷升高 DOPA、HVA。鸟嘌呤降低多巴胺水平。黄嘌呤使多巴胺和 DOPAC 同时发生减少。次黄嘌呤和尿酸对 PC12 细胞的 DOPA、多巴胺、DOPAC、HVA 无明显影响。提示尿酸和次黄嘌呤并非直接通过对多巴胺代谢的各级酶及产物本身发挥作用,而腺苷、腺嘌呤、鸟苷、鸟嘌呤、黄嘌呤对其有一定的影响④。

---

① 王丽君,罗蔚锋,王恒会,等.帕金森病患者血尿酸水平[J].中华神经科杂志,2008,41(03):157-158.

② JONES DC,GUNASEKAR PG,BOROWITZ JL,et al. Dopamine-induced Apoptosis is Mediated by Oxidative Stess and is Enhanced by Cyanide in Differentiated PC12 Cells[J].*J Neurochem*,2000,74(06):2296-2304.

③ DUAN W,LADENHEIM B,CUTLER RG,et al.Dietary Folate Deficiency and Elevated Homocysteine Levels Endanger Dopaminergic Neurons in Models of Parkinson's Disease[J].*J Neurochem*,2002,80(01):101-110.

④ LOEFFLER DA,CAMP DM,JUNEAU PL,et al. Purine-induced Alterations of Dopamine Metabolism in Rat Pheochromocytoma PC12 Cells[J].*Brain Res Bull*,2000,52(06):553-558.

五、展望

尿酸与 PD 相关性的进一步研究有利于 PD 更为有效合理的治疗。什么水平的尿酸血浓度既有助于减慢甚至预防 PD 的发生发展，又有利于痛风、糖脂代谢紊乱、高血压、冠心病等疾病的防治，急需从基因、分子、细胞、组织等不同角度进行深入的研究和探讨。体内尿酸血浓度过高如高尿酸血症，常合并糖脂代谢紊乱、高血压、冠心病等，且增加其病死率。尿酸水平的升高是引起这些疾病的一个原因，还是机体为了维护自身，减轻损伤而发生的自身调节保护性反应？或许两者兼有？有待于进一步研究。

（罗蔚锋　刘春风）

（本文原载于《中华神经科杂志》2008 年第 41 卷第 8 期）

尿酸转运体与帕金森病研究进展①

摘要：尿酸是生理性的抗氧化剂，流行病学及临床资料显示，低尿酸水平与帕金森病(PD)发病率增高密切相关，PD患者的血尿酸水平显著降低，高血尿酸水平能够降低PD的发病以及减慢PD的进展速度。尿酸转运体在尿酸分泌和重吸收过程中发挥关键作用，从而影响尿酸水平。本文将从尿酸转运体的角度介绍尿酸转运体与PD的研究进展。

关键词：尿酸；转运体；基因；帕金森病

Research Advances in the Association of Urate Transporters and Parkinson's Disease

Abstract：Uric acid is a kind of physiological antioxidants. The epidemiology and clinical studies indicate that its lower level is closely related to the higher incidence of Parkinson's disease. The serum urate concentrations of PD patients are much lower. Lower incidence and better prognosis have been observed on PD patients with higher serum urate. Urate transporters affect urate secretion and reabsorption, which have a strong and apparent impact on urate concentrations. This review discusses current information on the characteristics of urate transporters, with specific focus on their association with PD.

Key words：uric acid；transporter；gene；Parkinson's disease.

帕金森病是第二大中枢神经系统退行性病变，以中脑黑质多巴胺能神经元变性、缺失和路易体形成为病理特征，临床主要表现为锥体外系症状，包括运动迟缓、肌强直、静止性震颤和姿势或步态异常等。PD具有隐性起病，缓慢进展的特征，预计到2030年我国PD患者人数将达到

① 本文系江苏省科技项目(项目编号：BK2010229)；江苏省苏州市科学技术局、江苏省苏州市财政局科技计划项目合同财政拨款项目(项目编号：SS201112)。

近 500 万人①②。虽然帕金森病的发病机制仍不十分清楚,但目前研究认为,帕金森病的发生、发展是遗传和环境因素共同作用的结果。目前已有多项研究表明,本病与 LRRK2、PARKIN、PINKI 等基因的突变有关③④⑤。

尿酸可作为 PD 临床和影像学进展的标志物⑥,是帕金森病防治的潜在新靶点,研究发现尿酸对 PD 动物模型具有保护作用,尿酸可减少 6-羟基多巴胺对神经元的毒性作用,提高细胞活力,稳定细胞膜电位,表明尿酸能通过抗氧化应激活性发挥其对多巴胺能神经元的保护作用⑦⑧⑨。PD 动物模型实验表明,尿酸可以改善其学习记忆能力,其机制可能是尿酸发挥了抗氧化应激、保护多巴胺能神经元作用⑩。

一、尿酸的产生及其影响因素

尿酸通过嘌呤代谢通路由黄嘌呤氧化酶分解嘌呤产生,主要在肝脏产生,2/3 由肾脏排泄,其余 1/3 由肠道和皮肤等排泄⑪⑫。体内尿酸浓度由嘌

①　DORSEY ER, CONSTANTINESCU R, THOMPSON JP, et al. Projected Number of People with Parkinson Disease in the Most Populous Nations, 2005 through 2030[J]. *Neurology*, 2007, 68(05): 384-386.

②　WRIGHT WILLIS A, EVANOFF BA, LIAN M, et al. Geographic and Ethnic Variation in Parkinson Disease: A Population-Based Study of US Medicare Beneficiaries[J]. *Neuroepidemiology*, 2010, 34(03): 143-151.

③　ZIMPRIEH A, BISKUP S, LEITNER P, et al. Mutations in LRRK2 Cause Autosomal-dominant Parkinsonism with Pleomorphic Pathology[J]. *Neuron*, 2004, 44(04): 601-607.

④　PERIQUET M, LATOUEHE M, LOHMANN E, et al. Parkin Mutations are Frequent in Patients with Isolated Early-onset Parkinsonism[J]. *Brain*, 2003, 126(06): 1271-1278.

⑤　VALENTE EM, ABOU-SLEIMAN PM, CAPUTO V, et al. Hereditary Early-onset Parkinson's Disease Caused by Mutations in PINKI[J]. *Science*, 2004, 304(5674): 1158-1160.

⑥　SCHWARZSCHILD MA, SCHWID SR, MAREK K, et al. Serum Urate as a Predictor of Clinical and Radiographic Progression in Parkinson Disease[J]. *Arch Neurol*, 2008, 65(06): 716-723.

⑦　王丽君, 罗蔚锋, 王恒会, 等. 尿酸对 6-羟基多巴胺致大鼠黑质纹状体系毒性的影响[J]. 中华医学杂志, 2010, 90(19): 1362-1365.

⑧　朱红灿, 蔡春生, 耿利娇, 等. 尿酸对帕金森病模型大鼠多巴胺能神经元氧化应激的影响[J]. 中华老年医学杂志, 2010, 29(04): 319-323.

⑨　王晓君, 罗蔚锋, 王丽君, 等. 帕金森病患者认知功能与尿酸及相关因素分析[J]. 中华医学杂志, 2009, 89(23): 1633-1635.

⑩　朱红灿, 耿利娇, 蔡春生, 等. 尿酸对帕金森病大鼠学习记忆能力的影响及其机制[J]. 中华实验外科杂志, 2010, 27(02): 227-229.

⑪　LI S, SANNA S, MASCHIO A, et al. The GLUT9 gene is Associated with Serum Uric Acid Levels in Sardinia and Chianti Cohorts[J]. *PLoS Genet*, 2007, 3(11): 2156-2162.

⑫　SICA DA, SCHOOLWERTH AC. Renal Handling of Organic Anions and Cations: Excretion of Uric Acid. In: Brenner BM, Editor. *The Kidney*[M]. 6th ed. Philadelphia: WB Saunders, 2000: 680-700.

吟的摄入量、尿酸的生物合成及其排泄速率决定,基因编码的酶的异常会导致过度的内源性嘌呤合成。血尿酸水平主要受肾小球滤过作用、重吸收作用及分泌作用调节。研究表明,脑脊液中的尿酸水平与血尿酸水平呈线性相关,约为血尿酸水平的1/10。尿酸盐是尿酸存在的主要形式,主要分布于细胞外液,主要通过 hUTP 进行细胞内外的跨膜转运,hUTP 是具有高选择性的贯穿细胞膜脂质的离子通道,其3种亚型可见于人体内多种组织细胞,故其基因编码异常会显著影响人体尿酸水平。

近年来,全基因组相关性研究(genome-wide association studies,GWAS)已经证实尿酸浓度与9个基因位点的单核苷酸多态性有显著联系,其中包括编码尿酸盐转运体基因 ABCG2(BCRP)、SLC2A9(GLUT9)、SLC16A9(MCT9)、SLC17A1(NPT1)、SLC17A3(NPT4)、SLC17A4(NPT5)、SLC22A11(OAT4)、SLC22A12(URAT1),以及尿酸盐转运体相关支架蛋白 PDZK1①②③④⑤⑥⑦⑧⑨⑩⑪。

① LI S,SANNA S,MASCHIO A,et al.The GLUT9 Gene is Associated with Serum Uric Acid Levels in Sardinia and Chianti Cohorts[J].PLoS Genet,2007,3(11):2156-2162.

② DEHGHAN A,KOTTGEN A,YANG Q,et al. Association of Three Genetic Loci with Uric Acid Concentration and Risk of Gout: a Genome-wide Association Study[J].Lancet,2008,372(9654):1953-1961.

③ CAULFIELD MJ,MUNROE PB,O'NEILL D,et al.SLC2A9 is a High-capacity Urate Transporter in Humans[J]. PLoS Med,2008,5(10):e197.

④ WALLACE C,NEWHOUSE SJ,BRAUND P,et al.Genome-wide Association Study Identifies Genes for Biomarkers of Cardiovascular Disease: Serum Urate and Dyslipidemia et al[J]. Am J Hum Genet,2008,82(01):139-149.

⑤ STARK K,REINHARD W,NEUREUTHER K,et al.Association of Common Polymorphisms in GLUT9 Gene with Gout but not with Coronary Artery Disease in a Large Case-control Study[J].PLoS One,2008,3(04):e1948.

⑥ VITART V,RUDAN I,HAYWARD C,et al. SLC2A9 is a Newly Identified Urate Transporter Influencing Serum Urate Concentration,Urate Excretion and Gout[J]. Nat Genet,2008,40(04):437-442.

⑦ DORING A,GIEGER C,Mehta D,et al.SLC2A9 Influences Uric Acid Concentrations with Pronounced sex-Specific Effects[J].Nat Genet,2008,40(04):430-436.

⑧ BRANDSTATTER A,KIECHL S,KOLLERITS B,et al. Sex-specific Association of the Putative Fructose Trans-porter SLC2A9 Variants with Uric Acid Levels is Modified by BMI[J]. Diabetes Care,2008,31(08):1662-1667.

⑨ KOLZ M,JOHNSON T,SANNA S,et al. Meta-analysis of 28,141 Individuals Identifies Common Variants within Five New Loci that Influence Uric Acid Concentrations[J].Plos Genet,2009,5(06):1-10.

⑩ TU HP,CHEN CJ,TOVOSIA S,et al.Associations of a Nonsynonymous Variant in SLC2A9 with Gouty Arthritis and Uric Acid Levels in Han Chinese and Solomon Islanders[J]. Ann Rheum Dis,2010,69(05):887-890.

⑪ HOLLIS-MOFFATT JE,XU X,DALBETH N,et al.Role of the Urate Transporter SLC2A9 Gene in Susceptibility to Gout in New Zealand M ā ori,Pacific Island,and Caucasian Case-control Sample Sets[J]. Arthritis Rheum,2009,60(11):3485-3492.

二、影响人体尿酸水平的主要尿酸转运体

1. BCRP（ABCG2）

乳腺癌耐药相关蛋白（breast cancer resistance protein，BCRP）由 ATP-结合盒（ATP-binding cassette，ABC）半转运蛋白超家族的著名成员 ABCG2 编码。基因定位于 4q22，在胎盘、脑、肝脏、咽、肾脏、膀胱及小肠表达。ABCG2 主要表达于肾近曲小管的管腔膜侧，形成同型二聚体的 ABCG2 才具有发挥转运尿酸作用的活性，该转运体属于分泌型尿酸转运体[①]。在 GWA 研究中，ABCG2 单核苷酸多态性已经被证实与血尿酸浓度相关[②][③]。另外，ABCG2 也是高尿酸血症的候选基因之一[④]。考虑到 BCRP 蛋白在血脑屏障（the blood-brain barrier，BBB）内皮细胞上的表达，以及脑脊液（cerebrospinal fluid，CSF）尿酸水平由血尿酸水平及血脑屏障完整性决定[⑤]，很明显，BCRP 尿酸转运体与脑脊液尿酸水平是紧密相关的。目前研究表明，血尿酸已经可以被当作 PD 临床和影像学进展的可靠指标[⑥]。尽管脑脊液平均尿酸水平只有血尿酸水平的 1/10，但是脑脊液尿酸作为中枢神经系统抗氧化剂在 PD 发病及其进程中必然发挥着举足轻重的作用[⑦]。以中枢神经系统转运体包括 BCRP 转运体为治疗靶点的新技术已经被发现可以减少大脑病理改变及神经退行性疾病，如 PD 和 AD[⑧]。由此可见，中枢神经系统转运体 BCRP 与 PD 密切相关，可以为 PD 提供可靠和稳定的治疗或缓解的方向。

[①]　WOODWARD OM，KOTTGEN A，CORESH J，et al.Identification of a Urate Transporter，ABCG2，with a Common Functional Polymorphism Causing Gout[J].*Proc Natl Acad Sci USA*，2009，106（25）：10338−10342.

[②]　DEHGHAN A，KOTTGEN A，YANG Q，et al. Association of Three Genetic Loci with Uric Acid Concentration and Risk of Gout：a Genome-wide Association Study[J].*Lancet*，2008，372（9654）：1953−1961.

[③]　KOLZ M，JOHNSON T，SANNA S，et al. Meta-analysis of 28，141 Individuals Identifies Common Variants within Five New Loci that Influence Uric Acid Concentrations[J].*PloS Genet*，2009，5（06）：1−10.

[④]　DEHGHAN A，KOTTGEN A，YANG Q，et al. Association of Three Genetic Loci With Uric Acid Concentration and Risk of Gout：a Genome-wide Association Study[J].*Lancet*，2008，372（9654）：1953−1961.

[⑤]　BOWMAN GL，SHANNON J，FREI B，et al.Uric Acid as a CNS Antioxidant[J].*J Alzheimers Dis*，2010，19（04）：1331−1336.

[⑥]　SCHWARZSCHILD MA，SCHWID SR，MAREK K，et al.Serum Urate as a Predictor of Clinical and Radiographic Progression in Parkinson Disease[J].*Arch Neurol*，2008，65（06）：716−723.

[⑦]　BOWMAN GL，SHANNON J，FREI B，et al.Uric Acid as a CNS Antioxidant[J].*J Alzheimers Dis*，2010，19（04）：1331−1336.

[⑧]　JEDLITSCHKY G，GRUBE M，MOSYAGIN I，et al. Targeting CNS Transporters for Treatment of Neurodegenerative Diseases[J]. *Curr Pharm Des*，2014：20（10）：1523−1533.

2. MRP1（ABCC1），MRP3（ABCC3）和 MRP4（ABCC4）

多重耐药蛋白（multidrug resistance protein，MRP）是由 ABC 家族 ABCC 基因编码，由 ABCC4 编码的 MRP4 主要表达于肾脏、睾丸、卵巢、肝脏、小肠、肺等器官的细胞膜上，该基因位于 13 号染色体长臂上。MRP4 属于分泌型尿酸转运体，位于肾小管管腔膜上的 MRP4 将肾小管上皮细胞内的尿酸分泌入小管腔。另外，表达于肝细胞基侧膜上的 MRP4 参与肝脏对尿酸的转运。而 ABCC1 编码的 MRP1 及 ABCC3 编码的 MRP3 则主要表达于肝细胞的基侧膜参与尿酸的转运，其编码基因分别定位于 16 号染色体的短臂和 17 号染色体的长臂上。

3. GLUT9（SLC2A9）

由基因 SLC2A9 编码的葡萄糖转运体 9（glucose transporter 9，GLUT9）属于葡萄糖转运蛋白（glucose transporter，GLUT）家族成员，该转运体主要以易化扩散的方式转运葡萄糖，高度表达于肾脏和肝脏。Vitart 等[1]对非洲爪蛙卵母细胞的研究发现，GLUT9 具有转运尿酸和果糖的作用。Caulfield 等[2]的研究则表明 GLUT9 是高效的尿酸转运体，其转运尿酸的能力远远高于转运葡萄糖的能力，并且可通过对葡萄糖的转运而加速对尿酸的重吸收，因而摄入高糖或糖尿病均会影响尿酸水平。依据氨基端在胞内剪接部位的不同，GLUT9 可以分为两种异构体：GLUT9L（长型异构体）主要位于肾小管基底膜侧，主要发挥将尿酸从上皮细胞分泌入血液的作用；GLUT9S（短型异构体）则主要位于肾小管的管腔膜侧，起将尿酸分泌入管腔的作用。

近年来，研究表明 SLC2A9 是最有效的尿酸转运体，SLC2A9 主要表达在人类肾小管细胞的基底外侧膜[3]，尿酸盐通过其表达的转运体流向血液。

① VITART V, RUDAN I, HAYWARD C, et al. SLC2A9 is a Newly Identified Urate Transporter Influencing Serum Urate Concentration, Urate Excretion and Gout[J]. *Nat Genet*, 2008, 40(04)：437–442.

② CAULFIELD MJ, MUNROE PB, O'NEILL D, et al. SLC2A9 is a High-capacity Urate Transporter in Humans[J]. *PLoS Med*, 2008, 5(10)：e197.

③ SCHWARZSCHILD MA, SCHWID SR, MAREK K, et al. Serum Urate as a Predictor of Clinical and Radiographic Progression in Parkinson Disease[J]. *Arch Neurol*, 2008, 65(06)：716–723.

目前,几乎所有的 GWAS 研究已经证实,SLC2A9 与血尿酸水平有很强的相关性①②③④⑤⑥⑦⑧⑨⑩。欧洲研究者对位于 4p16.1 的 SLC2A9 区域的 4 个多态性位点进行了较大规模的研究,研究发现 SLC2A9 基因单核苷酸多态性影响了 PD 的发病年龄,其中 rs1014290 与 PD 发病年龄相关性最强⑪。

4. UAT

尿酸转运蛋白(urate transporter,UAT)属于一种特异性的分泌型尿酸转运体。研究表明,UAT 广泛表达于人体多种组织,主要存在于肾脏和肠道⑫。由 322 个氨基酸组成的 UAT 主要表达于 17 号染色体短臂上,含有 11 个外显子,全长 18 kb。UAT 是一种高选择性的离子通道,贯穿整个细胞膜,将肾小管上皮细胞内的尿酸分泌至肾小管腔中。尿酸主要是通过 UAT 跨

①　DEHGHAN A, KOTTGEN A, YANG Q, et al. Association of Three Genetic Loci with Uric Acid Concentration and Risk of Gout: a Genome-wide Association Study[J]. *Lancet*, 2008, 372(9654): 1953-1961.

②　CAULFIELD MJ, MUNROE PB, O'NEILL D, et al. SLC2A9 is a High-capacity Urate Transporter in Humans[J]. *PLoS Med*, 2008, 5(10): e197.

③　WALLACE C, NEWHOUSE SJ, BRAUND P, et al. Genome-wide Association Study Identifies Genes for Biomarkers of Cardiovascular Disease: Serum Urate and Dyslipidemia et al.[J]. *Am J Hum Genet*, 2008, 82(01): 139-149.

④　STARK K, REINHARD W, NEUREUTHER K, et al. Association of Common Polymorphisms in GLUT9 Gene with Gout but not with Coronary Artery Disease in a Large Case-control Study[J]. *PLoS One*, 2008, 3(04): e1948.

⑤　DORING A, GIEGER C, MEHTA D, et al. SLC2A9 Influences Uric Acid Concentrations with Pronounced Sex-specific Effects[J]. *Nat Genet*, 2008, 40(04): 430-436.

⑥　BRANDSTATTER A, KIECHL S, KOLLERITS B, et al. Sex-specific Association of the Putative Fructose Trans-porter SLC2A9 Variants with Uric Acid Levels is Modified by BMI[J]. *Diabetes Care*, 2008, 31(08): 1662-1667.

⑦　TU HP, CHEN CJ, TOVOSIA S, et al. Associations of a Nonsynonymous Variant in SLC2A9 with Gouty Arthritis and Uric Acid Levels in Han Chinese and Solomon Islanders[J]. *Ann Rheum Dis*, 2010, 69(05): 887-890.

⑧　HOLLIS-MOFFATT JE, XU X, DALBETH N, et al. Role of the Urate Transporter SLC2A9 Gene in Susceptibility to Gout in New Zealand M ā ori, Pacific Island, and Caucasian Case-control Sample Sets[J]. *Arthritis Rheum*, 2009, 60(11): 3485-3492.

⑨　KOLZ M, JOHNSON T, SANNA S, et al. Meta-analysis of 28,141 Individuals Identifies Common Variants within Five New Loci that Influence Uric Acid Concentrations[J]. *Plos Genet*, 2009, 5(06): 1-10.

⑩　VITART V, RUDAN I, HAYWARD C, et al. SLC2A9 is a Newly Identified Urate Transporter Influencing Serum Urate Concentration, Urate Excretion and Gout[J]. *Nat Genet*, 2008, 40(04): 437-442.

⑪　MAURIZIO F, FACHERIS ANDREW A. Variation in the Uric Acid Transporter Gene SLC2A9 and its Association with AAO of Parkinson's Disease[J]. *J Mol Neurosci*, 2011, 43(03): 246-250.

⑫　ENOMOTO A, KIMURA H, CHAIROUNGDUA A, et al. Molecular Identification of a Renal Urate Anion Exchanger that Regulates Blood Urate Levels[J]. *Nature*, 2002, 417(6887): 447-452.

膜区域之间的尿酸结合位点分泌入管腔的。肠道中的 UAT 发挥着排泄尿酸的作用,将肠黏膜上皮细胞中的尿酸分泌至肠腔,尿酸盐再经肠道细菌的酶解后排出体外。由此可见,UAT 在调节全身尿酸水平的稳态中起重要作用。

5. URAT1（SLC22A12）

尿酸阴离子转运体 1（urate anion transporter 1,URAT1）是最主要的尿酸重吸收转运体,属于有机阴离子转运体（organic anion transporter,OAT）家族的成员,在肾近曲小管上皮细胞的管腔膜侧被发现①,该转运体在尿酸转运中处于举足轻重的地位。由 555 个氨基酸构成的 URAT1 定位于 11 号染色体长臂上,全长 2 642 bp,含 10 个外显子,由基因 SLC22A12 编码,含有 12 个跨膜区域。URAT1 是调节全身尿酸水平的关键离子通道,该转运体发挥着将尿酸从肾小管管腔内重吸收至肾小管上皮细胞内的作用。在临床上,多种尿酸排泄剂均是主要通过与 URAT1 结合而影响对尿酸的重吸收从而发挥排泄尿酸的功能,以此来降低血尿酸水平,因此,URAT1 是治疗高尿酸血症的一个有效的靶点。反之,临床上那些抗尿酸排泄药则主要是通过增加细胞内与小管腔之间的有机阴离子浓度差和电位梯度来提高 URAT1 重吸收尿酸的能力,从而升高血尿酸水平。研究表明,低尿酸血症患者 SLC22A12 第 1639～1643 位置上的 5 个碱基对缺失,使 URAT1 末端的 7 个氨基酸变成 8 个新氨基酸,证实该区域对 URAT1 功能改变影响很大②。此外,另有研究表明,SLC22A12 基因单核苷酸多态性 rs893006 位点 GG 基因型与高尿酸血症密切相关③

6. NPT1（SLC17A1）和 NPT4（SLC17A3）

钠依赖的磷酸转运蛋白（sodium-dependent phosphate transport protein,NPT）中的 NPT 1 由 SLCl7A1 编码,该基因定位于 6p22.2,该转运体主要存在于肾近曲小管的管腔膜侧,是第一个被克隆的钠依赖的磷酸转运蛋白。研究表明该转运体是电压敏感性离子通道,属于分泌型尿酸转运体,发挥了

① ENOMOTO A, KIMURA H, CHAIROUNGDUA A, et al. Molecular Identification of a Renal Urate Anion Exchanger that Regulates Blood Urate Levels[J]. *Nature*,2002,417(6887)：447-452.

② ICHIDA K,HOSOYAMADA M,HISATOME I,et al.Clinical and Molecular Analysis of Oatients with Renal Hypouricemia in Japan Influence of URATl Gene Cnuirnary Urate Excretion[J]. *J Am Soc Nephrol*,2004,15(01)：164-173.

③ SHIMA Y,TEMYA K,OHTA H.Association between Intronic SNP in Urate-anion Exchanger Gene, SLC22A12 and Scram Uric Acid Levels in Japanese[J]. *Life Sci*,2006,79(23)：2234-2237.

转运尿酸等多种有机阴离子的作用①。由基因 SLCl7A3 编码的 NPT4 也主要在肾脏表达,该基因定位于 6p21.3,NPT4 的生物学效应还不明确。

7. OAT4(SLC22A11)和 OAT10（SLC22A13）

有机阴离子转运体(organic anion transporters,OATs)属于 SLC22A 家族(solute carrier family)成员,高度表达于肾小管上皮细胞管腔膜及基底外侧膜上,主要起调节内源性及外源性有机阴离子的排泄和重吸收的作用。目前已发现的 OAT 有 10 余种②。其中,OAT4 由基因 SLC22A11 编码,该基因位于 3 号染色体短臂上,主要表达于肾近曲小管上皮细胞的管腔膜及胎盘组织。该转运体通过尿酸与 OH-交换从而重吸收肾小管腔中的尿酸发挥调节尿酸水平的作用,但其重吸收尿酸的能力比 URAT1 弱③。而 OAT10 则由基因 SLC22A13 编码,高度表达于肾脏和肠道,该转运体重吸收尿酸的原理与 OAT4 相似。基因定位于 3p21.3,主要在肾和肠上表达,其重吸收尿酸原理同 OAT4。

8. OAT1(SLC22A6)、OAT2（SLC22A7）和 OAT3（SLC22A8）

在 OATs 中,主要位于肾小管上皮细胞基底膜上的 OAT1、OAT2 和 OAT3 主要承担从血液中摄取尿酸的任务。OAT1、OAT3 编码基因均位于 11 号染色体的长臂上,OAT2 编码基因则定位于 6 号染色体短臂上。其中,OAT1 由基因 SLC22A6 编码,主要在肾小管上皮细胞膜基底侧表达;OAT2 由基因 SLC22A7 编码,主要表达于肾脏及肝脏;OAT3 则由基因 SLC22A8 编码,主要表达于肾脏及眼部。OAT1 和 OAT3 两尿酸转运体均是阴离子-酮戊二酸交换体,因而具有非常相似的功能,能够转运多种相似的阴离子,并且两者转运的底物也类似,但是 OAT3 在与底物的亲和力方面高于 OAT1。OAT2 则主要通过谷氨酸盐与尿酸盐交换发挥转运机制。OAT1、OAT2 和 OAT3 将肾间质中的尿酸通过肾上皮细胞基底膜逆电化学梯度转运入肾小管上皮细胞内,同时肾小管上皮细胞内的酮戊二酸及谷氨酸盐被排入肾间质中。OAT1 和 OAT3 转运尿酸盐的动力来自肾小管上皮细胞内

① UCHINO H, TAMAI I, YAMASHITA K, et al. P-aminohippuric Acid Transport at Renal Apical Membrane Mediated by Human Inorganic Phosphate Transporter NPTl[J]. *Bioehem Biophys Res Commun*,2000,270(01):254-259.

② BUREKHARDT G,BUREKHARDT BC.In Vitro and in Viva Evidence of the Importance of Organic Anion Transporters(OATs)in Drug Therapy[J]. *Handb Exp Pharmacol*,2011,201:29-104.

③ HAGOS Y,STEIN D,UGELE B, et al. Human Renal Organic Anion Transporter 4 Operates as an Asymmetric Urate Transporter[J]. *J Am Soc Nephrol*,2007,18(02):430-439.

与肾间质内酮戊二酸的浓度梯度,上皮细胞内的酮戊二酸则主要来源于上皮细胞基底膜上 Na^+-酮戊二酸同向转运体对肾间质内酮戊二酸的摄取。同理,OAT2 转运尿酸的动力则可能来自胞内与间质谷氨酸盐的浓度梯度。

三、结论

　　鉴于尿酸作为抗氧化剂在 PD 患者发病及其病情进展中发挥着重要作用,尿酸转运体与人体尿酸水平息息相关,因此有必要进一步研究尿酸对 PD 的治疗作用及其与尿酸转运体作用的分子机制,为临床应用尿酸这个可干预因素防治 PD 提供一定的理论基础。由于目前尚缺乏治愈 PD 的方法,因此及早开展保护性治疗,以及寻找新的有效的干预手段,具有重要的临床意义,尿酸转运体可能成为有效的诊断和治疗 PD 的研究切入靶点。

（缪江芳　罗蔚锋）

（本文原载于《中国医药科学》2014 年第 4 卷第 16 期）

尿酸——帕金森病防治的潜在新靶点

关键词：尿酸；帕金森病；氧化应激；神经保护。

Potential Novel Target in Preventing Parkinson's Disease：Uric Acid

Key words：uric acid；Parkinson's disease；oxidative stress；neuroprotection.

帕金森病是中老年人常见的运动障碍疾病,氧化应激和线粒体功能障碍与 PD 患者黑质多巴胺能神经元变性、丢失密切相关。近年来的研究发现,尿酸水平的高低对 PD 的发病及发病后疾病的进展快慢有显著影响。本文将就尿酸的生物学特性及其与 PD 的关系做一综述。

一、尿酸的代谢、生理作用及影响体内尿酸水平的因素

尿酸是体内腺苷、鸟苷和饮食中细胞内核糖核酸嘌呤代谢的终产物,70%的尿酸经肾脏排泄,30%的尿酸经胆道和肠道排出体外。尿酸主要通过 hUTP 在人体细胞内外进行跨膜运动。hUTP 基因位于第 17 号染色体的短臂上,含有 11 个外显子。hUTP 可分为 3 种亚型,属于贯穿细胞膜脂质的离子通道,具有高度的选择性,广泛存在于体内多种组织细胞膜中①。

尿酸是人体内生理性的抗氧化剂,抑制过亚硝酸盐介导的硝化反应,具有清除氧自由基和其他活性自由基的作用,比抗坏血酸有更显著的增强红细胞膜脂质抗氧化能力、防止细胞溶解凋亡的作用。尿酸还能增强超氧化物歧化酶活性,延长其生存,防止细胞过氧化。Fe^{2+} 能够促使更多的活性氧自由基产生,加重氧化损伤,尿酸与 Fe^{2+} 具有很强的结合能力。

饮食和生活习惯对体内尿酸水平的高低有一定的影响。食用蔬菜、水

---

① LIPKOWITZ MS, LEAL-PINTO E, RAPPOPORT JZ, et al. Functional Reconstitution, Membrane Targeting, Genomic Structure, and Chromosomal Localization of a Human Urate Transporter［J］. *J Clin Invest*, 2001,107(09)：1103-1105.

果、巧克力及饮茶、饮葡萄酒会不同程度地提高人体血浆中的尿酸水平①。Ma 等②通过对 16 488 例中国受试者进行流行病学研究发现,肉食消费与 PD 发病风险存在负相关性,而肉食富含嘌呤可增高尿酸水平。牛奶能通过增加肾小管尿酸的分泌而降低尿酸水平,习惯性饮牛奶可增加 PD 的发病风险③。体育活动时由于机体排汗增加,血容量、肾血流量减少,故尿酸排泄减少,血尿酸则相对升高。Chen 等④针对 48 574 例男性和 77 254 例女性进行研究,调查其成年早期的体育锻炼情况,结果发现,体育活动基线水平在高四分位的男性人群比在低四分位的男性人群 PD 发病率低。

二、尿酸保护多巴胺能神经元的体外细胞水平的研究

通过体外实验研究发现尿酸具有很强的抗氧化活性,可以保护氧化应激导致的细胞损伤,对神经元具有保护作用⑤。对来源于 SD 大鼠胚胎的海马神经元进行体外培养研究发现,尿酸可以显著减轻兴奋性氨基酸-谷氨酸和氰化物——NaCN 对海马神经元的损害,具体机制与尿酸抑制氧化应激产物——活性氧簇(过氧化氢、过氧化亚硝酸盐)和脂质过氧化大量产生有关⑥。以胎鼠的脊髓神经细胞为研究对象,发现联合应用星形胶质细胞和尿酸可以保护兴奋性氨基酸-谷氨酸对其的毒性作用⑦。尿酸与多巴胺能神经元共培养,对多巴胺能神经元有明确的保护作用,在高钾轻度去极化,增

① LOTITO SB,FREI B.Consumption of Flavonoid-rich Foods and Increased Plasma Antioxidant Capacity in Humans:Cause,Consequence,or Epiphenomenon? [J].*Free Radio Biol Med*,2006,41(12):1727-1746.

② MA L,ZHANG L,GAO XH,et al.Dietary Factorsand Smoking as Risk Factors for PD in a Mral Population in China:a Nested Case-control Study[J].*Acta NeumI Stand*,2006,113(04):278-281.

③ CHOI HK,LIU S,CURHAN G.Intake of Purine——Rich Foods,Protein,and Dairy Products and Relationship to Serum Levels of Uric Acid:the Third National Health and Nutrition Examination Survey[J].*Arthritis Rheum*,2005,52(01):283-289.

④ Chen H,Zhang SM,Schwarzschild MA,et al.Physical Activity and the Risk of Parkinson Disease[J].*Neurology*,2005,64(04):664-669.

⑤ AMES BN,CATHCART R,SCHWIERS E,et al.Uric Acid Provides an Antioxidant Defense in Humans against Oxidant and Radical Caused Aging and Cancer a Hypothesis[J].*Proc NailAcad Sci USA*,1981,78(11):6858-6862.

⑥ YU ZF,BRUCE-KELLER AJ,GOODMAN Y,et al.Uric Acid Protects Neurons against Excitotoxic and Metabolic Insults in Cell Culture,and against Focal Ischemic Brain Injury In Vivo[J].*J Neurosci Res*,1998,53(05):613-625.

⑦ DU Y,CHEN CP,TSENG CY,et al.Astroglia-mediated Effects of Uric Acid to Protect Spinal Cord Neurons from Glutamate Toxicity [J].*Glia*,2007,55(05):463-472.

加钙内流的条件下,这种保护作用进一步提高①。

PC12 细胞富含多巴胺受体及合成、分解多巴胺所需的各种酶,被广泛应用于多巴胺能神经元毒性损害和死亡方式的研究。Keller 等②证实,尿酸能保护 PC12 细胞免受 Fe^{2+}、β-淀粉样物质等诱导的过亚硝酸盐、脂质过氧化反应对其的损害。本课题组的实验结果亦提示尿酸能够减轻 6-OHDA 对 PC12 细胞的毒性作用:尿酸可显著改善 6-OHDA 作用 6、12、24 h 后造成的 PC12 细胞生存率下降现象($P<0.05$);以及减少 6-OHDA 导致的 PC12 细胞 caspase-3 激活,降低 6-OHDA 导致的凋亡率上升($P<0.05$)]③。

三、尿酸对 PD 动物模型的保护作用

MPTP 可选择性引起黑质致密区多巴胺能神经元损伤,黑质-纹状体内多巴胺递质排空。MPTP 转变为 MPP^+ 后经多巴胺能神经元的转运蛋白摄取,聚集在线粒体内,产生过量的自由基,导致多巴胺能神经元的变性死亡④。6-OHDA 是多巴胺类似物,其结构与多巴胺相类似,常被误作为多巴胺神经递质摄入多巴胺能神经元,选择性造成多巴胺能神经元死亡⑤。

本课题组以 C57B1/6 小鼠为研究对象,利用微透析技术,分别给予小鼠左侧脑室持续灌注 24 h 人工脑脊液和不同剂量的尿酸后,腹腔注射 MPTP,再维持相同的干预治疗 24 h,发现适当提高脑组织中的尿酸水平能够减轻 MPTP 对小鼠多巴胺能神经元的损害⑥。以 SD 大鼠为研究对象的结果提示:腹腔注射尿酸可提高血、脑纹状体组织中的尿酸水平,显著减轻

① GUERREIRO S,PONCEAU A,TOULORGE D,et al.Protection of Midbrain Dopaminergic Neurons by the End-product of Purine Metabolism Uric Acid:Potentiation by Low-level Depolarization [J].*J Neurochem*,2009,109(04):1118-1128.

② KELLER JN,KINDY MS,HOLTSBERG FW,et al.Mitochondrial Manganese Superoxide Dismutase Prevents Neural Apoptosis and Reduces Ischemic Brain Injury:Suppression of Peroxynitrite Production,Lipid Peroxidation,and Mitochondrial Dysfunction[J].*J Neurosci*,1998,18(02):687-697.

③ 叶艳,罗蔚锋,朱婷鸽,等.尿酸减轻 6-羟基多巴胺对 PC12 细胞的毒性作用[J].中国临床神经科学,2010,18(02):135-139.

④ LEE DW,RAJAGOPALAN S,SIDDIQ A,et al.Inhibition of Prolyl Hydroxylase Protects against 1-methyl-4-phenyl-1,2,3,6-tetrahydropyridine-induced Neurotoxicity:Model for the Potential Involvement of the Hypoxia-inducible Factor Pathway in Parkinson Disease[J].*J Biol Chem*,2009,284(42):29065-29076.

⑤ MARIN C,AGUILAR E,MENGOD G,et al.Effects of Early vs Late Initiation of Levodopa Treatment in Hemiparkinsonian Rats[J].*Eur J Neurosci*,2009,30(05):823-832.

⑥ 王晓君,罗蔚锋,王丽君,等.帕金森病患者认知功能与尿酸及相关因素分析[J].中华医学杂志,2009,89(23):1633-1635.

6-OHDA 对黑质纹状体系统多巴胺能神经元的毒性作用,改善大鼠的自主活动,前肢运动功能等①。

四、体内尿酸水平对 PD 发病率影响的流行病学研究

对 8 000 例男性人群在进行常规的血尿酸水平测定后,进行长达 30 年的跟踪随访,有 92 例相继被诊断为 PD,经年龄、吸烟危险因素调整后发现,入组时血清尿酸水平高于平均值的人群其 PD 发病率降低 40%②。对 4 695 例 55 岁以上(包括 55 岁)人群进行前瞻性研究,平均随访 9.4 年,有 68 例被诊断为 PD。发现血清尿酸水平升高可以明显降低 PD 的发病率,且存在显著的剂量相关性($P<0.05$)③。对 18 000 例的男性人群进行前瞻性的流行病学研究,8 年后发现血浆尿酸水平处于高五分位值范围的人群相对于尿酸水平处于低五分位值范围人群,其 PD 发病率降低 55%。经年龄、吸烟、饮咖啡及其他与 PD 和血尿酸水平有关的因素调整后,尿酸与 PD 的发病率仍呈显著的负相关性。对年龄 65 岁以上 56 199 例无痛风的人群和 7 482 例痛风患者进行长期的跟踪随访(1991—2004 年,平均随访时间 8 年),结果提示有痛风患者人群的 PD 患病风险降低 30%。调整了年龄、性别、高血压、糖尿病、高脂血症等并发症,应用利尿剂和非甾体抗炎等因素之后,这种负相关性仍存在。进一步分析发现,对于没有应用利尿剂的观察对象,无论男性还是女性,结论相同,也就是说血尿酸水平越高,PD 的发病率越低④。Winquist 等⑤进行的横向社区流行病学调查发现,无论是男性还是女性,血尿酸水平处于平均值或高于平均值人群 PD 的患病率显著低于血尿酸水平处于平均值以下的人群。

① 王丽君,罗蔚锋,王恒会,等.尿酸对 6-羟基多巴胺致大鼠黑质纹状体系毒性的影响[J].中华医学杂志,2010,90(19):1362-1365.

② DAVIS JW,GRANDINETTI A,WASLIEN CI,et al.Observations on Serum Uric Acid Levels and the Risk of Idiopathic Parkinson Disease[J].Am J Epidemiol,1996,144(05):480-484.

③ DE LAU LM,KOUDSTAAL PJ,HOFMAN A,et al.Serum Uric Acid Levels and the Risk of Parkinson Disease[J].Am Neurol,2005,58(05):797-800.

④ WEISSKOPF MG,O'REILLY E,CHEN H,et al.Plasma Urate and Risk of Parkinson's Disease[J].Am J Epidemiol,2007,166(05):561-567.

⑤ WINQUIST A,STEENLAND K,SHANKAR A.Higher Serum Uric Acid Associated with Decreased Parkinson's Disease Prevalence in a Large Community-based Survey [J].Mov Disord,2010,25(07):932-936.

五、尿酸水平与 PD 的临床研究

1. PD 患者尿酸水平的变化

临床资料证实 PD 患者的黑质纹状体系统、脑脊液、血尿酸水平有明显变化。Church 等[1]对死亡后 PD 患者的黑质和尾状核组织中的尿酸、多巴胺进行测定，发现其尿酸、多巴胺的水平显著地低于年龄相匹配的健康对照组。在黑质中两者分别降低 54%、85%。PD 患者组尾状核组织匀浆液中的多巴胺氧化速度常数是 $4.20 \times 10^{-2}/min$，健康对照组仅为 $0.34 \times 10^{-2}/min$。黑质匀浆液中多巴胺氧化速度常数在 PD 患者组和健康对照组中分别是 $4.57 \times 10^{-2}/min$、$2.82 \times 10^{-2}/min$。于 PD 患者组尾状核中加入尿酸或过氧化氢酶，会使黑质组织匀浆液中的多巴胺氧化速度常数降低。Annanmaki 等[2]以 40 例 PD 患者和 29 例正常人为研究对象，对其血浆尿酸、血清铁蛋白、体重指数及乳制品饮食等进行检测评价，结果提示 PD 患者的血浆尿酸水平显著降低，尿酸水平的改变与血清铁蛋白变化密切联系。本课题组对 PD 患者的血尿酸水平进行对比性分析，发现其较健康对照组显著降低[3][4]。

尿酸转运体 SLC2A9 对于调节血尿酸水平的高低起着重要的作用。SLC2A9 包含有 rs733175、rs737267、rs1014290 和 rs6449213 等 4 个变异体。Facheris[5] 等对 664 例 PD 患者进行 SLC2A9 基因多态性、血尿酸水平和 PD 的发病年龄分析发现，rs1014290 与低尿酸水平、PD 发病年龄相对较早密切相关。对于女性 PD 患者血尿酸水平的改变有不同的报道，1990—2004 年，O'Reilly 及其同事进行了一项女性护理工作者参加的病例对照研究，发现 101 例女性 PD 患者的血尿酸水平（5.04 mg/dL）与 504 例正常女性患者的血尿酸水平（4.86 mg/dL）无显著性差异。其原因可能是单次测量血尿酸无法代表长时期内的尿酸水平。虽然男性尿酸和 PD 这种显著的反比关系也

①　CHURCH WH,WARD VL.Uric Acid is Reduced in the Substantia Nigra in Parkinson Disease：Effect on Dopamine Oxidation[J].*Brain Res Bull*,1994,33(04)：419-425.

②　ANNANMAKI T,MUURONEN A,MURROS K.Low Plasma Uric Acid Level in Parkinson's Disease[J].*Mov Disord*,2007,22(08)：1133-1137.

③　王丽君,罗蔚锋,王恒会,等.帕金森病患者血尿酸水平[J].中华神经科杂志,2008,41(03)：157-158.

④　罗蔚锋,王丽君,王晓君,等.老年男性帕金森病患者血尿酸水平的研究[J].中华老年医学杂志,2009,28(01)：60-61.

⑤　FACHERIS MF,HICKS AA,MINELLI C,et al.Variation in the Uric Acid Transporter Gene SLC2A9 and its Association with AAO of Parkinson's Disease[J].*J Mol Neurosci*,2011,43(03)：246-250.

是以单次测量为基础,但是女性标准可能多因绝经和绝经后激素的使用而改变。调查中另一项结果显示,绝经后妇女的尿酸水平高于绝经前妇女,绝经后未曾使用激素者高于曾经使用者,暗示绝经后使用激素可能改变了尿酸和 PD 之间的关联①。本课题组选择自 2007 年 9 月至 2008 年 10 月在苏州大学附属第二医院神经内科门诊就诊的 81 例女性 PD 患者,和同期 81 名在该院进行常规体检,性别、年龄(±3 岁)、体质量(±2 kg)匹配的健康者进行对比性研究,发现女性 PD 患者的血尿酸水平[(244.63±67.47 μmol/L)]显著低于健康对照组[(302.17±49.18)μmol/L]②。所以女性 PD 患者血尿酸水平的改变特点尚需进一步的研究。

2. 尿酸水平对 PD 患者认知功能的影响

PD 患者中 40%～50%会伴发认知功能障碍。Annanmaki 等③通过测定 40 例 PD 患者血尿酸浓度,然后对每个患者进行神经心理方面的测试,结果发现血尿酸水平较低的 PD 患者评分较低,即低的血尿酸水平同 PD 患者的认知功能下降相关。本课题组对 PD 患者进行认知功能评分,观察 PD 患者的认知功能与血尿酸等因素的关系,结果显示伴有认知功能障碍的 PD 患者的血尿酸水平低于无认知功能障碍的患者;PD 患者的认知功能障碍与其受教育水平、血尿酸水平呈正相关,而与年龄、H-Y 分期和抑郁程度呈负相关。进一步的分析发现,血尿酸水平与认知域中的记忆力、抽象概括力相关,高尿酸水平 PD 患者的记忆力、抽象概括力相对较好④⑤。其确切机制还有待于进一步探讨。结合《蒙特利尔认知评估量表(MoCA)(北京版)》,尿酸有可能成为 PD 早期认知功能障碍的预测因素之一,从而有助于早期发现 PD 患者的 MCI 症状,并通过饮食调整或药物治疗等途径,在一定范围内提高其尿酸水平,有望减缓 PD 患者由 MCI 向 PD 痴呆的发展。

既往人们对于高尿酸血症引起的损害已予以重视,如高尿酸血症会出

① O'REILLY EJ,GAO X,WEISSKOPF MG,et al.Plasma Urate and Parkinson's Disease in Women[J]. *Am J Epidemiol*,2010,172(05):666-670.

② 王晓君,罗蔚锋,王丽君,等.女性帕金森病患者血尿酸水平的研究[J].中国神经精神疾病杂志,2009,35(05):306-307.

③ ANNANMAKI T,PESSALA-DRIVER A,HOKKANEN L,et al.Uric Acid Associates with Cognition in Parkinson's Disease[J].*Parkinsenism Relat D*,2008,14(07):576-578.

④ 李丹,王晓君,罗蔚锋,等.尿酸对帕金森病患者不同认知功能域影响分析[J].中华神经科杂志,2010,43(06):400-402.

⑤ 王晓君,罗蔚锋,王丽君,等.帕金森病患者认知功能与尿酸及相关因素分析[J].中华医学杂志,2009,89(23):1633-1635.

现痛风的症状。在一般人群中,高尿酸血症还预测高血压病的发展,而尿酸水平与高血压病的发生率之间呈独立的正相关关系已被报道①。Bos 等②发现血尿酸水平与心脏病及卒中的发病风险呈显著正相关,已经发现确诊冠心病患者的血尿酸水平显著高于健康者。本课题组的临床研究结果表明,PD 患者的血尿酸水平为(261±90)μmol/L,处于正常生理尿酸水平范围,但显著低于正常对照人群的(337±60)μmol/L。

综上所述,相对高尿酸水平能够有效降低 PD 发病风险,延缓 PD 患者进展速度,这些均提示在一定范围内提高尿酸水平是 PD 保护性治疗的潜在靶点。但存在的问题在于,通过增加血尿酸水平是否能够有效延缓多巴胺能神经元的进行性变性,进而延缓 PD 病程和改善预后,并且这种有益性的神经保护作用是否超过由于机体总尿酸水平的增加而带来的负面影响,即什么水平的血尿酸浓度既有助于减慢甚至预防 PD 的发生发展,又有利于痛风、糖脂代谢紊乱、高血压、冠心病等疾病的防治。这些问题都急需从基因、分子、细胞及组织等不同角度进行深入的研究和探索。

(黄婷婷 罗蔚锋 刘春风)

(本文原载于《中华神经医学杂志》2012 年第 11 卷第 11 期)

---

① JOSSA F,FARINARO E,PANICO S,et al.Serum Uric Acid and Hypert-ension:the Olivetti Heart Study[J].*J Hum Hypertens*,1994,8(09):677-681.

② BOS MJ,KOUDSTAAL PJ,HOFINAN A,et al.Uric Acid is a Risk Factor for Myocardial Infarction and Stroke:the Rotterdam Study[J].*Stroke*,2006,37(06):1503-1507.

帕金森病脑脊液生物指标研究进展①

摘　要：帕金森病以黑质纹状体系统多巴胺能神经元进行性变性缺失和路易小体的出现为病理特征。研究发现脑脊液中尿酸、黄嘌呤和高草香酸水平以及它们的比值、a-synuclein、DJ-1、Aβ1-42、8-羟基脱氧鸟苷、超氧化物歧化酶等脑脊液生物学指标在 PD 患者发生了有意义的变化。

关键词：帕金森病；脑脊液；尿酸；a-synuclein；8-羟基脱氧鸟苷。

Study on the Cerebrospinal Fluid Biomarkers in the Patients with Parkinson's Disease

Abstract：Parkinson's disease is a common neurodegenerative disorder characterized by progressive degeneration of the dopaminergic neurons in the substantia nigra pars compacta and generation of Lewy body. Several studies suggest that uric acid, xanthine, homovanillic acid and their ratio, a-synuclein, DJ-1, Aβ1-42, 8-hydroxy-2'-deoxyguanosine, Superoxide Dismutase and other biomarkers of cerebrospinal fluid（CSF）in patients with PD have been significantly changed.

Key words：Parkinson's disease；cerebrospinal fluid；uric acid；α-Synuclein；8-Hydroxy -2'-deoxyguanosine.

帕金森病是中老年人常见的神经系统退行性疾病之一。PD 产生的运动功能障碍主要有静止性震颤、肌强直、运动迟缓和姿势或步态异常等。病程中常合并嗅觉减退、神经心理障碍等非运动症状，晚期残障严重，生活不能自理，给社会和家庭带来沉重负担。目前认为，PD 是受遗传因素、环境因

① 本文系江苏省自然科学基金（项目编号：BK2010229）；江苏省高校自然科学基金（项目编号：O8KJB320012）；苏州市科技发展计划（社会发展及医药）项目（项目编号：SSO8015）、苏州市科技支撑计划项目（项目编号：SS201112）。

素共同影响,并在年龄老化等作用下的结果。其主要病理特征为黑质纹状体系统多巴胺能神经元进行性变性缺失和路易小体的出现。帕金森病的诊断主要依赖临床症状及体征、对左旋多巴制剂治疗的反应等,目前尚无特异敏感的生化指标可作为临床确定的依据。因此,研究此类退行性疾病的生物标志物是该领域的研究热点之一,目的是希望发现稳定性和重复性均佳的生物标志物来帮助临床早期诊断。由于受大脑取材的限制,能够反映大脑病理生理改变的脑脊液(cerebrospinal fluid,CSF)成为常用的研究对象。近年来有关 PD 的脑脊液生物学指标的研究取得较大进展,发现尿酸、黄嘌呤和高草香酸水平及它们的比值、a-synuclein、DJ-1、Aβ1-42、8-羟基脱氧鸟苷、超氧化物歧化酶等脑脊液生物学指标在 PD 患者中发生了有意义的变化。

一、脑脊液尿酸水平与帕金森病

UA 是体内腺苷、鸟苷和饮食中细胞内核糖核酸嘌呤代谢的终末产物,腺苷在腺苷脱氨酶、嘌呤核苷磷酸化酶、黄嘌呤氧化酶的作用下生成黄嘌呤和尿酸。UA 是一种生理性的抗氧化剂,能够清除人体内 60% 的自由基。UA 能够清除超氧化物、羟基及单态氧。通过阻止超氧歧化酶的降解清除超氧化物,阻止其与一氧化氮结合生成过氧化亚硝酸盐的作用,阻止蛋白的硝化作用;螯合铁离子,抑制铁依赖的维生素的氧化,阻止增多的自由基进一步造成氧化损伤。

高尿酸水平的个体具有明显低的 PD 发病风险,高尿酸导致的痛风病人有明显低的 PD 发病率[1][2];相反,血尿酸水平降低会增加 PD 发生的风险[3][4][5]。

① WEISSKOPF MG,O'REILLY E,CHEN H,et al.Plasma Urate and Risk of Parkinson's Disease[J].*Am Epidemiol*,2007,166(05):561-567.

② ALONSO A, RODRIGUEZ LA, LOGROSCINO G, et al. Gout and Risk of Parkinson Disease:a Prospective Study[J].*Neurology*,2007,69(17):1696-1700.

③ HUANG YX,LUO WF.Potential Role of Uric Acid as a Biomarker for Parkinson's Disease[J].*Med Hypotheses*,2010,75(02):273.

④ ANDREADOU E, NIKOLAOU C, GOURNARAS F, et al.Serum Uric Acid Levels in Patients with Parkinson's Disease:their Relationship to Treatment and Disease Duration[J].*Clin Neurol Neurosurg*,2009,111(09):724-728.

⑤ 罗蔚锋,王丽君,王晓君,等.老年男性帕金森病患者血尿酸水平的研究[J].中华老年医学杂志,2009,28(01):60-61.

王丽君等①比较了 121 例 PD 患者及 121 例健康体检者的血 UA 水平,按照年龄、性别配对,发现 PD 患者血 UA 水平(260.76±90.42 μmol/L)显著低于健康体检人群组(336.95±59.64 μmol/L,$P<0.01$)。Ascherio 等②对病程小于 5 年的 713 名 PD 患者进行了研究,结果发现高的脑脊液 UA 可以明显降低 PD 的发病率,并且可以减慢 PD 病人的临床进展。

二、脑脊液中黄嘌呤、高草香酸及它们的比值与帕金森病

黄嘌呤(xanthine,X)是腺苷、鸟苷和饮食中细胞内核糖核酸嘌呤代谢过程的产物,腺苷在腺苷脱氨酶、嘌呤核苷磷酸化酶、黄嘌呤氧化酶的作用下生成黄嘌呤,黄嘌呤也是尿酸的直接前体。HVA 是中枢神经系统中多巴胺的主要代谢产物,通常被作为判断多巴胺活性的主要指标。

Le Witt 等③对 217 名未进行药物治疗的 PD 患者及 26 名健康对照者进行了研究。结果在对 PD 患者组和健康对照组脑脊液含量的分析中发现,二者的 X 和 HVA 没有显著性差异,但是 X 与 HVA 的比值却有显著性差异,在健康对照组,脑脊液中 X/HVA 为 13.1±5.5,在 PD 患者组,脑脊液中 X/HVA 为 17.4±6.7($P=0.001\ 7$),24 个月后再次收集 PD 患者的脑脊液,发现 X/HVA 为 19.7±8.7($P<0.001$),这两次收集 PD 患者脑脊液中的 X/HVA 和健康对照组比较,都有显著性差异。同时作者通过研究还发现,脑脊液中的 X/HVA 也与 PD 患者疾病的严重程度有关。但是也有学者④在与健康对照组的比较中发现,PD 患者脑脊液中的 HVA 水平是降低的。脑脊液中 X/HVA 水平的增高及 HVA 水平的降低,可能是黑质纹状体多巴胺能神经元的丢失所致,由此可将之作为 PD 的生物指标之一。

① 王丽君,罗蔚锋,王恒会,等.帕金森病患者血尿酸水平[J].中华神经科杂志,2008,41(03):157-158.

② ASCHERIO A,LEWITT PA,XU K,et al.Urate as a Predictor of the Slower Rate of Clinical Decline in Parkinson Disease[J].*Arch.Neurol*,2009,66(12)1460-1468.

③ LEWITT P,SCHULTZ L,AUINQER P,et al.CSF Xanthine,Homovanillic Acid,and their Ratio as Biomarkers of Parkinson's Disease[J].*Brain Research*,2011,1408(08):88-97.

④ GOLDSTEIN DS,HOLMES C,BENTHO O,et al.Biomarkers to Detect Central Dopamine Deficiency and Distinguish Parkinson Disease from Multiple System Atrophy[J].*Parkinsonism Relat Disord*,2008,14(08):600-607.

三、脑脊液中 a-synuclein 及 DJ-1 与帕金森病

a-突触核蛋白(a-snynuclein)是一种由 140 个氨基酸构成的蛋门质,在脑中含量丰富,主要分布于大脑皮质、海马、纹状体、杏仁核、黑质等部位。研究结果表明,a-synuclein 与神经退行性疾病尤其是帕金森病的发病具有密切关系。路易体是帕金森病的主要病理特征,而异常折叠的 a-synuclein 被证明是其主要成分。a-synuclein 基因突变导致家族遗传性帕金森病的发病;另外,a-synuclein 转基因小鼠和果蝇复制出帕金森病的主要病理变化和运动障碍。DJ-1 蛋白在体内广泛分布,包括在基底节不同类型细胞的胞核、胞质中均有表达。目前已报道的 DJ-1 基因功能包括:参与细胞周期的调节,控制基因转录,调节 mRNA 稳定性和参与细胞应激反应。目前对其突变后致病的机制还知之甚少,它可能与 a-synuclein 和 Parkin 一样,通过影响氧化应激和使蛋白酶体降解系统失调而导致 PD 的发生。

Heng 等[1]对 117 名 PD 患者、132 名健康对照者、50 名 AD 患者进行了研究,结果表明,与健康对照组和 AD 组相比,PD 患者脑脊液中的 DJ-1 和 a-synuclein 水平是降低的,PD 患者脑脊液中 DJ-1 降低的敏感度和特异度分别是 90% 和 70%,a-synuclein 降低的敏感度与特异度分别是 92% 和 58%。但是作者在研究中也发现,PD 患者脑脊液中的这两种蛋白只能协助 PD 的诊断,与 PD 的严重程度没有明显的相关性。Shi 等[2]对 122 名健康对照者、126 名 PD 患者、33 名 AD 患者脑脊液中的 DJ-1 和 a-synuclein 水平进行了研究。结果发现,与对照组比较,PD 患者与 AD 患者的 DJ-1 和 a-synuclein 水平有下降趋势。近年有多名学者[3][4][5][6]通过研究也发现 PD 患者脑脊液

①　HONG Z,SHI M,CHUNG KA. et al. DJ-1 and Alpha-synuclein in Human Cerebrospinal Fluid as Biomarkers of Parkinson's Disease[J].*Brain*,2010,133(Pt3):713-726.

②　SHI M,ZABETIAN CP,HANCOCK AM,et al. Significance and Confounders of Peripheral DJ-1 and Alpha-synuclein in Parkinson's Disease[J].*Neurosci Lett*,2010,480(01):78-82.

③　WARAGAI M,SEKIYAMA K.SEKIGAWA A,et al. Alpha-synuclein and DJ-1 as Potential Biological Fluid Biomarkers for Parkinson's Disease[J].*Int J Mol Sci*,2010,11(11):4257-4266.

④　MOLLENHAUER B, LOCASCIO JJ, SCHULZ-SCHAEFFER W, et al. a-Synuclein and Tau Concentrations in Cerebrospinal Fluid of Patients Presenting with Parkinsonism:a Cohort Study[J].*Lancet Neurol*,2011,10(03)230-240.

⑤　TOKUDA T,SALEM SA,ALLSOP D,et al. Decreased Alpha-synuclein in Cerebrospinal Fluid of Aged Individuals and Subjects with Parkinson's Disease[J].*Biochem Biophys Res Commun*,2006,349(01):162-166.

⑥　PETER LW. Recent Advances in CSF Biomarkers for Parkinson's Disease[J].*Parkinsonism Relat Disord*,2012,18(Suppl 1):S49-51.

中的 DJ-1 和 a-synuclein 水平是下降的,并且 a-synuclein 水平的升高或降低
与 PD 的严重程度有关。

四、脑脊液中总 Tau 蛋白、磷酸化的 Tau 蛋白、Aβ1−42、Flt3 ligand 及 fractalkine 水平与帕金森病

Tau 蛋白是含量最高的微管相关蛋白,具有稳定微管系统、调控神经细胞生长发育的功能,并在神经系统形成和轴突通讯传导中起重要作用。过度磷酸化的 Tau 蛋白聚集形成的神经纤维缠结是许多神经退行性疾病的病理特征。配对螺旋样纤维螺旋丝为神经纤维缠结的主要成分,研究发现螺旋丝与启动氧化自由基系统导致神经细胞的死亡有关。因此,Tau 蛋白异常与各类神经退行性疾病中的神经细胞死亡有密切的关系。Aβ 是老年斑形成的始动因子,也是老年斑核中的核心成分。Flt3 ligand 和 fractalkine 是与 PD 相关的炎症因子。

Shi 等[1]研究发现,脑脊液中总 Tau 蛋白、磷酸化的 Tau 蛋白、Aβl−42、Flt3 ligand 及 fracta-lkine 水平不仅可以区分 PD 患者和健康对照组,而且可以鉴别 PD 患者和 AD 患者与多系统萎缩患者。尤其是 Flt3 ligand,在 PD 患者脑脊液检测中过度表达,而且敏感性和特异性都非常高。而且作者也发现,fractalkine/Aβ1-42 的比值与 PD 的严重程度和疾病的进展都有相关性。Siderowf 等[2]通过研究也发现,与对照组相比,PD 患者脑脊液中的 Aβ1-42 水平降低。在有认知功能障碍的 PD 患者中,Aβ1-42 水平更低。Aβ1-42 水平为认知功能损伤的指标。Aasly 等[3]对 26 名 LRRK2 突变的 PD 患者脑脊液中的 Aβ1-42 水平、总 Tau 蛋白及磷酸化 Tau 蛋白进行检查发现,三者水平的降低与纹状体多巴胺功能减退有关。

五、脑脊液中 8-羟基脱氧鸟苷与氧化型辅酶 Q10

8-羟基脱氧鸟苷(8-hydroxy-2-deoxyguanosine,8-OHdG)是活性氧自由基

① SHI M, BRADNER J, HANCOCK AM, et al. Cerebrospinal Fluid Biomarkers for Parkinson Disease Diagnosis and Progression[J]. *Ann Neurol*, 2011, 69(03): 570−580.

② SIDEROWF A, XIE SX, HURTIG H, et al. CSF Amyloid Api-42-42 Predicts Cognitive Decline in Parkinson Disease[J]. *Neurology*, 2010, 75(12): 1055−1061.

③ AASLY JO, SHI M, SOSSI V, et al. Cerebrospinal Fluid Amyloid β and Tau in LRRK2 Mutation Carriers[J]. *Neurology*, 2012, 78(01): 55−61.

如羟自由基、单线态氧等攻击 DNA 分子中的鸟嘌呤碱基第 8 位碳原子产生的一种氧化性化合物。羟自由基和超氧阴离子能直接与 DNA 分子反应,导致 DNA 链断裂、碱基修饰和 DNA 蛋白交联等氧化性 DNA 损伤,其中最主要的致突变性损伤反应是八位碳上鸟嘌呤与胸腺嘧啶碱基置换性突变,从而产生 8-OHdG。它是一种内源性诱变剂,具有突变倾向(G：C—T：A 置换),通常认为它是活性氧引起突变的一个可能原因[1]。辅酶 Q10 是生物体内广泛存在的脂溶性醌类化合物,具有促进氧化磷酸化反应和保护生物膜结构完整性的功能。CoQl0 在细胞线粒体内呼吸链质子转移及电子传递中起重要作用,是细胞呼吸和细胞代谢的激活剂,也是重要的抗氧化剂和非特异性免疫增强剂。

Isobe 等[2]对 20 名 PD 患者及年龄匹配 20 名的健康对照组研究发现,PD 患者脑脊液中氧化型辅酶 Q10 与总辅酶 Q10 的比值及 8-羟基脱氧鸟苷是增高的。测定脑脊液中 8-OHdG 的含量,发现 PD 患者组显著高于同年龄健康对照组,并且 8-OHdG 的含量与病情进展速度呈线性相关。通过检测 8-OHdG 和氧化型辅酶 Q10 与总辅酶 Q10 的比值的水平可以评估体内氧化损伤和修复的程度,氧化应激与 DNA 损伤的相互关系,对于研究 PD 与氧化应激的关系具有重要意义。

六、脑脊液中 SOD 与帕金森病

SOD 是机体主要的抗氧化酶之一,它能够清除超氧化物,保护细胞免受氧化损伤。它通过催化超氧化物歧化成 H_2O_2 和 O_2,这些 H_2O_2 再通过过氧化氢酶(CAT)和谷胱甘肽过氧化物酶(GSH—PX)等的催化转化成无毒的 H_2O_2[3]。

① WU LL,CHIOU CC,CHANG PY,et al.Urinary 8-OHDG：a Marker of Oxidative Stress to DNA and a Risk Factor for Cancer Atherosclerosis and Diabetics[J].*Clin Chim Acta*,2004,339(1-2)：1-9.

② ISOBE C,ABE T,TERAYAMA Y.Levels of Reduced and Oxidized CoenzymeQ-10 and 8-hydroxy-20-deoxyguanosine in the Cerebrospinal Fluid of Patients with Living Parkinson's Disease Demonstrate that Mitochondrial Oxidative Damage and/or Oxidative DNA Damage Contributes to the Neurodegenerative Process [J].*Neurosci Lett*,2010,469(01)：159-163.

③ CUONG DV,KIM N,YOUM JB,et al.Nitric Oxide-cGMP-Protein Kinase G Signaling Pathway Induces Anoxic Preconditioning through Activation of ATP-sensiti ve K+channels in Rat Hearts [J].*Am J Physiol Heart circ Physiol*,2006,290(05)：1808-1817.

Boll 等①通过研究发现,PD 患者脑脊液中的 Cu/Zn 依赖性 SOD 水平是降低的。因此,检查 PD 患者脑脊液中的 Cu/Zn 依赖性 SOD 水平,可能有助于 PD 的诊断。

七、展望

对于 PD 的生物指标的研究是非常必要的,不仅可以有效地追踪 PD 高危人群的健康状况,比如有 PD 家族史的人们,有助于 PD 的早期诊断,而且有助于在治疗中监测病情进展,从而为新的治疗手段提供可能。

（郑丽霞　罗蔚锋）
（本文原载于《国际老年医学杂志》2012 年第 33 卷第 3 期）

---

① BOLL MC,CARAZ-ZUBELDIA M,MONTES S,et al.Free Copper,Ferroxidase and SOD1 Activities,Lipid Peroxidation,and NO(x)Content in the CSF:a Different Marker profile in Four Neurodegenerative Diseases[J].*Neurochem Res*,2008,33(09):1717-1723.

帕金森病的血生物学指标研究进展①

摘 要： 帕金森病以黑质多巴胺能神经元变性、缺失和路易小体形成为病理特征,其发生机制与黑质纹状体系统氧化应激反应增强、自由基增多损害多巴胺能神经元等密切相关。研究发现尿酸、8-羟基脱氧鸟苷、谷胱甘肽、铁和白介素-6等血生物学指标在帕金森病患者中发生了有意义的变化,本文就此做一综述。

关键词 帕金森病;生物学指标;研究进展。

Advances in the Study on the Blood Biomarkers of Parkinson's Disease

Abstract：Parkinson's disease is a common neurodegenerative disorder, characterized by progressive degeneration of the dopaminergic neurons in the substantia nigra pars compacts and generation of Lewy body. The exact mechanisms remain unknown. However oxidative stress and free radical are generally thought to play a prominent role in the etiology of PD.Several studies suggest that uric acid, 8-hydroxy-2'-deoxyguanosine, glutathione, iron, interleukin-6 and other biomarkers of blood in PD patients have been significantly changed.

Key words Parkinson's disease;biomarkers;research.

帕金森病是老年人常见的神经系统退行性疾病之一,其主要病理特征为中脑黑质致密部多巴胺能神经元的进行性变性减少,导致黑质纹状体系统多巴胺水平降低。其发生机制与黑质纹状体系统氧化应激反应增强,自由基增多损害多巴胺能神经元等密切相关。临床表现分为运动障碍症状和非运动障碍症状两大类,运动障碍症状包括静止性震颤、运动迟缓、肌强直

① 本文系江苏省自然科学基金项目(项目编号:BK2010229);江苏省高校自然研究计划项目(项目编号:08KJB320012);苏州市科技发展计划(社会发展及医药)资助项目(项目编号:200815404)。

和姿势或步态异常等。当临床出现运动障碍症状时,黑质多巴胺能神经元的数目已经减少 50% 以上,纹状体 DA 水平减少达 80% 以上。近年来有关 PD 的血生物学指标的研究取得了长足的进展,发现尿酸、8-羟基脱氧鸟苷、谷胱甘肽、铁和白介素-6 等血生物学指标在 PD 患者中发生了有意义的变化。

一、血尿酸与 PD

尿酸,是体内腺苷、鸟苷和饮食中细胞内核糖核酸嘌呤代谢的终末产物,腺苷在腺苷脱氨酶、嘌呤核苷磷酸化酶、黄嘌呤氧化酶的作用下生成黄嘌呤和尿酸。UA 是一种生理性的抗氧化剂,清除人体内 60% 的自由基。UA 能够清除超氧化物,羟基及单态氧,通过阻止超氧歧化酶的降解清除超氧化物,阻止其与一氧化氮结合生成过氧化亚硝酸盐的作用,阻止蛋白的硝化作用;螯合铁离子,抑制铁依赖的维生素的氧化,阻止增多的自由基进一步造成氧化损伤。

流行病学和临床研究①②③④⑤⑥⑦⑧⑨⑩发现,血 UA 水平可以影响 PD 的发生,血尿酸水平高的人群 PD 的发生率显著降低,PD 患者的血 UA 水平

① WEISSKOPF MG,O'REILLY E,CHEN H,et al.Plasma Urate and Risk of Parkinson's Disease[J].*Am Epidemiol*,2007,166(05):561-567.

② HUANG YX,LUO WF.Potential Role of Uric Acid as a Biomarker for Parkinson's Disease[J].*Med Hypotheses*,2010,75(02):273.

③ GAO X,CHEN H,CHOI HK,et al.Diet,Urate and Parkinson's Disease Risk in Men[J].*Am Epidemiol*,2008,167(07):831-83&

④ DE LAU LM,KOUDSTAAL PJ,HOFMAN A,et al.Serum Uric Acid Levels and the Risk of Parkinson Disease[J].*Ann Neurol*,2005,58(05):797-800.

⑤ DE VERA M,RAHMAN MM,RANKIN J,et al.Gout and the Risk of Parkinson's Disease:a Cohort Study[J].*Arthritis Rheum*,2008,59(11):1549-1554.

⑥ ALONSO A,RODRFGUEZ LA,LOGROSCINO G,et al.Gout and Risk of Parkinson Disease:a Prospective Study[J].*Neurology*,2007,69(17):1696-1700.

⑦ 罗蔚锋,王丽君,王晓君,等.老年男性帕金森病患者血尿酸水平的研究[J].中华老年医学杂志,2009,28(01):60-61.

⑧ ANNANMAKI T,MUURONEN A,MURROS K.Low Plasma Uric Acid Level in Parkinson's Disease[J].*Mov Disord*,2007,22(08):1133-1137.

⑨ 王丽君,罗蔚锋,王恒会,等.帕金森病患者血尿酸水平[J].中华神经科杂志,2008,41(03):157-158.

⑩ 王晓君,罗蔚锋,王丽君,等.帕金森病患者认知功能与尿酸及相关因素分析[J].中华医学杂志,2009,89(23):1633-1635.

显著低于健康对照组,伴有认知功能损害患者的血 UA 水平更低。我们曾对 18 000 例的男性人群进行前瞻性的研究①,8 年后发现血浆 UA 水平处于高五分位值范围的人群相对于 UA 水平处于低五分位值范围人群,PD 发病率降低 55%,经年龄、吸烟、饮咖啡及其他与 PD 和血浆 UA 水平有关的因素纠正后,UA 与 PD 的发病率仍呈显著的负相关性。对 11 258 例痛风患者,与年龄、性别等配对的 56 199 名对照者进行对比性研究②,平均随访 8 年,共有 1182 例新发 PD 患者,痛风组 PD 的发生率显著低于对照组。王丽君等③比较了 121 例 PD 患者及 121 例健康体检者的血 UA 水平,按照年龄、性别配对,发现 PD 患者组的血 UA 水平(260.76±90.42 μmol/L)显著低于健康体检人群组(336.95±59.64 μmol/L,$P<0.01$),说明低血 UA 水平可能是 PD 发病的危险因素。

二、8-羟基脱氧鸟苷与 PD

8-OHdG 是活性氧自由基如羟自由基、单线态氧等攻击 DNA 分子中的鸟嘌呤碱基第 8 位碳原子产生的一种氧化性化合物。羟自由基和超氧阴离子能直接与 DNA 分子反应,导致 DNA 链断裂、碱基修饰和 DNA 蛋白交联等氧化性 DNA 损伤,其中最主要的致突变性损伤反应是第 8 位碳上鸟嘌呤与胸腺嘧啶碱基置换性突变,从而产生 8-OHdG。它是一种内源性诱变剂,具有突变倾向(G:C—T:A 置换),通常认为它是活性氧引起突变的一个可能原因④。

对 211 例 PD 患者及 135 例健康对照者进行血白细胞中 8-OHdG 的测定,发现 PD 患者的 8-OHdG 含量较健康对照者显著升高,H-Y 分期后期与病情呈平行关系⑤。PD 患者中过量的活性氧基的形成损害神经元、脂质、

① WEISSKOPF MG,O'REILLY E,CHEN H,et al.Plasma Urate and Risk of Parkinson's Disease[J].Am Epidemiol,2007,166(05):561-567.

② DE VERA M,RAHMAN MM,RANKIN J,et al.Gout and the Risk of Parkinson's Disease:a Cohort Study[J].Arthritis Rheum,2008,59(11):1549-1554.

③ 王丽君,罗蔚锋,王恒会,等.帕金森病患者血尿酸水平[J].中华神经科杂志,2008,41(03):157-158.

④ WU LL,CHIOU CC,CHANG PY,et al.Urinary 8-OHDG:A Marker of Oxidative Stess to DNA and a Risk Factor for Cancer Athemelerosis and Diabetics[J].Clin Chim Acta,2004,330(06):1-9.

⑤ CHEN CM,LIU JL,WU YR,et al.Increased Oxidative Damage in Peripheral Blood Correlates with Severity of Parkinson's Disease[J].Neurobiol Dis,2009,33(03):429-435.

蛋白和 DNA 的氧化损伤水平增高,其标志物 8-OHdG、丙二醛(malondialdehyde,MDA)和活性羰基在基底节区的水平显著升高。另外,PD 患者尿液中的 8-OHdG 含量在疾病早期已有升高[1]。有研究者[2]比较了尚未接受过药物治疗的 66 名 PD 患者和 25 名健康人的血液样本,与健康对照者相比,PD 患者存在高水平的 8-OHdG。有学者[3]研究了 20 例 PD 患者和 20 例健康对照者,测定其脑脊液中 8-OHdG 的含量,发现 PD 组显著高于同年龄健康对照组,并且 8-OHdG 的含量与病情进展速度呈线性相关。通过检测 8-OHdG 的水平可以评估体内氧化损伤和修复的程度,以及氧化应激与 DNA 损伤的相互关系,对于研究 PD 与氧化应激的关系具有重要意义。

三、谷胱甘肽与 PD

谷胱甘肽是人类细胞中自然合成的一种三肽,由谷氨酸、半胱氨酸和甘氨酸组成,含有巯基(SH),以还原型(GSH)和氧化型(GSSG)两种形式存在,并且在体内 90% 以上以还原形式存在,是细胞抗氧化系统中的主要成分。它既可以非酶促反应的形式直接与氧自由基结合,达到清除氧自由基的目的,又可以作为谷胱甘肽过氧化物酶(glutathione peroxidase,GPx)催化反应中的底物,起到清除氧自由基的作用。GPX 虽不能直接清除自由基,但可清除过氧化氢(H_2O_2)和脂质过氧化物(LPO),减少自由基的生成。GSH 可通过各种氧化反应使超氧阴离子(O_2^-)、H_2O_2 和 LPO 变成低毒性物质,从而保护生物膜及生物大分子免受自由基损伤。另外,研究[4][5]发现,黑

① SEET RC,LEE CY,LIM EC,et al.Oxidative Damage in Parkinson Disease:Measurement Using Accurate Biomarkers[J].*Free Radic Biol Med*,2010,48(04):560-566.

② BOGDANOV M,MATSON WR,WANG L,et al.Metabolomic Profiling to Develop Blood Biomarkers for Paricinson's Disease[J].*Brain*,2008,131(Pt2):389-396.

③ ISOBE C,ABE T,TERAYAMA Y,et al.Levels of Reduced and Oxidized Coenzyme Q-10 and 8-hydroxy-2'-deoxyguanosine in the Cerebrospinal Fluid of Patients with Living Parkinson's Disease Demonstrate that Mitochondrial Oxidative Damage and/or Oxidative DNA Damage Contributes to the Neurodegenerative Process[J].*Neurosci Lett*,2010,469(01):159-163.

④ BURWELL LS,NADTOCHIY SM,TOMPKINS AJ,et al.Direct Evidence for S-nitrosylation of Mitochondrial Complex I[J].*Biochem J*,2006,394:627-634.

⑤ CHINTA SJ,KUMAR MJ,HSU M,et al.Inducible Alterations of Glutathione Levels in Adult Dopaminergie Midbrain Neurons Result in Nogrostriatal Degeneration[J].*J NeUrosci*,2007,27(51):13997-14006.

质部位 GSH 水平下降可通过亚硝化作用抑制呼吸链酶合体 Ⅰ 的活性,从而导致中脑 DA 神经元受损乃至死亡。

PD 患者临床症状出现之前,黑质内 GSH 水平已有下降,因此 GSH 可以作为诊断早期 PD 的生物学指标之一[1][2]。Younes-Mhenni 等[3]经严格筛选 80 例 PD 患者和 29 例健康对照者,按年龄、性别配对,将 PD 患者的病情按 H-Y 分期划分(Ⅰ、Ⅱ为轻度,Ⅲ、Ⅳ为中度),发现 PD 患者组较对照组总谷胱甘肽及还原性谷胱甘肽含量减少,而氧化性谷胱甘肽含量增加。对死亡的 PD 患者、进行性核上性麻痹(PSP)及多系统萎缩(MSA)患者,进行黑质谷胱甘肽水平的测定,发现各病例组的谷胱甘肽含量较对照组显著降低[4]。有研究者[5]比较了尚未接受过药物治疗的 66 名 PD 患者和 25 名健康人的血液样本,与健康对照者相比,PD 患者的氧化性谷胱甘肽水平显著增高。对 211 例 PD 患者及 135 例健康对照者进行红细胞中的 GPx 含量测定,与健康对照者相比,PD 患者的 GPx 含量显著下降,并且 PD 患者的 GPx 含量与病情进展速度呈正相关[6]。

四、铁与PD

铁(Iron,Fe)是人体所必需的一种金属元素,在脑内分布非常广泛,基底神经节中含量最高,它一般有两种价态—— Fe^{2+} 和 Fe^{3+},并且随着电子的得失而相互转化。Fe 在脑内氧的运输、电子传递、神经递质和髓鞘合成等功能活动中具有重要作用。Fe 必须经过血脑屏障才能进入大脑,转铁蛋白(transferrin,Tf)-转铁蛋白受体(transferrin receptor,TfR)转运系统是 Fe 进入

① BHARATH S, ANDERSEN JK. Glutathione Depletion is a Midbrain-derived Immortalized Dopaminergic Cell Line Results in Limited Tyrosine nitration of Mitochondrial Complex I Subunits: Implications for Parkinson's Disease[J].Antioxid Redos Signal,2005,7(7-8):900-910.

② MAHER P.The Effects of Stress and Aging on Glutathione Metabolism[J]. Ageing Res Rev,2005,4(2):288-314.

③ YOUNES-MHENNI S, FRIH-AYED M.KERKENI A, et al. Peripheral Blood Markers of Oxidative Stress in Parkinson's Disease[J].Eur Neurol,2007,58(02):78-83.

④ FITZMAURICE PS, ANG L, GUTTMAN M, et al. Nigral Glutathione Deficiency is not Specific for Idiopathic Parkinson's Disease[J].Mov Disord,2003,18(09):969-976.

⑤ BOGDANOV M,MATSON WR, WANG L,et al.Metabolomic Profiling to Develop Blood Biomarkers for Parkinson's Disease[J].Brain,2008,131(Pt2):389-396.

⑥ CHEN CM,LIU JL,WU YR,et al.Increased Oxidative Damage in Peripheral Blood Correlates with Severity of Parkinson's Disease[J].Neurobiol Dis,2009,33(03):429-435.

血脑屏障血管内皮细胞的主要途径。三价金属离子转运蛋白 1（ferroportin 1，FP1）和二价金属离子转运蛋白 1（divalent metal transport 1，DMT1）是具有转运铁功能的因子。黑质内 DA 能神经元的 DMT1 表达异常会引起脑内 Fe 平衡的紊乱，使得 Fe 在该部位特异性聚积①，高浓度 Fe 可以导致细胞内羟自由基和 MDA 水平的升高，继而引起细胞损伤甚至死亡。

高浓度 Fe 可增加黑质 DA 能神经元对毒性氧自由基的易感性，在 PD 患者中尤为明显②。过量游离的 Fe 可以通过 Fenton 反应产生羟自由基，后者作用于蛋白质、核酸和含有大量不饱和脂肪酸的细胞膜，从而引起细胞损伤。对 91 例 PD 患者及 18 例健康对照者进行全血、脑脊液及尿液中 Fe 的含量测定，发现③与健康对照者相比，PD 患者全血和尿液中 Fe 的含量增加，而脑脊液中 Fe 的含量减少。Forte 等④的研究结果与之类似。Fukushima 等⑤最近报道，将影响 Fe 水平有关的因素纠正后，在 PD 患者临床症状出现之前，其血清 Fe 水平显著高于性别、年龄配对的健康对照者。

五、人白介素-6 与 PD

人白介素-6（interleukin-6，IL-6）是一种多功能细胞因子，其前体为 212 肽，包括一段 28 肽的信号肽，成熟的 IL-6 含有 184 个氨基酸残基，分子量为 26 kD。IL-6 来源于机体的多种细胞，包括免疫系统细胞、骨骼肌细胞、内皮细胞、脂肪细胞、肝细胞等。正常状态下，血液中的 IL-6 主要由脂肪组织分泌，约占 1/3。此外，胰岛 β 细胞也可自分泌少量 IL-6。IL-6 必须与其受体结合才具有生物学活性。天然存在的 IL-6 受体有两种：一种是膜结合受体，另一种是可溶性受体。IL-6 可激活星形胶质细胞合成一定的神经营养

① SALAZAR J, MENA N, HUNOT S, et al. Divalent Metal Transporter 1（DMT1）Contributes to Neurodegeneration in Animal Models of Parkinson's Disease［J］. *Proc Natl Acad Sci USA*, 2008, 105（47）：18578-18583.

② DONOVAN A, BROWNLIE A, ZHOU Y, et al. Positional Cloning of Zebrafish Ferroportinl Identifies a Conservedvertebrateiron Exporter［J］. *Nature*, 2000, 403（6771）：776-781.

③ BOCCA B, ALIMONTI A, SENOFONTE O, et al. Metal Changes in CSF and Peripheral Compartments of Parkinsonian Patients［J］. *J Neurol Sci*, 2006, 248（1-2）：23-30.

④ FORTE G, BOCCA B, SENOFONTE O, et al. Trace and Major Elements in Whole Blood, Serum, Cerebrospinal Fluid and Urine of Patients with Parkinson's Disease［J］. *J Neural Transm*, 2004, 111（08）：1031-1140.

⑤ FUKUSHIMA T, TAN X, LUO Y, et al. Relationship between Blood Levels of Heavy Metals and Parkinson's Disease in China［J］. *Neuroepidemiology*, 2010, 34（01）：18-24.

因子,从而起到一定的营养神经和促进神经再生的作用①。另外,它还是免疫调节剂细胞因子,通过抑制 IL-lβ 和 TNF-α 的产生起到免疫保护作用。最后,IL-6 还参与人体的其他生物学过程,如参与免疫应答、炎性反应及诱导肝细胞的急性期反应等。其中,炎症因素与中枢系统变性疾病特别是黑质纹状体部位受损的关系已日益受到关注②。

　　Scalzo 等③通过测定 44 例 PD 患者和 22 例健康对照者血清中的 IL-6 水平,发现 PD 患者血清中的 IL-6 水平较健康对照者显著增高,然而 IL-6 水平与病情严重性无相关性。Chen 等④随访 84 例 PD 患者及 165 例健康对照者,发现血清中 IL-6 含量增高将增加发生 PD 的危险性,并且其含量在 PD 尚未达到诊断标准时已有升高。推测在 PD 临床症状出现前较长一段时间内,血清中 IL-6 的含量已有变化,这将有助于 PD 的早期诊断。

六、展望

　　对于 PD 生物指标的研究是非常必要的,不仅可以有效地追踪 PD 高危人群的健康状况,比如有 PD 家族史的人们,有助于对 PD 的早期症状作出判断,而且有助于在治疗中监测病情进展,从而为新的治疗手段提供可能。

(朱婷鸽　罗蔚锋)

(本文原载于《国际老年医学杂志》2011 年第 32 卷第 4 期)

---

①　JURIC DM,CARMAN-KRZAN M.Cytokine-regulated Secretion of Nerve Growth Factor from Cultured Rat Neonatal Astrocytes[J]. *Pflugers Arch*,2000,440[Suppl 5]:R96-98.

②　ANNA L,BARTELS MD,KLAUS L,et al.Neuroinflammation in the Pathophysiology of Parkinson's Disease:Evidence from Animal Models to Human in Vivo Studies with[(11)C]PK11195 PET[J].*Mov Disord*,2007,22(13):1852-1856.

③　SCALZO P,KAMMER A,CARDOSO F,et al.Serum Levels of Interleukin-6 are Elevated in Patients with Parkinson's Disease and Correlate with Physical Performance[J].*Neurosci Lett*,2010,468(01):56-58.

④　CHEN H,O'REILLY EJ,SCHWARZSCHILD MA,et al. Peripheral Inflammatory Biomarkers and Risk of Parkinson's Disease[J].*Am J Epidemiol*,2008,167(01):90-95.